Psychosis in Youth

Editors

JEAN A. FRAZIER
YAEL DVIR

CHILD AND ADOLESCENT PSYCHIATRIC CLINICS OF NORTH AMERICA

www.childpsych.theclinics.com

Consulting Editor
HARSH K. TRIVEDI

October 2013 • Volume 22 • Number 4

ELSEVIER

1600 John F. Kennedy Boulevard • Suite 1800 • Philadelphia, Pennsylvania, 19103-2899

http://www.theclinics.com

CHILD AND ADOLESCENT PSYCHIATRIC CLINICS OF NORTH AMERICA Volume 22, Number 4
October 2013 ISSN 1056–4993, ISBN-13: 978-0-323-22712-4

Editor: Joanne Husovski
Developmental Editor: Donald Mumford

Child and Adolescent Psychiatric Clinics of North America (ISSN 1056-4993) is published quarterly by Elsevier Inc., 360 Park Avenue South, New York, NY 10010-1710. Months of issue are January, April, July, and October. Business and Editorial Offices: 1600 John F. Kennedy Boulevard, Suite 1800, Philadelphia, PA 19103-2899. Periodicals postage paid at New York, NY and additional mailing offices. Subscription prices are $297.00 per year (US individuals), $471.00 per year (US institutions), $149.00 per year (US students), $343.00 per year (Canadian individuals), $567.00 per year (Canadian institutions), $189.00 per year (Canadian students), $408.00 per year (international individuals), $567.00 per year (international institutions), and $189.00 per year (international students). International air speed delivery is included in all *Clinics* subscription prices. All prices are subject to change without notice. **POSTMASTER:** Send address changes to *Child and Adolescent Psychiatric Clinics of North America*, Elsevier Health Sciences Division, Subscription Customer Service, 3251 Riverport Lane, Maryland Heights, MO 63043. **Customer Service: 1-800-654-2452 (U.S. and Canada); 314-447-8871 (outside U.S. and Canada). Fax: 314-447-8029. E-mail: JournalsCustomer Service-usa@elsevier.com (for print support) or journalsonlinesupport-usa@elsevier.com (for online support).**

Reprints. For copies of 100 or more of articles in this publication, please contact the Commercial Reprints Department, Elsevier Inc., 360 Park Avenue South, New York, New York 10010-1710 Tel.: (212) 633-3812; Fax: (212) 462-1935, e-mail: reprints@elsevier.com.

Child and Adolescent Psychiatric Clinics of North America is covered in *MEDLINE/PubMed (Index Medicus), ISI, SSCI, Research Alert, Social Search, Current Contents,* and *EMBASE/Excerpta Medica.*

Printed and bound by CPI Group (UK) Ltd, Croydon, CR0 4YY

Transferred to digital print 2012

Contributors

CONSULTING EDITOR

HARSH K. TRIVEDI, MD
Associate Professor of Psychiatry, Vanderbilt University School of Medicine; Executive
Medical Director, Chief of Staff, Vanderbilt Psychiatric Hospital, Nashville, Tennessee

CONSULTING EDITOR EMERITUS

ANDRÉS MARTIN, MD, MPH

FOUNDING CONSULTING EDITOR

MELVIN LEWIS, MBBS, FRCPSYCH, DCH

EDITORS

JEAN A. FRAZIER, MD
Robert M. and Shirley S. Siff Endowed Chair in Autism, Professor of Psychiatry and
Pediatrics, Vice Chair and Director, Division of Child and Adolescent Psychiatry,
Department of Psychiatry, University of Massachusetts Medical School, Worcester,
Massachusetts

YAEL DVIR, MD
Assistant Professor of Psychiatry, Division of Child and Adolescent Psychiatry,
Department of Psychiatry, University of Massachusetts Medical School, Worcester,
Massachusetts

AUTHORS

KELLY ALLOTT, PhD
Associate Professor, Orygen Youth Health Research Centre, Parkville, Victoria; Centre for
Youth Mental Health, The University of Melbourne, Melbourne, Australia

MARIO ALVAREZ-JIMENEZ, PhD
Associate Professor, Orygen Youth Health Research Centre, Parkville, Victoria; Centre for
Youth Mental Health, The University of Melbourne, Melbourne, Australia

ROBERT F. ASARNOW, PhD
Departments of Psychiatry and Biobehavioral Sciences, and Psychology, University of
California at Los Angeles, Los Angeles, California

SARAH BENDALL, PhD
Associate Professor, Orygen Youth Health Research Centre, Parkville, Victoria; Centre for
Youth Mental Health, The University of Melbourne, Melbourne, Australia

SHELDON BENJAMIN, MD
Professor, Departments of Psychiatry and Neurology, University of Massachusetts
Medical School, Worcester, Massachusetts

JOY L. BRASFIELD, BA
Mental Health and Development Program, Department of Psychology, Emory University,
Atlanta, Georgia

BENJAMIN K. BRENT, MD, MS
Harvard Medical School; Division of Public Psychiatry, Massachusetts Mental Health
Center; Department of Psychiatry, Beth Israel Deaconess Medical Center; Department of
Psychiatry, Massachusetts General Hospital, Boston, Massachusetts

GABRIELLE A. CARLSON, MD
Professor of Psychiatry and Pediatrics, Director, Child and Adolescent Psychiatry,
Stony Brook University School of Medicine, Stony Brook, New York

DAVID M. COCHRAN, MD, PhD
Assistant Professor of Psychiatry, Division of Child and Adolescent Psychiatry,
Department of Psychiatry, University of Massachusetts Medical School, Worcester,
Massachusetts

SARAH D. COHEN, MD
Assistant Clinical Professor of Psychiatry and Behavioral Sciences, Division of Child and
Adolescent Psychiatry, Department of Psychiatry, Albert Einstein College of Medicine,
Bronx, New York

BRIAN DENIETOLIS, PsyD
Department of Psychiatry, University of Massachusetts Medical School, Worcester,
Massachusetts

DAVID I. DRIVER, MD
Child Psychiatry Branch, National Institutes of Mental Health (NIMH), National Institutes
Health (NIH), Bethesda, Maryland

YAEL DVIR, MD
Assistant Professor of Psychiatry, Division of Child and Adolescent Psychiatry,
Department of Psychiatry, University of Massachusetts Medical School, Worcester,
Massachusetts

JENNIFER K. FORSYTH, MA
Department of Psychology, University of California at Los Angeles, Los Angeles, California

SOPHIA FRANGOU, MD, PhD
Professor of Psychiatry, Department of Psychiatry, Icahn School of Medicine at Mount
Sinai, New York, New York

JEAN A. FRAZIER, MD
Robert M. and Shirley S. Siff Endowed Chair in Autism, Professor of Psychiatry and
Pediatrics, Vice Chair and Director, Division of Child and Adolescent Psychiatry,
Department of Psychiatry, University of Massachusetts Medical School, Worcester,
Massachusetts

DANIELLE GOERKE, DO
Child and Adolescent Psychiatry Fellow, Division of Child and Adolescent Psychiatry,
University of Minnesota Medical School, Minneapolis, Minnesota

NITIN GOGTAY, MD
Child Psychiatry Branch, National Institutes of Mental Health (NIMH), National Institutes
Health (NIH), Bethesda, Maryland

SANDRA M. GOULDING, MPH, MA
Mental Health and Development Program, Department of Psychology, Emory University,
Atlanta, Georgia

CARRIE W. HOLTZMAN, MA
Mental Health and Development Program, Department of Psychology, Emory University,
Atlanta, Georgia

MATCHERI S. KESHAVAN, MD
Harvard Medical School; Division of Public Psychiatry, Massachusetts Mental Health
Center; Department of Psychiatry, Beth Israel Deaconess Medical Center, Boston,
Massachusetts

EÓIN KILLACKEY, D. Psych
Associate Professor, Orygen Youth Health Research Centre, Parkville, Victoria; Centre for
Youth Mental Health, The University of Melbourne, Melbourne, Australia

HARVEY N. KRANZLER, MD
Professor of Clinical Psychiatry and Behavioral Sciences, Division of Child and
Adolescent Psychiatry, Department of Psychiatry, Albert Einstein College of Medicine,
Bronx, New York

SANJIV KUMRA, MD
Associate Professor, Head of the Division of Child and Adolescent Psychiatry, University
of Minnesota Medical School, Minneapolis, Minnesota

MARGO D. LAUTERBACH, MD
Clinical Assistant Professor, Department of Psychiatry, University of Maryland School
of Medicine; Neuropsychiatry Program, Sheppard Pratt Health System, Baltimore,
Maryland

ALLISON N. MACDONALD, BA
Mental Health and Development Program, Department of Psychology, Emory University,
Atlanta, Georgia

PATRICK MCGORRY, MD, PhD
Professor, Orygen Youth Health Research Centre, Parkville, Victoria; Centre for Youth
Mental Health, The University of Melbourne, Melbourne, Australia

JUDITH L. RAPOPORT, MD
Child Psychiatry Branch, National Institutes of Mental Health (NIMH), National Institutes
Health (NIH), Bethesda, Maryland

ARTHUR T. RYAN, MA
Mental Health and Development Program, Department of Psychology, Emory University,
Atlanta, Georgia

LARRY J. SEIDMAN, PhD
Harvard Medical School; Division of Public Psychiatry, Massachusetts Mental Health
Center; Department of Psychiatry, Beth Israel Deaconess Medical Center; Department of
Psychiatry, Massachusetts General Hospital, Boston, Massachusetts

DANIEL I. SHAPIRO, MA
Mental Health and Development Program, Department of Psychology, Emory University, Atlanta, Georgia

LINMARIE SIKICH, MD
Director, ASPIRE Program, Associate Professor, University of North Carolina at Chapel Hill, Chapel Hill, North Carolina

AIMEE L. STANISLAWSKI, MD
Clinical Assistant Professor, Behavioral Health, VA Western NY Healthcare System; Department of Psychiatry, School of Medicine and Biomedical Sciences, State University of New York at Buffalo, Buffalo, New York

HEIDI W. THERMENOS, PhD
Harvard Medical School; Division of Public Psychiatry, Massachusetts Mental Health Center; Department of Psychiatry, Beth Israel Deaconess Medical Center; Department of Psychiatry, Massachusetts General Hospital, Boston, Massachusetts; Athinoula A. Martinos Imaging Center, Charlestown, Massachusetts

HANAN D. TROTMAN, PhD
Mental Health and Development Program, Department of Psychology, Emory University, Atlanta, Georgia

ELAINE F. WALKER, PhD
Mental Health and Development Program, Department of Psychology, Emory University, Atlanta, Georgia

Contents

The clinical severity, impact on development, and poor prognosis of child-hood onset schizophrenia may represent a more homogeneous group. Positive symptoms in children are necessary for the diagnosis and hallucinations are more often multimodal. In healthy children and children with a variety of other psychiatric illnesses, hallucinations are not uncommon and diagnosis should not be based on these alone. Childhood onset schizophrenia is an extraordinarily rare illness that is poorly understood but seems continuous with the adult onset disorder. Once a diagnosis is affirmed, aggressive medication treatment combined with family education and individual counseling may defer further deterioration.

The psychosis prodrome offers great promise for identifying neural mechanisms involved in psychotic disorders and offers an opportunity to implement empirical interventions to delay, and ultimately ameliorate, illness onset. This article summarizes the literature on individuals in the putatively prodromal phase of psychosis/deemed at clinical high risk (CHR) for psychosis onset. Standardized measurement and manifestation of the CHR syndromes are discussed, followed by empirical findings that highlight the psychological deficits and biological abnormalities seen in CHR syndromes and psychotic disorders. Current controversies surrounding the diagnosis of CHR syndromes and issues related to the treatment of CHR individuals are also presented.

The significance of psychosis has yet to be fully understood and research is complicated because psychosis is often a state rather than trait occurrence. In youth, psychoticlike phenomena are common. Rates of lifetime psychotic symptoms are higher than rates of psychosis during a current episode of mania or depression, at least in youth. Rates vary widely between studies. Hallucinations are also more common than delusions in youth. Psychotic phenomena can be mood congruent or incongruent. A good mental status examination requires close questioning. There are several interviews that structure how questions are asked, and rating scales that help anchor severity.

A review of the published literature found 60 congenital and acquired disorders with symptoms that include psychosis in youth. The prevalence, workup, genetics, and associated neuropsychiatric features of each disorder are described. Eighteen disorders (30%) have distinct phenotypes (doorway diagnoses); 18 disorders (30%) are associated with intellectual disability; and 43 disorders (72%) have prominent neurologic signs. Thirty-one disorders (52%) can present without such distinct characteristics, and are thus more easily overlooked. A systematic and cost-effective differential diagnostic approach based on estimated prevalence and most prominent associated signs is recommended.

Section 2: Differential Diagnosis and Comorbidities in Psychosis

Patients are often encountered clinically who have autism spectrum disorders (ASD) and also have symptoms suggestive of a comorbid psychotic disorder. A careful assessment for the presence of comorbid disorders is important. However, the core deficits seen in ASD, in social reciprocity, communication, and restricted behaviors and interests, can be mistaken for psychosis. Also, there is a subset of patients who present with a complex neurodevelopmental disorder with impairments that cross diagnostic categories. This article reviews the connections between ASD and psychosis, and highlights the key points to consider in patients who present with these "autism-plus" disorders.

Childhood trauma is a common occurrence and has been associated with psychosis and suggested as a risk factor leading to psychosis and schizophrenia in adulthood. This article introduces the scope of the problem and discusses the evidence for causal relationships between childhood adversities and increased risk for psychosis. The relationship between specific types of trauma and their association with specific psychotic symptoms is described, as well as the manifestations of co-occurring trauma effects and psychosis in adolescents. Clinical presentations and the use of diagnostic instruments, diagnostic comorbidities, and evidence-based psychotherapeutic interventions to treat effects of trauma in youth with psychotic illnesses are discussed.

This article reviews the literature for the most pressing diagnostic and treatment challenges faced in working with adolescents. Diagnosing the treatment interventions required for this population involve psychoeducation, engagement of the patient and family in the treatment process, and use of antipsychotic medications. Cannabis may be a causal risk factor in psychotic illness, and data support recommendations to reduce or cease cannabis use in this population. Treatment strategies are discussed that are effective in adult patients and that may be efficacious for youth to abstain from substances after the resolution of psychotic symptoms.

Section 3: Early Onset Psychosis Etiologies and Biomarkers

Recognizing positive psychotic symptoms and their diagnostic context in youth is challenging. A large minority say they "hear things others do not hear," though they seldom present with complaints of hallucinations or delusions. Few have schizophrenia spectrum disorders, but many have other psychiatric disorders. Frequently, they have psychotic symptoms for an extended period before diagnosis. Clinicians should understand psychotic symptoms and their differential diagnoses. This article reviews the epidemiology, associated diagnoses, and prognosis of hallucinations and delusions in youth. Strategies for optimizing the clinical diagnostic interview, appropriate laboratory tests, indications for psychological testing, and rating scales are reviewed.

Schizophrenia is a heritable disorder. The genetic architecture of schizophrenia is complex and heterogeneous. This article discusses genetic studies of childhood-onset schizophrenia (COS) and compares findings in familial aggregation, common allele, and rare allele studies of COS with those for adult-onset schizophrenia (AOS). COS seems to be a rare variant of AOS with greater familial aggregation of schizophrenia spectrum disorders and higher occurrence of rare allelic variants. The usefulness of genetic screening for diagnosis and individualized treatment is limited; however, identifying common pathways through which multiple genes adversely affect neural systems offers great promise toward developing novel pharmacologic interventions.

This article reviews the literature on structural magnetic resonance imaging findings in pediatric and young adult populations at clinical or genetic high-risk for schizophrenia and early-onset schizophrenia. The implications of this research are discussed for understanding the pathophysiology of schizophrenia and for early intervention strategies. The evidence linking brain structural changes in prepsychosis development and early-onset schizophrenia with disruptions of normal neurodevelopmental processes during childhood or adolescence is described. Future directions are outlined for research to address knowledge gaps regarding the neurobiological basis of brain structural abnormalities in schizophrenia and to improve the usefulness of these abnormalities for preventative interventions.

Cognitive impairment is recognized as a central feature of schizophrenia. Early-onset schizophrenia (EOS) represents a more severe variant of the disorder associated with onset in childhood or adolescence. Examination of the cognitive abnormalities of EOS offers the opportunity to explore how disease-related mechanisms may affect facets of cognitive development. This article summarizes and synthesizes available data with regards to the profile of cognitive impairments in EOS, their severity, and their evolution over the course of the disorder.

Section 4: Evidence Based Interventions for Psychosis

The efficacy of antipsychotic use in children and adolescents with psychosis has been shown in an increasing number of randomized controlled trials. Chronic use of second-generation and third-generation antipsychotics has the potential for significant side effects, especially metabolic syndrome. A review of the literature on side effect profiles of antipsychotic medications used in children and adolescents is provided to help clinicians develop treatment plans for their patients. Clozapine has the best efficacy of all antipsychotic medications in adults as well as children and adolescents who are treatment resistant. Guidance is provided for the management of clozapine side effects.

During recovery, young people with psychosis need attention paid not only to their psychotic symptoms but also to the areas of functioning that restrict their capacity to live a fulfilled life in the community. Despite improvements in medications and psychological therapies, people with psychosis still have poor outcomes in functional domains such as vocation, physical health, housing, and imprisonment. This article reviews 2 of these areas: vocational functioning and physical health. It examines the extent of each of these issues, provides guidance as to what evidence there exists on which to base interventions, and describes such evidence.

CHILD AND ADOLESCENT PSYCHIATRIC CLINICS

RELATED INTEREST

Journal of the American Academy of Child & Adolescent Psychiatry,
April 2010 (Vol. 49, No. 4)
Cognitive and Psychiatric Predictors to Psychosis in Velocardiofacial Syndrome: A 3-Year Follow-Up Study
Kevin M. Antshel, Robert Shprintzen, Wanda Fremont, Anne Marie Higgins,
Stephen V. Faraone, Wendy R. Kates

AACAP Members: Please go to www.jaacap.org for information on access to the Child and Adolescent Psychiatric Clinics. *Resident* Members of AACAP: Special access information is available at www.childpsych.theclinics.com.

DOWNLOAD Free App!

Review Articles
THE CLINICS

NOW AVAILABLE FOR YOUR iPhone and iPad

CHILD AND ADOLESCENT PSYCHIATRIC CLINICS

Preface
Psychotic Disorders in Youth: Diagnostic and Treatment Challenges

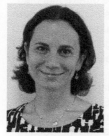 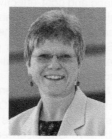

Yael Dvir, MD   Jean A. Frazier, MD
Editors

Psychotic symptoms in children and adolescents are among the most challenging symptoms for clinicians to identify, interpret, and treat; much of this is because of their emergence during a critical time of cognitive and language development. Onset of such symptoms during childhood has significant effects on normal development. While primary psychotic disorders are not as common in prepubertal children, their prevalence, including that of prodromal symptoms, increases significantly during adolescence and the transitional age period (15–25 years). In addition, psychotic symptoms and psychotic-like symptoms can be part of many other more common psychiatric conditions in youth. This issue was designed to help practicing child and adolescent psychiatrists and mental health providers become informed about the most recent scientific advances in this area of neuroscience, so that the providers feel more comfortable with identifying, assessing, and treating youth with psychosis. Accordingly, this issue is organized into 4 sections.

The first section provides an overview of the different clinical presentations of psychosis in children and adolescents and includes 4 articles, reviewing (1) childhood-onset schizophrenia (COS), a rare form of childhood psychosis, which provides an opportunity to study a more homogenous form of schizophrenia; (2) the psychosis prodrome and clinical risk for psychotic disorders, a topic of great importance to the child psychiatrist/mental health provider, aiming at identifying and intervening early in the illness process in an effort to delay and even prevent the development of psychosis; (3) the presentation of psychotic symptoms within the context of the much more common affective disorders in youth; and finally, (4) a clinically useful guide to the diagnosis and evaluation of psychotic disorders in children and adolescents, which includes the use of standardized assessments.

Child Adolesc Psychiatric Clin N Am 22 (2013) xiii–xiv
http://dx.doi.org/10.1016/j.chc.2013.04.008
1056-4993/13/$ – see front matter © 2013 Published by Elsevier Inc.

childpsych.theclinics.com

The second section reviews common comorbidities, which cause diagnostic confusion, either as a differential diagnosis or as comorbid conditions. These include (1) autism and the intersection with psychosis and the schizophrenia spectrum; (2) childhood trauma and psychosis; and (3) the etiologic contributions and clinical considerations of substance abuse and psychosis.

The third section provides an overview of the cause of the clinically diverse early-onset psychotic disorders in youth and biomarkers of early-onset psychoses, and includes 4 articles: (1) congenital and acquired disorders presenting as psychosis in children and young adults, providing a systematic and cost-effective differential diagnostic approach to the psychiatrists, neurologists, and pediatricians evaluating youth with psychotic symptoms for possible medical, neurologic, or neurodevelopmental causes; (2) a review of the genetics of COS, which discusses genetic studies of COS and compares findings in familial aggregation, common allele and rare allele studies of COS to those for adult-onset schizophrenia (AOS); (3) a clinically relevant review of neuroimaging findings (structural MRI) in schizophrenia high-risk youth and early-onset schizophrenia (EOS); and (4) neurocognition in EOS.

Finally, the fourth and last section provides an overview of the use of medication and rehabilitation in the treatment of youth with psychotic disorders and includes reviews of (1) psychopharmacology, including the role of clozapine and adjunctive therapies; and (2) an overview of community rehabilitation and psychosocial interventions for psychotic disorders in youth.

This is the first issue of the *Child and Adolescent Psychiatric Clinics of North America* that brings together this broad array of clinical and diagnostic considerations, a state-of-the-art review of the advances in neuroscience/biomarkers regarding these disorders, and applicable evidence-based treatment interventions. It is our hope that you will find the result informative and useful. We would like to thank our authors for their valued contributions, and Joanne Husovski at Elsevier for her guidance and support.

Yael Dvir, MD
Department of Psychiatry
University of Massachusetts Medical School
55 Lake Avenue North
Worcester, MA 01655, USA

Jean A. Frazier, MD
Department of Psychiatry
University of Massachusetts Medical School
Biotech I, Suite 100, 365 Plantation Street
Worcester, MA 01605, USA

E-mail addresses:
yael.dvir@umassmed.edu (Y. Dvir)
jean.frazier@umassmed.edu (J.A. Frazier)

Childhood Onset Schizophrenia and Early Onset Schizophrenia Spectrum Disorders

David I. Driver, MD, Nitin Gogtay, MD, Judith L. Rapoport, MD*

KEYWORDS

- Schizophrenia • Childhood onset schizophrenia • Childhood psychosis

KEY POINTS

- Childhood onset schizophrenia (COS) is an extraordinarily rare illness with an incidence less than 0.04%. In both healthy children and children with a variety of other psychiatric illnesses, hallucinations are not uncommon; diagnosis should not be based on these alone.
- The evaluation of a child with suspected COS includes collecting extensive collateral information, observing patients/families over several visits, excluding underlying medical illnesses and evaluating, with a high index of suspicion, for speech/language/educational deficits and comorbid mood or anxiety disorders.
- Once the diagnosis is established and other comorbidities are addressed, treatment planning should encompass aggressive psychopharmacologic, psychotherapeutic, and psychosocial interventions.
- Clozapine is an excellent third-line medication for use in COS. Epidemiologic studies demonstrate that its use often occurs much later than recommended by the clinical guidelines.

INTRODUCTION

The clinical severity, impact on development, and poor prognosis of childhood onset schizophrenia (COS) may represent more homogeneous forms of the disorder.[1,2] In addition, the deleterious effects of incorrectly diagnosing COS are equally important to recognize. Despite the relatively high (up to 5%) prevalence of psychotic symptoms in otherwise healthy children,[3,4] COS is very rare and so epidemiologic incidence data with diagnoses based on standardized clinical assessments are lacking. It is generally accepted that the incidence of COS is less than 0.04% based on the observations

The authors declare no conflicts of interest.
Child Psychiatry Branch, National Institutes of Mental Health (NIMH), National Institutes Health (NIH), Building 10, Room 3N202, 10 Center Drive, MSC 1600, Bethesda, MD 20892-1600, USA
* Corresponding author.
E-mail address: rapoporj@mail.nih.gov

Child Adolesc Psychiatric Clin N Am 22 (2013) 539–555
http://dx.doi.org/10.1016/j.chc.2013.04.001
1056-4993/13/$ – see front matter Published by Elsevier Inc.
childpsych.theclinics.com

from the National Institutes of Mental Health (NIMH) cohort. Approximately 30% to 50% of patients with affective or other atypical psychotic symptoms are misdiagnosed as COS,[5–9] and greater than 90% of the initial referrals to the NIMH study of COS to date received alternate diagnoses. Because the attempt of this work is to study schizophrenia in its most homogeneous form, children with a diagnosis of schizoaffective disorder are excluded. In general, very few schizoaffective children have been seen by the authors over the years, precluding any meaningful data analyses.

Although neurobiologically and phenomenologically continuous with its adult counterpart, COS represents a more severe form of the disorder,[10,11] with more prominent prepsychotic developmental disorders, brain abnormalities, and genetic risk factors.[2,9] The use of various screening and diagnostic tools has not proven to be as valuable as the longitudinal assessment by a judicious clinician. A unique benefit of the NIMH COS study is the washout period, whereby patients are observed inpatient, medication free for up to 3 weeks. If a provisional diagnosis of COS is appropriate based on the screening process (clinical interview, records review, structured interview), the patient is admitted to the unit and begins the rigorous process of tapering all medications (up to 4 weeks). During this period, and the subsequent medication-free phase (up to 3 weeks), patients are observed by staff, receive weekly ratings, and have the support of up to 2 individually assigned staff members (ie, 2:1 staffing). This process has ruled out COS in almost 40% of the children provisionally diagnosed as COS.

Realizing the framework and limitations of the environment in which psychiatric providers operate,the authors' model is not feasible outside of the NIMH. However, the keys to attaining accurate diagnoses and optimizing treatment planning lie in evaluating children suspected of having COS for speech/language/educational deficits, obtaining extensive collateral information, and observing patients and their families over several visits. Furthermore, COS carries with it a commitment to use a class of medications with a significant side-effect profile and significant long-term health risks.[12] Given the implications of the diagnosis, it is important for clinicians to exercise a considerable amount of caution and care when evaluating children with COS, being careful not to focus solely on addressing the psychotic symptoms and subsequently overlooking common comorbidities, such as receptive and expressive language disorders.

Research on the effects of a delayed diagnosis in COS is sparse, and this study design excludes children whose diagnosis may have been delayed, occurring after the age of 13. In addition, even the adult literature is limited by the lack of a standardized measurement.[13,14] However, in adults, it has been shown that a delay in diagnosis results in a longer duration of untreated psychosis, having a robust but moderate effect on clinical outcome.[14,15] Although a measured, thoughtful approach to diagnosis is advocated, making a timely diagnosis is also important.

Premorbid Phenotype

Of children with COS, 67% show premorbid disturbances in social, motor, and language domains as well as demonstrate learning disabilities and have what seem to be comorbid mood or anxiety disorders. In addition, although not reported in studies of the premorbid history of adult onset schizophrenia,[16,17] 27% have met criteria for autism/autism spectrum disorders before the onset of their psychotic symptoms.[18] Outcome and prognosis have been positively correlated with the presence and severity of these developmental abnormalities,[19–21] with some studies suggesting the severity of these deficits may actually represent a premorbid phenotype for COS.[22–27]

The data on the premorbid functioning and symptomatology of the NIMH patients confirm and extend these findings. A review of the authors' cohort (n = 47) in 2000 showed that 55% had language abnormalities, 57% had motor abnormalities, and 55% had social abnormalities several years before the onset of psychotic symptoms. There was also a high rate of failed grades and special education placement.[24,28] Gender, familial psychopathology, and familial eye-tracking dysfunction have shown significant relationships with at least some aspect of the probands' premorbid development (**Table 1**).[24]

These results have been strengthened by a 2012 review of the authors' cohort (n = 118). Of the 118 children in the cohort, 65 (55.08%) had premorbid academic impairments, 85 (72.03%) had premorbid social/behavioral impairments, 60 (50.85%) had premorbid language impairments, 52 (44.07%) had premorbid motor impairments, and 24 (20.34%) screened positive for pervasive developmental disorder (**Table 2**). The average number of abnormalities (15 domains) in each child was 3.89, and 103 (87.29%) children had premorbid impairment in at least one domain. In addition, 47% of children who did not have a pervasive developmental disorder (eg, autism, Asperger, pervasive developmental disorder not otherwise specified) received prepsychotic mental health treatment and/or a psychiatric or psychological evaluation.

DEFINITION/SYMPTOM CRITERIA

Since Kolvin's classic studies, it is generally agreed on that COS can be diagnosed with the unmodified Diagnostic and Statistical Manual of Mental Disorders, Fourth Edition Text Revision (DSM IV-TR) criteria for schizophrenia (**Table 3**).[29] In addition, the NIMH study has defined COS whereby the onset of psychotic symptoms is before the 13th birthday, combined with a premorbid Intelligence Quotient of 70 or above, and absence of any significant neurologic problem. The DSM V proposes a reorganization to reflect a gradient of psychopathology, from least to most severe, and updated severity dimensions.[30]

Table 1			
Relation of premorbid impairments to schizophrenia risk factors for 49 patients with COS			
Premorbid Impairment and Risk Factor	Present (N)	Absent (N)	P Value
Speech and language impairment			
Sex	27	22	.57
Score for family loading for schizophrenia spectrum disorders	27	21	.04
Mean family score for eye tracking	22	17	.04
Motor impairment			
Sex	28	21	.009
Score for family loading for schizophrenia spectrum disorders	28	20	.50
Mean family score for eye tracking	22	17	.25
Social impairment			
Sex	27	22	.56
Score for family loading for schizophrenia spectrum disorders	27	21	.15
Mean family score for eye tracking	19	20	.37

Table 2 Realms of premorbid developmental problems based on 2012 chart review	
	N (%)
Social/behavioral	85 (72.03%)
Academic	65 (55.08)
Language	60 (50.85%)
Motor	52 (44.07%)
Pervasive developmental disorder	24 (20.34%)

CLINICAL FINDINGS
Physical Examination

The diagnosis of COS requires exclusion of an underlying medical or psychiatric illness. It is only after all other identifiable causes of "organic psychosis" have been excluded that a diagnosis of COS can appropriately be considered. Details regarding the components of the physical examination of individuals suspected of having a primary psychiatric illness are discussed in this issue by Kumra and Goerke entitled, "Substance Abuse and Psychosis: Etiologic Contribution and Clinical Considerations." A physical and thorough neurologic examination is essential to the diagnostic process and clinicians should be vigilant to any abnormal physical and/or neurologic findings because COS is a diagnosis of exclusion. It is also important to have in mind the rare medical causes and frequently missed diagnoses during the evaluation. Although discussed elsewhere in this issue, a select summary list is provided in **Table 4**.

Rating Scales and Diagnostic Modalities

Frequently used rating scales are discussed in subsequent articles in this issue. For the NIMH COS study the Social Communication Questionnaire, previously known as the Autism Screening Questionnaire, and Kiddie-Sads-Present and Lifetime Version (K-SADS-PL), are used, with the supplemental ratings as indicated by the results of the K-SADS-PL, for all probands. The Schedule for Affective Disorders and Schizophrenia and the Structured Interview for DSM-III Personality are used to evaluate all family members for axis I and axis II disorders, respectively. During follow-up visits the probands are evaluated using the Scale for the Assessment of Positive Symptoms, Scale for the Assessment of Negative Symptoms, Brief Psychiatric Rating Scale for Children, Clinical Global Impressions Scale, Children's' Global Impressions Scale, Bunny-Hamburg Global Ratings, Simpson-Angus Scale, and Abnormal Involuntary Movement Scale.[34]

As previously mentioned, it is simply not feasible to apply what is done at NIMH in the community. In clinical practice, it is routinely recommended to outpatient providers that they use the Scale for the Assessment of Positive Symptoms and Scale for the Assessment of Negative Symptoms to monitor clinical progress and the Abnormal Involuntary Movement Scale to monitor for potential side effects of the medication regimen (**Table 5**).

Imaging

Structural brain abnormalities are an established feature of schizophrenia, characterized by decreased total gray matter (GM) volume reduction in cortex, hippocampus, and amygdala.[35–43] The number of imaging studies of childhood and early onset

Table 3
DSM IV-TR criteria for schizophrenia

A. Characteristic symptoms: Two (or more) of the following, each present for a significant portion of time during a 1-month period (or less if successfully treated) Note: Only one Criterion A symptom is required if delusions are bizarre or hallucinations consist of a voice keeping up a running commentary on the person's behavior or thoughts, or 2 or more voices conversing with each other.	1. Delusions 2. Hallucinations 3. Disorganized speech (eg, frequent derailment or incoherence) 4. Grossly disorganized or catatonic behavior 5. Negative symptoms (ie, affective flattening, alogia, or avolition)
B. Social/occupational dysfunction	For a significant portion of the time since the onset of the disturbance, one or more major areas of functioning, such as work, interpersonal relations, or self-care, are markedly below the level achieved before the onset (or when the onset is in childhood or adolescence, failure to achieve expected level of interpersonal, academic, or occupational achievement).
C. Duration	Continuous signs of the disturbance persist for at least 6 mo. This 6-month period must include at least 1 mo of symptoms (or less if successfully treated) that meet Criterion A (ie, active-phase symptoms) and may include periods of prodromal or residual symptoms. During these prodromal or residual periods, the signs of the disturbance may be manifested by only negative symptoms or 2 or more symptoms listed in Criterion A present in an attenuated form (eg, odd beliefs, unusual perceptual experiences).
D. Schizoaffective and mood disorder exclusion	Schizoaffective disorder and mood disorder with psychotic features have been ruled out because either (1) no major depressive, manic, or mixed episodes have occurred concurrently with the active-phase symptoms; or (2) if mood episodes have occurred during active-phase symptoms, their total duration has been brief relative to the duration of the active and residual periods.
E. Substance/general medical condition exclusion	The disturbance is not due to the direct physiologic effects of a substance (eg, a drug of abuse, a medication) or a general medical condition.
F. Relationship to a pervasive developmental disorder	If there is a history of autistic disorder or another pervasive developmental disorder, the additional diagnosis of schizophrenia is made only if prominent delusions or hallucinations are also present for at least a month (or less if successfully treated).

Table 4
Differential diagnoses of childhood onset schizophrenia

Medical etiologies	• Seizure disorder • Anti-*N*-methyl-D-aspartate receptor encephalitis • Herpes simplex encephalitis • Lysosomal storage diseases • Neurodegenerative disorders • Central nervous system tumors • Progressive organic central nervous system disorder (eg, sclerosing panencephalitis) • Metabolic disorders • Chromosomal disorders: 22q11 deletion syndrome[a]
Misdiagnosed psychiatric illnesses	• Psychotic depression • Bipolar disorder • Autism-spectrum disorders pervasive developmental disorders • Obsessive–compulsive disorder • Generalized anxiety disorder • Posttraumatic stress disorder • "Multidimensionally impaired" (not a formal DSM diagnosis, but discussed further below): individuals with multiple language or learning disorders, mood lability, and transient psychotic symptoms

[a] Rates significantly higher than expected.[31–33]

schizophrenia is growing with most them coming from the NIMH cohort. Advances in computational image analysis permit regional GM density, or cortical thickness measurements, which, when automated, can be applied to large samples, increasing statistical power,[44–47] which provides unprecedented anatomic detail of cortical GM change across both the entire cortex and the age (**Fig. 1**).[43,47] Prospective longitudinal brain magnetic resonance imaging rescan measures for the NIMH COS sample show progressive changes in COS, particularly during adolescence, highlighting this period as critical, and particularly vulnerable to treatment influences. These changes occur only during a limited period because the rate and degree of cortical loss if continued would resemble the extreme loss seen in some dementias.[43,47] As it is, the GM volume of COS is 8% to 10% less than that of age-matched controls.

Longitudinal analysis of quantitative brain imaging data suggests the rate of GM loss slows as these COS patients reach age 20, as shown in refs.[50–52] These studies also support the previous findings that, although representing a more severe form, COS is continuous with its adult-onset counterpart. The total, frontal, temporal, and parietal GM loss, not seen in healthy children and adolescents nor in those with atypical psychosis, seems to be diagnostically specific for COS.[50]

PATHOLOGIC CONDITION

Identifying the neurobiological basis and pathophysiology of schizophrenia is an essential future goal for establishing its diagnostic validity, delineating meaningful subtypes or alternate diagnoses, and finding causative mechanisms and novel targets for drug development.[53,54] To date, the cause of schizophrenia is unknown. There is general agreement that this is a brain disease, with alterations of white and gray matter, disconnectivity, and in vivo brain function. Research measures, such as neural synchrony, sleep architecture, smooth pursuit eye movements (SPEM), and prepulse inhibition, all reflect widespread disorder. The few narrower models are discussed in

Table 5
Tools used by the NIMH child branch in the evaluation of COS

Tool	Description
Initial evaluation	
Social Communication Questionnaire previously known as the Autism Screening Questionnaire	Brief instrument helps evaluate communication skills and social functioning in children who may have autism or autism spectrum disorders. Completed by a parent or other primary caregiver in less than 10 min
Kiddie-Sads-Present and Lifetime Version (K-SADS-PL)	A semi-structured diagnostic interview designed to assess current and past episodes of psychopathology in children and adolescents according to DSM-III-R and DSM-IV criteria
Psychotic Disorders Supplement[a] Affective Disorders Supplement[a] Anxiety Disorders Supplement[a] Behavioral Disorders Supplement[a] Substance abuse and other disorders supplement[a]	Supplements to the K-SADS-PL used for diagnostic exploration and clarification; administered in the order in which symptoms appeared
Follow-up	
Scale for the Assessment of Positive Symptoms[b]	Assessment of positive symptoms of psychosis devised primarily to focus on schizophrenia
Scale for the Assessment of Negative Symptoms[b]	Assessment of negative symptoms of psychosis devised primarily to focus on schizophrenia
Brief Psychiatric Rating Scale for Children	A 21-item, clinician-based rating scale designed for use in evaluating psychiatric problems of children and adolescents
Clinical Global Impressions Scale[b]	A primary outcome frequently used in medical care and clinical research to measure in studies evaluating the efficacy of treatments
Children's Global Impressions Scale[b]	An adaptation of the Clinical Global Impressions Scale for children
Bunny-Hamburg Global Ratings Psychosis subscale[b] Depression subscale[b]	Two subscales that, when used together, best exclude COS as a viable diagnosis (62% accuracy at screening, 85% accuracy at the medication-free period)[c]
Simpson-Angus Scale	An established instrument for neuroleptic-induced parkinsonism
Abnormal Involuntary Movement Scale	12-item clinician administered and scored anchored scale used to detect and follow the occurrence of tardive dyskinesia in patients receiving neuroleptic medications

[a] Used as indicated by the results of the K-SADS-PL.
[b] Available in the Handbook of Psychiatric Measures (Book with CD-ROM for Windows) by the American Psychiatric Association.
[c] Ref.[34]

this issue by Frazier, Dvir, and Cochran in "Autism and Schizophrenia" and by Dvir, Frazier, and Deneitolis in "Trauma and Psychosis."

The general model of schizophrenia as a neurodevelopmental disorder is widely held. One version focused on schizophrenia as a static lesion, occurring during fetal brain development,[55] whereas others argued that schizophrenia occurs as a result of a second "hit" in the form of abnormal brain development during adolescence,

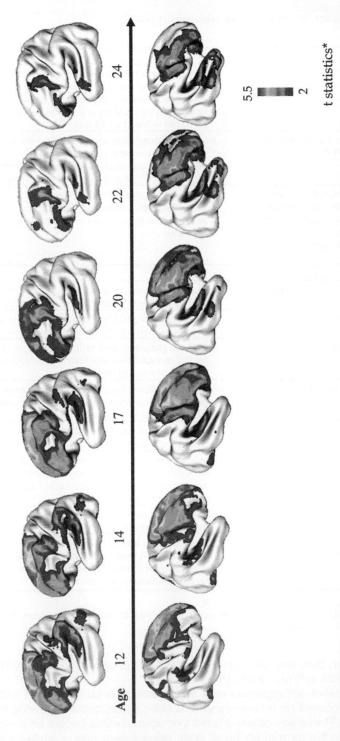

Fig. 1. Progression of cortical gray matter (GM) loss in childhood onset schizophrenia (COS) (n = 70, 162 scans) relative to age-, sex-, and scan interval–matched healthy controls (n = 72, 168 scans) from adolescence to young adulthood (age, 12–24 years).[48,49] Analyses were performed using mixed model regression statistics and co-varied from mean cortical thickness. Side bar shows t statistic with threshold to control for multiple comparisons using the false discovery rate procedure with q = 0.05. Differences are from mixed model regression with age centered at approximate 3-year intervals for middle 80% of the age range; colors represent areas of statistically significant thinning in COS.81.[43]

such as excessive synaptic and/or dendritic elimination resulting in aberrant neuronal connectivity.[9,56,57] These theories have merged and it is now generally understood that COS is a multifactorial illness, characterized by multiple genetic elements, each contributing a modest degree of risk[58] and interacting with the environment. There are also various other hypotheses focused on the cortical amino acid neurotransmitter systems (ie, dopamine, glutamate, GABA, serotonin).[59,60]

Alterations in genetics, neurodevelopment, and neurotransmitter systems[61] remain among the most promising directions for further research. Schizophrenia risk genes are associated with transcripts that are enriched in, or unique to, the human brain. Some also show preferential expression in the fetal brain.[62] Studies have revealed aberrant neuronal development, specifically localized to prefrontal and temporal cortices.[56] Alterations in timing of developmental disruption of GABAergic interneurons as the basis for several different neurodevelopmental disorders are gaining increasing support.[63] It is almost certain that both dopamine and glutamate transmission are abnormal in this disorder[64–66] and striatal dopamine overactivity may be critical to conversion to psychosis or psychotic symptoms generally.[56,67,68]

Not only does the cause of COS elude us, several roadblocks to progress toward finding the cause remain. First, the phenotypic, biologic, and etiologic heterogeneity of schizophrenia may account for the fact that the effect size of these individual risks does not support any single neurobiological finding as a core deficit in the illness.[54,69,70] Second, the difficulty in studying the human brain and the lack of good animal models continue to be a handicap. Recent postmortem studies indicate time-specific developmental genetic effects. It remains clear however that schizophrenia, including COS, has no clearly definable neuropathologic markers (eg, demyelinated neurons in multiple sclerosis).[54] Although the study of COS suggests it may have more salient genetic effects,[71] there is no finding of even a rare form of genetic dominant transmission for COS.

DIAGNOSTIC DILEMMAS

The diagnosis of COS is a difficult, time-consuming process. Although early developmental abnormalities in social, motor, and language domains in COS are more striking compared with the later onset cases,[22–24,28,72] they are not diagnostic and do not cumulatively represent a reliable premorbid phenotype. In addition, not only do healthy children experience hallucinations, but also children with various other psychiatric and behavioral disturbances present with positive symptoms.[73,74] Pressure from families, the severity of the clinical picture, and time limitations placed on providers coalesce to make the diagnosis of COS a tedious process fraught with pitfalls. The most common disorders misdiagnosed as COS are affective disorders, organic psychosis, pervasive developmental disorders, and a group referred to as "atypical psychosis" or "multidimensionally impaired (MDI)." Details regarding these disorders, the latter of which is an important differential and is described in detail in later discussion, and achieving diagnostic clarity are described elsewhere in this issue.

The NIMH cohort has been going on since 1990, using nationwide recruitment. Over the past 22 years, over 3000 charts have been reviewed. Of these, 90% are rejected from further consideration as they fail to meet the criteria for COS. Over 300 children have been screened in person, of whom approximately 60% receive other psychiatric diagnoses, such as affective disorders, anxiety, or behavioral disorders. More than 200 children who seemed likely to meet criteria for COS were admitted to the research unit and underwent an initial observation period followed by complete medication washout. After being observed off medications for up to 3 weeks, an additional

20% of children did not meet criteria for COS and received an alternative diagnosis. A 4-year to 6-year follow-up study of the ruled-out cases indicated good stability of the alternative diagnoses and nonschizophrenic status.[75] The most frequent alternative diagnoses have been affective disorders and anxiety disorders. A subgroup of children has also shown a form of atypical psychosis provisionally labeled as "MDI"[28,76,77] based on a unique set of features, which warrants further description.

The "Multidimensionally Impaired (MDI)" Group

To date, 33 children have been given the provisional diagnosis of "MDI" after the medication washout period and have been followed prospectively along with the COS children. This heterogeneous group of children, in general, has severe functional impairment associated with transient psychotic symptoms, multiple developmental abnormalities, abnormal neuropsychological test profiles, eye movement abnormalities, and familial risk factors that are not adequately characterized by existing DSM-IV categories.[76,78,79] Despite the presence of overlapping symptoms with childhood and early-onset schizophrenia, there are distinct features that have been used as the "operational diagnostic criteria" by the NIMH group to distinguish these individuals[76,78]:

1. Brief, transient episodes of psychosis and perceptual disturbance, typically in response to stress.
2. Nearly daily periods of emotional lability disproportionate to precipitants.
3. Impaired interpersonal skills despite the desire to initiate peer friendships (distinction from COS).
4. Cognitive deficits as indicated by multiple deficits in information processing.
5. No clear thought disorder (clinically can be difficult to define, especially in the presence of communication disorder).

Attention deficit hyperactivity disorder is highly comorbid in the MDI group.

At first glance, the symptom cluster these patients present suggests these children will likely progress to develop schizophrenia spectrum disorders; in the current DSM these patients could be considered psychosis NOS. These children are similar in some way to some of the other syndromes described, such as the multiple complex developmental disorder, borderline syndrome of childhood, or other borderline disorders of childhood.[79–82] However, contrary to MDI, these other syndromes have more predominant symptoms of pervasive developmental disorder, greater evidence of formal thought disorder, and onset before age 5.[79,83,84] The MDI group seems to have a distinct course, with none progressing to schizophrenia at long-term follow-up,[85] but strikingly, 38% developing bipolar disorder, type I.[86] This long-term data emphasize that when diagnosing a child with schizophrenia, there are significant short-term and long-term implications, including the potential for neglecting other disorders, because psychosis often becomes the primary focus.

PROCESS OF ELIMINATION

It has long been known that hallucinations, delusions, and disordered thoughts can occur in healthy nonpsychotic children[87] but usually diminish after age 6.[88] Transient anxiety-related and stress-related visual hallucinations are also occasionally reported in preschool children,[89] and the prognosis of these phenomena is benign. However, when psychotic phenomena occur in school-aged children, they generally tend to be more persistent and associated with drug toxicity or more significant mental illness.[1,90–92]

Box 1
Select comorbidities for childhood onset schizophrenia

Psychiatric comorbidities

- Obsessive–compulsive Disorder

- Attention Deficit Hyperactivity Disorder

- Expressive language disorders

- Receptive language disorders

- Auditory processing deficits

- Executive functioning deficits

- Mood disorder; primarily Major Depressive Disorder

Medical comorbidities associated with treatment

- Diabetes[a]

- Hyperlipidemia[a]

- Cardiovascular disease[a]

- Obesity[a]

- Hyperprolactinemia[a]

- Dyskinesia

   [a] Highly correlated with the treatment of schizophrenia.[94]

COMORBIDITIES

COS is highly correlated with other illnesses and disorders (**Box 1**).[24] During the evaluation of a child with suspected COS, it is imperative they are screened, with a high index of suspicion, for other comorbid illnesses and disorders, both psychiatric[18] and medical[93] (see **Table 5**),[94] the latter of which accounts for almost 60% of premature deaths not related to suicide in adult schizophrenia patients.[93,95]

SUMMARY: IMPLICATIONS FOR CLINICAL PRACTICE

Schizophrenia is a devastating illness, particularly when presenting in childhood or adolescence. Despite the presence of premorbid characteristics, a reliable premorbid phenotype has not been defined and research into the pathophysiology of the syndrome remains ongoing without a substantial target demonstrated in a systematic way. The frequency and duration of psychotic episodes have deleterious neuropsychological, neurophysiological, and neurostructural effects,[96–100] making prompt, aggressive treatment an important component of care. Once the diagnosis is established and other comorbid conditions are adequately assessed, clinicians should treat this illness aggressively. Treatment planning should encompass psychopharmacologic, psychotherapeutic, and early psychosocial intervention, such as support and education of the family about the disorder, particularly during the first years of the evolution of the disease, as these can actually improve the course of illness.[101] In addition, clinicians should not avoid using Clozapine, as evidenced by the epidemiologic studies demonstrating that its use occurs even much later than that recommended by the clinical guidelines.[101]

REFERENCES

1. Schreier HA. Hallucinations in nonpsychotic children: more common than we think? J Am Acad Child Adolesc Psychiatry 1999;38(5):623–5.
2. Childs B, Scriver CR. Age at onset and causes of disease. Perspect Biol Med 1986;29(3 Pt 1):437–60.
3. Kelleher I, Cannon M. Psychotic-like experiences in the general population: characterizing a high-risk group for psychosis. Psychol Med 2011;41(1):1–6.
4. Kelleher I, Connor D, Clarke MC, et al. Prevalence of psychotic symptoms in childhood and adolescence: a systematic review and meta-analysis of population-based studies. Psychol Med 2012;42(9):1857–63.
5. Werry JS. Child and adolescent (early onset) schizophrenia: a review in light of DSM-III-R. J Autism Dev Disord 1992;22(4):601–24.
6. McKenna K, Gordon CT, Rapoport JL. Childhood-onset schizophrenia: timely neurobiological research. J Am Acad Child Adolesc Psychiatry 1994;33(6):771–81.
7. Gordon CT, Frazier JA, McKenna K, et al. Childhood-onset schizophrenia: an NIMH study in progress. Schizophr Bull 1994;20(4):697–712.
8. Gogtay N, Weisinger B, Bakalar JL, et al. Psychotic symptoms and gray matter deficits in clinical pediatric populations. Schizophr Res 2012;140(1–3):149–54.
9. Rapoport JL, Gogtay N. Childhood onset schizophrenia: support for a progressive neurodevelopmental disorder. Int J Dev Neurosci 2011;29(3):251–8.
10. Nicolson R, Malaspina D, Giedd JN, et al. Obstetrical complications and childhood-onset schizophrenia. Am J Psychiatry 1999;156(10):1650–2.
11. Nicolson R, Giedd JN, Lenane M, et al. Clinical and neurobiological correlates of cytogenetic abnormalities in childhood-onset schizophrenia. Am J Psychiatry 1999;156(10):1575–9.
12. De Hert M, Dobbelaere M, Sheridan EM, et al. Metabolic and endocrine adverse effects of second-generation antipsychotics in children and adolescents: a systematic review of randomized, placebo controlled trials and guidelines for clinical practice. Eur Psychiatry 2011;26(3):144–58.
13. Large M, Nielssen O, Slade T, et al. Measurement and reporting of the duration of untreated psychosis. Early Interv Psychiatry 2008;2(4):201–11.
14. Singh SP. Outcome measures in early psychosis; relevance of duration of untreated psychosis. Br J Psychiatry Suppl 2007;50:s58–63.
15. Black K, Peters L, Rui Q, et al. Duration of untreated psychosis predicts treatment outcome in an early psychosis program. Schizophr Res 2001;47(2–3):215–22.
16. Done DJ, Crow TJ, Johnstone EC, et al. Childhood antecedents of schizophrenia and affective illness: social adjustment at ages 7 and 11. BMJ 1994;309(6956):699–703.
17. Jones P, Rodgers B, Murray R, et al. Child development risk factors for adult schizophrenia in the British 1946 birth cohort. Lancet 1994;344(8934):1398–402.
18. Rapoport J, Chavez A, Greenstein D, et al. Autism spectrum disorders and childhood-onset schizophrenia: clinical and biological contributions to a relation revisited. J Am Acad Child Adolesc Psychiatry 2009;48(1):10–8.
19. Gupta S, Rajaprabhakaran R, Arndt S, et al. Premorbid adjustment as a predictor of phenomenological and neurobiological indices in schizophrenia. Schizophr Res 1995;16(3):189–97.
20. Gupta S, Andreasen NC, Arndt S, et al. Neurological soft signs in neuroleptic-naive and neuroleptic-treated schizophrenic patients and in normal comparison subjects. Am J Psychiatry 1995;152(2):191–6.

21. Gupta SK, Kunka RL, Metz A, et al. Effect of alosetron (a new 5-HT3 receptor antagonist) on the pharmacokinetics of haloperidol in schizophrenic patients. J Clin Pharmacol 1995;35(2):202–7.
22. Hollis C. Child and adolescent (juvenile onset) schizophrenia. A case control study of premorbid developmental impairments. Br J Psychiatry 1995;166(4): 489–95.
23. Alaghband-Rad J, McKenna K, Gordon CT, et al. Childhood-onset schizophrenia: the severity of premorbid course. J Am Acad Child Adolesc Psychiatry 1995;34(10):1273–83.
24. Nicolson R, Lenane M, Singaracharlu S, et al. Premorbid speech and language impairments in childhood-onset schizophrenia: association with risk factors. Am J Psychiatry 2000;157(5):794–800.
25. Asarnow JR, Ben-Meir S. Children with schizophrenia spectrum and depressive disorders: a comparative study of premorbid adjustment, onset pattern and severity of impairment. J Child Psychol Psychiatry 1988;29(4):477–88.
26. Russell A, Bott L, Sammons C. The phenomena of schizophrenia occurring in childhood. J Am Acad Child Adolesc Psychiatry 1989;28:399–407.
27. Watkins JM, Asarnow RF, Tanguay PE. Symptom development in childhood onset schizophrenia. J Child Psychol Psychiatry 1988;29(6):865–78.
28. Nicolson R, Rapoport JL. Childhood-onset schizophrenia: rare but worth studying. Biol Psychiatry 1999;46(10):1418–28.
29. Kolvin I. Studies in the childhood psychoses. I. Diagnostic criteria and classification. Br J Psychiatry 1971;118(545):381–4.
30. Association, A.P. Recent Updates to Proposed Revisions for DSM-5. 2012; Recent Updates to Proposed Revisions for DSM-5. Available at: http://www.dsm5.org/Pages/RecentUpdates.aspx. Accessed November 28, 2012.
31. Murphy KC, Jones LA, Owen MJ. High rates of schizophrenia in adults with velo-cardio-facial syndrome. Arch Gen Psychiatry 1999;56(10):940–5.
32. Arinami T, Ohtsuki T, Takase K, et al. Screening for 22q11 deletions in a schizophrenia population. Schizophr Res 2001;52(3):167–70.
33. Green T, Gothelf D, Glaser B, et al. Psychiatric disorders and intellectual functioning throughout development in velocardiofacial (22q11.2 deletion) syndrome. J Am Acad Child Adolesc Psychiatry 2009;48(11):1060–8.
34. Gochman P, Miller R, Rapoport JL. Childhood-onset schizophrenia: the challenge of diagnosis. Curr Psychiatry Rep 2011;13(5):321–2.
35. Lawrie SM, Abukmeil SS. Brain abnormality in schizophrenia. A systematic and quantitative review of volumetric magnetic resonance imaging studies. Br J Psychiatry 1998;172:110–20.
36. Wright IC, Rabe-Hesketh S, Woodruff PW, et al. Meta-analysis of regional brain volumes in schizophrenia. Am J Psychiatry 2000;157(1):16–25.
37. Shenton ME, Dickey CC, Frumin M, et al. A review of MRI findings in schizophrenia. Schizophr Res 2001;49(1–2):1–52.
38. Pantelis C, Yucel M, Wood SJ, et al. Structural brain imaging evidence for multiple pathological processes at different stages of brain development in schizophrenia. Schizophr Bull 2005;31(3):672–96.
39. Mathalon DH, Sullivan EV, Lim KO, et al. Progressive brain volume changes and the clinical course of schizophrenia in men: a longitudinal magnetic resonance imaging study. Arch Gen Psychiatry 2001;58(2):148–57.
40. Gur RE, Cowell P, Turetsky BI, et al. A follow-up magnetic resonance imaging study of schizophrenia. Relationship of neuroanatomical changes to clinical and neurobehavioral measures. Arch Gen Psychiatry 1998;55(2):145–52.

41. Lieberman J, Chakos M, Wu H, et al. Longitudinal study of brain morphology in first episode schizophrenia. Biol Psychiatry 2001;49(6):487–99.
42. DeLisi LE. Regional brain volume change over the life-time course of schizophrenia. J Psychiatr Res 1999;33(6):535–41.
43. Gogtay N. Cortical brain development in schizophrenia: insights from neuroimaging studies in childhood-onset schizophrenia. Schizophr Bull 2008;34(1): 30–6.
44. Luders E, Narr KL, Thompson PM, et al. Mapping cortical gray matter in the young adult brain: effects of gender. Neuroimage 2005;26(2):493–501.
45. Thompson PM, Mega MS, Vidal C, et al. Detecting Disease Specific Patterns of Brain Structure using Cortical Pattern Matching and a Population-Based Probabilistic Brain Atlas, IEEE Conference on Information Processing in Medical Imaging (IPMI), UC Davis 2001. In: Insana M, Leahy RM, editors. Lecture Notes in Computer Science (LNCS), vol. 2082. Berlin, Heidelberg: Springer-Verlag; 2001. p. 488–501.
46. Thompson PM, Giedd JN, Woods RP, et al. Growth patterns in the developing brain detected by using continuum mechanical tensor maps. Nature 2000; 404(6774):190–3.
47. Gogtay N, Giedd JN, Lusk L, et al. Dynamic mapping of human cortical development during childhood through early adulthood. Proc Natl Acad Sci U S A 2004;101(21):8174–9.
48. Greenstein D, Lerch J, Shaw P, et al. Childhood onset schizophrenia: cortical brain abnormalities as young adults. J Child Psychol Psychiatry 2006;47(10): 1003–12.
49. Gogtay N, Greenstein D, Lenane M, et al. Cortical brain development in nonpsychotic siblings of patients with childhood-onset schizophrenia. Arch Gen Psychiatry 2007;64(7):772–80.
50. Gogtay N, Sporn A, Clasen LS, et al. Comparison of progressive cortical gray matter loss in childhood-onset schizophrenia with that in childhood-onset atypical psychoses. Arch Gen Psychiatry 2004;61(1):17–22.
51. Sporn AL, Greenstein DK, Gogtay N, et al. Progressive brain volume loss during adolescence in childhood-onset schizophrenia. Am J Psychiatry 2003;160(12): 2181–9.
52. Gogtay N, Sporn A, Clasen LS, et al. Structural brain MRI abnormalities in healthy siblings of patients with childhood-onset schizophrenia. Am J Psychiatry 2003;160(3):569–71.
53. Keshavan MS, Berger G, Zipursky RB, et al. Neurobiology of early psychosis. Br J Psychiatry Suppl 2005;48:s8–18.
54. Keshavan MS, Tandon R, Boutros NN, et al. Schizophrenia, "just the facts": what we know in 2008. Part 3: neurobiology. Schizophr Res 2008;106(2–3):89–107.
55. Weinberger DR. Implications of normal brain development for the pathogenesis of schizophrenia. Arch Gen Psychiatry 1987;44(7):660–9.
56. Rapoport JL, Giedd JN, Gogtay N. Neurodevelopmental model of schizophrenia: update 2012. Mol Psychiatry 2012;17(12):1228–38.
57. Feinberg I. Schizophrenia: caused by a fault in programmed synaptic elimination during adolescence? J Psychiatr Res 1982;17(4):319–34.
58. Gogos JA, Gerber DJ. Schizophrenia susceptibility genes: emergence of positional candidates and future directions. Trends Pharmacol Sci 2006;27(4): 226–33.
59. Miyamoto S, LaMantia AS, Duncan GE, et al. Recent advances in the neurobiology of schizophrenia. Mol Interv 2003;3(1):27–39.

60. Weinberger DR. The biological basis of schizophrenia: new directions. J Clin Psychiatry 1997;58(Suppl 10):22–7.
61. Sawa A, Snyder SH. Schizophrenia: diverse approaches to a complex disease. Science 2002;296(5568):692–5.
62. Kleinman JE, Law AJ, Lipska BK, et al. Genetic neuropathology of schizophrenia: new approaches to an old question and new uses for postmortem human brains. Biol Psychiatry 2011;69(2):140–5.
63. Marin O. Interneuron dysfunction in psychiatric disorders. Nat Rev Neurosci 2012;13(2):107–20.
64. Henn FA. Dopamine: a marker of psychosis and final common driver of schizophrenia psychosis. Am J Psychiatry 2011;168(12):1239–40.
65. Lewis DA, Gonzalez-Burgos G. Neuroplasticity of neocortical circuits in schizophrenia. Neuropsychopharmacology 2008;33(1):141–65.
66. Beneyto M, Lewis DA. Insights into the neurodevelopmental origin of schizophrenia from postmortem studies of prefrontal cortical circuitry. Int J Dev Neurosci 2011;29(3):295–304.
67. Howes OD, Bose SK, Turkheimer F, et al. Dopamine synthesis capacity before onset of psychosis: a prospective [18F]-DOPA PET imaging study. Am J Psychiatry 2011;168(12):1311–7.
68. Howes OD, Kapur S. The dopamine hypothesis of schizophrenia: version III–the final common pathway. Schizophr Bull 2009;35(3):549–62.
69. Tandon R, Keshavan MS, Nasrallah HA. Schizophrenia, "just the facts" what we know in 2008. 2. Epidemiology and etiology. Schizophr Res 2008;102(1–3): 1–18.
70. Tsuang MT, Faraone SV. The case for heterogeneity in the etiology of schizophrenia. Schizophr Res 1995;17(2):161–75.
71. Walsh T, McClellan JM, McCarthy SE, et al. Rare structural variants disrupt multiple genes in neurodevelopmental pathways in schizophrenia. Science 2008; 320(5875):539–43.
72. Green WH, Padron-Gayol M, Hardesty AS, et al. Schizophrenia with childhood onset: a phenomenological study of 38 cases. J Am Acad Child Adolesc Psychiatry 1992;31(5):968–76.
73. Garralda ME. Hallucinations in children with conduct and emotional disorders: II. The follow-up study. Psychol Med 1984;14(3):597–604.
74. Garralda ME. Hallucinations in children with conduct and emotional disorders: I. The clinical phenomena. Psychol Med 1984;14(3):589–96.
75. Calderoni D, Wudarsky M, Bhangoo R, et al. Differentiating childhood-onset schizophrenia from psychotic mood disorders. J Am Acad Child Adolesc Psychiatry 2001;40(10):1190–6.
76. McKenna K, Gordon CT, Lenane M, et al. Looking for childhood-onset schizophrenia: the first 71 cases screened. J Am Acad Child Adolesc Psychiatry 1994;33(5):636–44.
77. Kumra S, Briguglio C, Lenane M, et al. Including children and adolescents with schizophrenia in medication-free research. Am J Psychiatry 1999;156(7): 1065–8.
78. Kumra S, Jacobsen LK, Lenane M, et al. "Multidimensionally impaired disorder": is it a variant of very early-onset schizophrenia? J Am Acad Child Adolesc Psychiatry 1998;37(1):91–9.
79. Towbin KE, Dykens EM, Pearson GS, et al. Conceptualizing "borderline syndrome of childhood" and "childhood schizophrenia" as a developmental disorder. J Am Acad Child Adolesc Psychiatry 1993;32(4):775–82.

80. Dahl EK, Cohen DJ, Provence S. Clinical and multivariate approaches to the nosology of pervasive developmental disorders. J Am Acad Child Psychiatry 1986;25(2):170–80.

81. Petti TA, Vela RM. Borderline disorders of childhood: an overview. J Am Acad Child Adolesc Psychiatry 1990;29(3):327–37.

82. Van der Gaag RJ, Buitelaar J, Van den Ban E, et al. A controlled multivariate chart review of multiple complex developmental disorder. J Am Acad Child Adolesc Psychiatry 1995;34(8):1096–106.

83. Cohen DJ, Paul R, Volkmar FR. Issues in the classification of pervasive and other developmental disorders: toward DSM-IV. J Am Acad Child Psychiatry 1986; 25(2):213–20.

84. Ad-Dab'bagh Y, Greenfield B. Multiple complex developmental disorder: the "multiple and complex" evolution of the "childhood borderline syndrome" construct. J Am Acad Child Adolesc Psychiatry 2001;40(8):954–64.

85. Nicolson R, Lenane M, Brookner F, et al. Children and adolescents with psychotic disorder not otherwise specified: a 2- to 8-year follow-up study. Compr Psychiatry 2001;42(4):319–25.

86. Gogtay N, Ordonez A, Herman DH, et al. Dynamic mapping of cortical development before and after the onset of pediatric bipolar illness. J Child Psychol Psychiatry 2007;48(9):852–62.

87. Lukianowicz N. Hallucinations in non-psychotic children. Psychiatr Clin (Basel) 1969;2(6):321–37.

88. Caplan R. Thought disorder in childhood. J Am Acad Child Adolesc Psychiatry 1994;33(5):605–15.

89. Rothstein A. Hallucinatory phenomena in childhood. A critique of the literature. J Am Acad Child Psychiatry 1981;20(3):623–35.

90. Abramowicz M. Drugs that cause psychiatric symptoms. Med Lett Drugs Ther 1993;35:65–70.

91. Davison K. Schizophrenia-like psychoses associated with organic cerebral disorders: a review. Psychiatr Dev 1983;1(1):1–33.

92. McGee R, Williams S, Poulton R. Hallucinations in nonpsychotic children. J Am Acad Child Adolesc Psychiatry 2000;39(1):12–3.

93. Lambert TJ, Velakoulis D, Pantelis C. Medical comorbidity in schizophrenia. Med J Aust 2003;178(Suppl):S67–70.

94. Colton CW, Manderscheid RW. Congruencies in increased mortality rates, years of potential life lost, and causes of death among public mental health clients in eight states. Prev Chronic Dis 2006;3(2):A42.

95. Goff DC, Cather C, Evins AE, et al. Medical morbidity and mortality in schizophrenia: guidelines for psychiatrists. J Clin Psychiatry 2005;66(2):183–94 [quiz: 147, 273–4].

96. Ienciu M, Romosan F, Bredicean C, et al. First episode psychosis and treatment delay–causes and consequences. Psychiatr Danub 2010;22(4):540–3.

97. Franz L, Carter T, Leiner AS, et al. Stigma and treatment delay in first-episode psychosis: a grounded theory study. Early Interv Psychiatry 2010;4(1): 47–56.

98. Norman RM, Mallal AK, Manchanda R, et al. Does treatment delay predict occupational functioning in first-episode psychosis? Schizophr Res 2007;91(1–3): 259–62.

99. Compton MT, Esterberg ML. Treatment delay in first-episode nonaffective psychosis: a pilot study with African American family members and the theory of planned behavior. Compr Psychiatry 2005;46(4):291–5.

100. Harrigan SM, McGorry PD, Krstev H. Does treatment delay in first-episode psychosis really matter? Psychol Med 2003;33(1):97–110.
101. Vera I, Rezende L, Molina V, et al. Clozapine as treatment of first choice in first psychotic episodes. What do we know? Actas Esp Psiquiatr 2012;40(5): 281–9.

The Prodrome and Clinical Risk for Psychotic Disorders

Sandra M. Goulding, MPH, MA*, Carrie W. Holtzman, MA,
Hanan D. Trotman, PhD, Arthur T. Ryan, MA,
Allison N. MacDonald, BA, Daniel I. Shapiro, MA,
Joy L. Brasfield, BA, Elaine F. Walker, PhD

KEYWORDS

- Psychosis • Prodrome • Schizophrenia • Clinical high risk

KEY POINTS

- Clinical high-risk (CHR) syndromes are associated with milder versions of psychological deficits and biological abnormalities observed in psychotic disorders, with those manifesting greater severity of deficits and abnormalities appearing to be at higher risk for conversion to psychosis.
- Evidence of changes in brain structure during the prodromal phase indicates a neuropathologic process that may be the focus of future preventive intervention efforts to target neural mechanisms involved in the emergence of psychosis.
- Justification for intervention efforts (ie, clinical trials) requires further empirical inquiry designed to enhance the predictive power of current algorithms used to identify individuals likely to develop a psychotic disorder.

INTRODUCTION
Nature of the Problem

Despite decades of research on causes and treatment, schizophrenia and other psychotic disorders are still among the most severe and debilitating mental illnesses.[1] With typical onset in late adolescence/young adulthood, psychoses often have a chronic and relapsing course with potentially devastating functional implications. Although studies have examined the life span, research on the period preceding the modal age of psychosis onset has intensified.[2] Referred to as the prodrome, this period involves increasing symptoms and gradual functional decline that begin several months to years before clinical onset. As a result, the prodrome may offer the greatest

Disclosures: This research was supported in part by grant U01MHMH081988 from the National Institute of Mental Health awarded to Dr Walker.
Mental Health and Development Program, Department of Psychology, Emory University, 36 Eagle Row, Room 270, Atlanta, GA 30322, USA
* Corresponding author.
E-mail address: sandra.m.goulding@emory.edu

Child Adolesc Psychiatric Clin N Am 22 (2013) 557–567
http://dx.doi.org/10.1016/j.chc.2013.04.002
1056-4993/13/$ – see front matter © 2013 Elsevier Inc. All rights reserved.

childpsych.theclinics.com

promise for identifying neural mechanisms involved in the emergence of psychosis and implementing preventive intervention trials.[3] This article provides an overview of (1) the manifestation and measurement of prodromal syndromes; (2) cognitive, environmental, and neurobiological factors associated with psychosis risk; and (3) diagnostic and treatments issues.

Definition

Although current diagnostic taxonomies draw boundaries among subtypes of psychotic disorders, accumulating findings suggest that (1) genetic risk factors are not specific to subtypes of psychosis and no single gene has a major impact on risk status,[4] (2) prenatal and perinatal complications increase risk for affective and nonaffective psychoses,[5] and (3) bioenvironmental risk factors (eg, substance abuse) are linked with risk for the full spectrum of psychoses.[6] Although future research will likely result in the identification of distinct causal subtypes, at present the natural diagnostic boundaries are unknown. Therefore psychoses and psychotic disorders are used in this article to refer to the spectrum of psychotic disorders, including affective and nonaffective disorders.

Although the psychosis prodrome is a retrospective construct, with the term prodromal suggesting inevitability of subsequent illness, contemporary research on the prodrome is prospective in nature. Such studies use standardized measures to index subclinical perceptual, ideational, and behavioral symptoms of psychosis, and individuals whose symptoms exceed a specified severity threshold are designated as clinical high risk (CHR).[7–10]

Prodromal Syndrome Criteria

Commonly used measures of CHR syndromes (**Table 1**) are based on empirical findings from retrospective research on symptoms and functional deficits that precede

Table 1
Measures of clinical high-risk symptoms/syndromes used in prospective investigations of CHR groups

	Format			Symptoms/Syndromes Measured		
Measure	Structured Interview	Clinical Checklist	Basic Symptoms[a]	Genetic Risk and Deterioration[b]	Brief Limited Psychotic Episode[c]	Attenuated Positive Symptoms[d]
BSIP	X			X	X	X
CAARMS	X			X	X	X
SIPS/SOPS	X			X	X	X
SPI-A/SPI-CY		X	X	X	X	X

Abbreviations: BSIP, Basel Screening Instrument for Psychosis[7]; CAARMS, Comprehensive Assessment of the At-risk Mental State[8]; SIPS/SOPS, Structured Interview for Prodromal Syndromes/Scale of Prodromal Symptoms[9]; SPI-A/SPI-CY, Schizophrenia Proneness Instrument, adult version/child and youth version.[10,11]
   [a] Basic symptoms include cognitive-perceptive symptoms and cognitive disturbances.
   [b] Genetic risk deterioration generally involves genetic risk/family history of psychosis and functional decline.
   [c] Brief limited psychotic episode includes transient psychotic symptoms at a specified frequency over a given period of time.
   [d] Attentuated positive symptoms are subthresholds for the frequency, severity, and duration required for a psychotic episode/disorder.

psychosis onset. Attenuated positive symptoms, pivotal in CHR criteria and indexed by all of these measures, include unusual perceptual experiences and ideations that do not meet the level of conviction and severity required for hallucinations and delusions. Likewise, the suspiciousness observed in the prodrome is not at the intensity of paranoid delusions, and the disorganized communication does not meet the threshold for diagnosis of a formal thought disorder. In addition to attenuated positive symptoms, measures also tap subclinical negative symptoms.

The Structured Interview for Prodromal Syndromes (SIPS) is the most widely used measure of prodromal syndromes in the United States. Like other measures that use standard CHR criteria, the SIPS enhances positive predictive power (ie, the ratio of true-positives to combined true-positives and false-positives) greater than the population prevalence rate for psychoses (ie, 1%–2%).[9] Among those identified as putatively prodromal, only a proportion goes on to develop a psychotic disorder. Current estimates suggest that only 20% to 40% of those who meet CHR criteria convert to psychosis within 2 to 4 years. Therefore, although superior to predictive power based solely on genetic high risk (GHR; ie, family history of psychosis) status,[11] the rates of false-positives (ie, those who do not develop psychosis) identified by current measures of prodromal syndromes remain substantial. As a result, to improve predictive power, researchers continue to refine and combine these measures with other indices.

Nonetheless, as summarized later, CHR syndromes are associated with abnormalities similar to those observed in psychoses, with the most pronounced found in those who later convert to psychosis. These studies are typically longitudinal and involve both CHR and healthy control (HC) groups. In addition to monitoring progression of clinical, behavioral, and neurobiological factors assessed at baseline, follow-up assessments also track progression to psychosis onset. For example, the North American Prodrome Longitudinal Study (NAPLS[12]) uses the Structured Clinical Interview for Diagnostic and Statistical Manual of Mental Disorders, Fourth Edition, axis I disorders to determine symptoms that indicate psychosis.[13]

CLINICAL FINDINGS
General and Social Cognitive Functioning

Cognitive deficits, particularly in memory and attentional functions, are among the most extensively documented aspects of psychosis.[14,15] Likewise, a recent meta-analysis concluded that CHR individuals have significant cognitive deficits relative to matched HCs, and that CHR participants who convert to psychosis have greater baseline impairment than nonconverters.[16] The severity of processing speed and verbal memory deficits also discriminates converters from nonconverters, with verbal memory impairment predicting faster conversion rates. In addition, cognitive impairments worsen over time, with those later in the developmental course of the prodrome displaying greater deficits in some domains than those in early phases.[17]

Considerable research has also shown pervasive social cognitive impairment, including deficits in social reasoning and processing of social and emotional information, in patients with chronic and first-episode psychosis (FEP).[18] Current evidence suggests that CHR groups exhibit performance on social cognitive tasks that is intermediate to HC and FEP groups.[19] Follow-up studies indicate that deficits are more pronounced in converters than nonconverters, and predict faster conversion rates even when controlling for general cognitive functioning at baseline.[20] In addition, evidence for temporal stability of impairment in those with recent onset of psychosis suggests that social cognitive deficits are traitlike rather than transient.[21]

Psychosocial Stress and Trauma

Although cross-sectional studies provide no consistent evidence that patients with psychosis experience more stressful life events (eg, death of loved one) than controls, longitudinal studies indicate that patients rate events as more stressful and have a significant increase in number of events before relapse.[22,23] Further, studies of minor stressors (eg, being stuck in traffic) have linked these daily hassles with positive and affective symptom severity in patient groups.[23] Although the numbers of stressful life events/daily stressors do not differ between CHR and HC groups, those at CHR experience them as more stressful when they occur.[24] Within CHR groups, chronic stress is a predictor of positive and depressive symptom severity.[25] In addition, CHR and patient groups report more emotional reactivity to daily stressors, with daily stress intensifying symptom severity.[26,27] Further, both groups also report greater exposure to childhood trauma, which has been linked with increased risk for psychosis conversion.[28] As discussed later, evidence also suggests greater biological sensitivity to stress in CHR groups.

Substance Abuse

Substance use, abuse, and dependence are common in patients with psychoses. CHR groups also show increased rates of substance use/abuse, and use of any illicit substance has been associated with increased risk of psychosis conversion.[12] Most research in the prodrome has focused on cannabis, which has been linked with increased risk of relapse and poorer clinical course in patient groups.[29] Interest in cannabis also stems from studies showing that administration of delta-9-tetrahydrocannabinol, the active ingredient in cannabis, can elicit positive, negative, and cognitive symptoms of psychoses.[30] Retrospective studies of the general population have linked cannabis use with earlier onset of the prodrome and greater risk of psychosis.[31,32] Although cannabis use is increased in CHR samples, prospective studies have not linked cannabis use and risk of psychosis conversion.[33] Further research is needed to determine whether use has a causal role in psychosis onset, or reflects self-medication of prodromal symptoms.

IMAGING
Neuroanatomy

A wide range of abnormalities in brain structure are associated with psychotic disorders. A recent review indicates decreases in intracranial and total brain volume, with the largest reductions in gray matter volume within cortical and subcortical regions.[34] White matter reduction has also been observed in both medication-naive and medicated groups, and has been linked with severity of illness progression. A review of research involving CHR groups similarly indicates cortical and hippocampal gray matter volume reductions,[35] with more pronounced reductions in converters than nonconverters.[36] Consistent with evidence of significant memory impairment, hippocampal volume seems to be reduced in patient and CHR groups.[37] Results suggest that brain volume reductions associated with psychosis precede illness onset. Further, increasing evidence of neuroplasticity in adolescents/young adults[22] suggests that these developmental brain abnormalities may prove to be targets for preventive intervention.

Neurophysiology

Among the most consistently reported biomarkers in psychoses, as measured with electroencephalogram and electromyogram, are abnormal neurophysiologic indices that include measures of response inhibition and deviance detection.[38–40] Measures of response inhibition include prepulse inhibition (PPI), P50 suppression, and antisaccade (AS) eye movement suppression. PPI is a reduction of the startle response that results when a startle stimulus is preceded by a nonstartling warning stimulus. In brief, PPI modulates the startle reflex, is associated with a smaller startle response, and enhances the ability to process stimuli. In contrast, P50 is a positive event-related potential (ERP), and decreases in P50 amplitude on presentation of repetitious stimuli reflect the ability to gate out redundant information. In addition, reflexive AS can be reduced by voluntarily focusing visual attention on a specific location or object. Errors and/or latencies indicate dysfunction in the frontal cortex, which controls saccadic eye movements.

With regard to deviance detection, measures include mismatch negativity (MMN) and P300 ERP. P300, a large positive component of the poststimulus ERP waveform, is more pronounced in response to novel stimuli and reflects capacity to attend to/detect a stimulus, update working memory, and attribute salience to a deviant stimulus. Reductions are associated with negative symptoms, declining attentional capacities, and gray matter volume deficits. However, MMN is a negative ERP waveform that is observed when repetitively alternating stimuli are periodically interrupted by a third distinctly different stimulus. Because MMN reflects greater capacity to detect differences among stimuli despite the distractor stimulus (ie, auditory discrimination), reductions indicate sensory-memory anomalies.

Although comparisons of PPI in HC and CHR groups have not revealed consistent differences,[41–43] few examine the association with psychosis conversion. There is more consistent evidence that CHR groups manifest reductions in P50 suppression relative to HCs,[44] with more pronounced reductions in those who also meet GHR criteria.[45] Likewise, comparisons of CHR and HC groups reveal trends for reduced AS suppression and MMN.[46–49] However, the most consistent findings concern P300 amplitude. In brief, CHR groups manifest reduced amplitude relative to HCs and the magnitude of reduction discriminates converters from nonconverters.[50] P300 amplitude is also linked to white and gray matter volume,[51] suggesting that functional brain impairments tapped by neurophysiologic indices reflect structural brain abnormalities.

PATHOLOGY
Neurotransmitters: Dopaminergic and Glutamatergic Systems

Theories of dopamine (DA) activity in psychosis have been prominent for decades, and substantial evidence indicates heightened DA in subcortical regions. Patients with psychosis manifest increased striatal DA activity and DA receptor density, and the extent of DA receptor occupancy (eg, D2 receptor) is associated with effectiveness of antipsychotics.[52] Dysregulated presynaptic DA activity results in excessive DA release from areas projecting to the striatum, especially in the associative striatum where cognitive and limbic cortical inputs are integrated.[53] CHR groups also show heightened DA activity (eg, increased DA synthesis),[54,55] with DA function in the brain stem recently linked to psychosis conversion.[56]

Antagonists of the N-methyl-D-aspartic acid (NMDA) glutamate receptor increase extracellular glutamate, a known cause of oxidative stress, excitotoxicity, and hallucinations.[57] CHR and FEP groups have recently been shown to have increased levels of glutamate in the dorsal caudate.[58] In addition, expression of the proteins required for proper functioning of the glutamate system are reduced in patient, GHR, and CHR groups,[59] and evidence indicating an inverse relationship between thalamic glutamate levels and frontal cortical activity not found in HCs[60] suggests that aberrant glutamate activity alters cortical function in CHR individuals.

DA and glutamate systems in the brain are intimately linked functionally, and it is likely that both have a role in the cause of psychosis.[61] In brief, negative symptoms and cognitive deficits are linked with glutamate dysfunction, whereas DA abnormalities are suggested to subserve positive symptoms. Interconnectedness of glutamate and DA systems also suggests that dysregulation in one can precipitate dysregulation in the other. Evidence of an inverse relationship between hippocampal glutamate and striatal DA activity in those at CHR but not HCs[62] suggests that relatedness of hippocampal glutamate and striatal DA activity is altered. Results also indicated a link between DA uptake and severity of abnormal beliefs, and for the interaction of hippocampal glutamate and DA uptake to predict psychosis conversion.

Biological Stress Response: the Hypothalamic-Pituitary-Adrenal Axis

Because of the hypothesized role of stress in triggering symptom expression, indices of the biological stress response are of interest in CHR samples. The few studies that have investigated hypothalamic-pituitary-adrenal (HPA) function in CHR groups suggest increased baseline cortisol that also discriminates converters from nonconverters.[63,64] Evidence suggests that converters have larger baseline pituitary volume than nonconverters, which also indicates increased HPA activity.[65] In addition, in a positron emission tomography study examining stress-induced cortisol and DA, those at CHR had more pronounced DA and cortisol responses than HCs, and increases in cortisol were positively associated with DA.[66] Results are consistent with the notion that stress exacerbates psychotic symptoms via augmentation of DA.

DIAGNOSTIC DILEMMAS

Significant controversies and challenges surround diagnoses of CHR syndromes.[67] With regard to inclusion of Attenuated Positive Syndrome (APS) as a formal diagnosis in diagnostic taxonomies, arguments in favor have included benefits for research and the observation that individuals who meet CHR syndrome criteria are typically seeking help and in distress. Arguments against involve concerns of overdiagnosis, stigmatization, and excessive medication of those who are false-positives. After considering proposals and preliminary data, it was decided that DSM-V will not include a provisional APS diagnosis.[68] Future research will decide whether APS is reconsidered for later DSM revisions, which will partly depend on enhancement of risk prediction beyond levels achieved with current measurement of CHR syndromes.

Meanwhile, practitioners are confronted with the need to diagnose CHR syndromes, and the range of nonspecific symptoms that tend to co-occur with the prodrome contributes to diagnostic complexity. A vignette of a typical CHR case is provided in **Box 1**.

Before prospective studies of CHR samples, retrospective studies documented the broad range of symptoms and syndromes (eg, depression, anxiety, obsessive-compulsive behavior, learning and attentional problems, personality disorders, and substance abuse) that precede psychosis. Prospective research in CHR samples yields similar findings, with many cases meeting criteria for at least 1 life-time/current diagnosis, and half having a life-time diagnosis of depressive or anxiety disorder.[12,69] Thus, as with psychotic disorders, the psychosis prodrome is characterized by a high rate of comorbid psychiatric syndromes. In the absence of a formal diagnostic category, those with attenuated positive symptoms will continue to be diagnosed from typically co-occurring symptoms or syndromes.

Box 1
Clinical Vignette: CHR

John is an 18-year-old college freshman who arrived for the interview with a disheveled appearance. He reported no history of psychiatric problems, although he did see a counselor in high school for depressive feelings. John described current sadness and distress about increasing problems with concentration and academic performance. Although enthusiastic at the beginning of the school year, John has experienced a decrease in academic and social motivation and greater preoccupation with interpersonal relationships. He has made no friends in college, and thinks that the other students are avoiding him and criticizing him behind his back. Although not sure about the nature of the criticism, John speculated that it might be caused by his increased interest and involvement in paranormal phenomena. John stated that moving on campus at the start of freshman year and being exposed to a new peer group has resulted in him thinking that there may be paranormal influences at work in what he once would have considered coincidental interactions with others. During the first semester he joined a campus meditation group to deal with stress, and shared his fascination with paranormal experiences with the members of the group. More specifically, John described his belief that most of what humans experience is through a sixth sense and that awareness of the sense is only achieved by a subgroup of individuals like him. Although he voluntarily admitted to the examiner that this could just be his imagination, John added that now, almost on a daily basis, he has transient feelings that he is receiving sixth-sense messages from others students when he passes by them on campus. Nonetheless, in hindsight, he thinks he should not have shared these ideas with the group, because it gave them the wrong impression.

Most of those meeting CHR criteria in research settings have been treated with psychotherapy or pharmacotherapy, with medications most commonly prescribed being antidepressants (49%), antipsychotics (24%), stimulants (14%), and mood stabilizers (11%).[70] Findings suggest that practitioners are treating mood syndromes and attenuated positive symptoms, but there are insufficient data to inform these interventions. For example, antipsychotics can reduce attenuated positive symptoms and delay psychosis onset, but there are no studies that show their effectiveness as preventive agents in CHR groups.[71] Likewise, antidepressants may reduce symptom severity (especially pronounced depressive symptoms), but support for their effectiveness as preventive agents in CHR samples is lacking.

Although evidence suggests that cognitive behavioral interventions and omega-3 fatty acids can reduce attenuated positive and mood symptoms, more clinical trials addressing symptom reduction and psychosis prevention are needed.[71] In the interim, there are 3 foci in CHR treatment. First, treatment should be designed to reduce current symptoms (eg, mood) that accompany CHR syndromes and cause significant distress. Second, treatment should augment protective factors (eg, improve family environment and social skills, and decrease substance use) to reduce the likelihood of psychosis conversion. Third, close monitoring increases the likelihood that positive symptoms will be rapidly and effectively treated if they reach psychotic threshold.

SUMMARY

Significant progress has been made in the characterization of CHR syndromes, and findings indicate that they are associated with milder versions of many psychological deficits and biological abnormalities observed in psychotic disorders. Moreover, those at CHR who manifest the most severe deficits and abnormalities seem to be at greatest risk for psychosis conversion. Findings indicating prodromal changes in brain structure suggest that this stage is characterized by neuroplasticity that can provide leverage for preventive intervention. Although a level of scientific understanding that supports specific interventions has not yet been reached, the present trajectory of research progress holds promise for the future. One of the main goals of ongoing research is development of better prediction algorithms with the goal of attaining levels of positive predictive power that can justify delivery of preventive interventions in clinical trials.

REFERENCES

1. Murray CJL, Lopez AD. The global burden of disease: a comprehensive assessment of mortality and disability from diseases, injuries, and risk factors in 1990 and projected to 2020. Cambridge (MA): Harvard University Press; 1996.
2. Yung AR, McGorry PD. The prodromal phase of first-episode psychosis: past and current conceptualizations. Schizophr Bull 1996;22:353–70.
3. Addington J, Heinssen R. Prediction and prevention of psychosis in youth at clinical high risk. Annu Rev Clin Psychol 2012;8:269–89.
4. O'Donovan MC, Craddock NJ, Owen MJ. Genetics of psychosis; insights from views across the genome. Hum Genet 2009;126:3–12.
5. Buka SL, Fan AP. Association of prenatal and perinatal complications with subsequent bipolar disorder and schizophrenia. Schizophr Res 1999;39:113–9.
6. Moore TH, Zammit S, Lingford-Hughes A, et al. Cannabis use and risk of psychotic or affective mental health outcomes: a systematic review. Lancet 2007; 370:319–28.
7. Riecher-Rössler A, Aston J, Ventura J, et al. The Basel Screening Instrument for Psychosis: development, structure, reliability and validity. Fortschr Neurol Psychiatr 2008;76:207–16.
8. Yung AR, Yuen HP, McGorry PD, et al. Mapping the onset of psychosis: the Comprehensive Assessment of At-Risk Mental States. Aust N Z J Psychiatry 2005;39:964–71.
9. Miller TJ, McGlashan TH, Rosen JL, et al. Prodromal assessment with the structured interview for prodromal syndromes and the scale of prodromal symptoms: predictive validity, interrater reliability, and training to reliability. Schizophr Bull 2003;29:703–15.
10. Schulze-Lutter F, Ruhrmann S, Fusar-Poli P, et al. Diagnosing schizophrenia in the initial prodromal phase. Arch Gen Psychiatry 2001;58:158–64.
11. Sorensen HJ, Mortensen EL, Reinisch JM, et al. Parental psychiatric hospitalisation and offspring schizophrenia. World J Biol Psychiatry 2009;10:571–5.
12. Cannon TD, Cadenhead K, Cornblatt B, et al. Prediction of psychosis in youth at high clinical risk. Arch Gen Psychiatry 2008;65:28–37.
13. First M, Spitzer RL, Gibbon M, et al. Structured clinical interview for DSM-IV axis I disorders, patient edition (SCID-I/P). New York: NYS Psychiatric Institute; 2002.
14. Mesholam-Gately RI, Guiliano AJ, Goff KR, et al. Neurocognition in first-episode schizophrenia: a meta-analytic review. Neuropsychology 2009;23:315–36.
15. Bora E, Yucel M, Pantelis C. Cognitive impairment in affective psychoses: a meta-analysis. Schizophr Bull 2010;36:112–25.
16. Giuliano AJ, Li H, Mesholam-Gately RI, et al. Neurocognition in psychosis risk syndrome: quantitative and qualitative review. Curr Pharm Des 2012;18: 399–415.
17. Schultze-Lutter F, Ruhrmann S, Picker H, et al. Relationship between subjective and objective cognitive function in the early and late prodrome. Br J Psychiatry Suppl 2007;191:s43–51.
18. Horan W, Olivier P, Kern R, et al. Neurocognition, social cognition and functional outcome in schizophrenia. In: Gaebel W, editor. Schizophrenia: current science

and clinical practice. Oxford (United Kingdom): John Wiley & Sons; 2011. p. 65–108.

19. Kim HS, Shin NY, Jang JH, et al. Social cognition and neurocognition as predictors to psychosis in individuals at ultra-high risk. Schizophr Res 2012;38: 865–72.

20. Green MF, Bearden CE, Cannon TD, et al. Social cognition in schizophrenia, part 1: performance across phase of illness. Schizophr Bull 2012;38:854–64.

21. Horan WP, Green MF, de Groot M, et al. Social cognition in schizophrenia, part 2: 12 month prediction of outcome in first-episode patients. Schizophr Bull 2012; 38:865–72.

22. Walker EF, Mittal V, Tessner K. Stress and the hypothalamic pituitary adrenal axis in the developmental course of schizophrenia. Annu Rev Clin Psychol 2008;4: 189–216.

23. Phillips LJ, Francey SM, Edwards J, et al. Stress and psychosis: towards the development of new models of investigation. Clin Psychol Rev 2007;27:307–17.

24. Holtzman CW, Shapiro DI, Trotman HD, et al. Stress and the prodromal phase of psychosis. Curr Pharm Des 2012;18:527–33.

25. Phillips LJ, Edwards J, McMurray N, et al. Comparison of experiences of stress and coping between young people at risk of psychosis and a non-clinical cohort. Behav Cogn Psychother 2012;40:69–88.

26. Pruessner M, Iyer SN, Faridi K, et al. Stress and protective factors in individuals at ultra-high risk for psychosis, first episode psychosis, and healthy controls. Schizophr Res 2011;129:29–35.

27. Palmier-Claus JE, Dunn G, Lewis SW. Emotional and symptomatic reactivity to stress in individuals at ultra-high risk of developing psychosis. Psychol Med 2012;42:1003–12.

28. Bechdolf A, Thompson A, Nelson B, et al. Experience of trauma and conversion to psychosis in an ultra-high-risk (prodromal) group. Acta Psychiatr Scand 2010; 121:377–84.

29. van der Meer FJ, Velthorst E, Meijer CJ, et al. Cannabis use in patients at clinical high risk of psychosis: impact on prodromal symptoms and transition to psychosis. Curr Pharm Des 2012;18:5036–44.

30. D'Souza DC, Perry E, MacDougall L, et al. The psychotomimetic effects of intravenous delta-9-tetrahydrocannabinol in healthy individuals: implications for psychosis. Neuropsychopharmacology 2004;29:1558–72.

31. van Os J, Bak M, Hanssen M, et al. Cannabis use and psychosis: a longitudinal population-based study. Am J Epidemiol 2002;156:319–27.

32. Compton MT, Broussard B, Ramsay CE, et al. Pre-illness cannabis use and the early course of nonaffective psychotic disorders. Schizophr Res 2011;126: 71–6.

33. Auther AM, McLaughlin D, Carrión RE, et al. Prospective study of cannabis use in adolescents at clinical high risk for psychosis: impact on conversion to psychosis and functional outcome. Psychol Med 2012;42:2485–97.

34. Hajima S, van Haren N, Cahn W. Brain volumes in schizophrenia: a meta-analysis in over 18,000 subjects. Schizophr Bull 2012. [Epub ahead of print].

35. Smieskova R, Fusar-Poli P, Allen P, et al. Neuroimaging predictors of transition to psychosis - systematic review and meta-analysis. Neurosci Biobehav Rev 2010; 34:1206–22.

36. Fusar-Poli P, Crossley N, Woolley J, et al. Gray matter alterations related to P300 abnormalities in subjects at high risk for psychosis: longitudinal MRI-EEG study. Neuroimage 2011;55:320–8.

37. Witthaus H, Mendes U, Brüne M, et al. Hippocampal subdivision and amygdalar volumes in patients in an at-risk mental state for schizophrenia. J Psychiatry Neurosci 2010;35:33–40.
38. Cadenhead KS. Vulnerability markers in the schizophrenia spectrum: implications for phenomenology, genetics, and the identification of the schizophrenia prodrome. Psychiatr Clin North Am 2002;25:837–53.
39. Turetsky BI, Calkins ME, Light GA, et al. Neurophysiological endophenotypes of schizophrenia: the viability of selected candidate measures. Schizophr Bull 2007;33:69–94.
40. van der Stelt O, Belger A. Application of electroencephalography to the study of cognitive and brain functions in schizophrenia. Schizophr Bull 2007;33:955–70.
41. Ziermans T, Schothorst P, Magnee M, et al. Reduced prepulse inhibition in adolescents at risk for psychosis: a 2-year follow-up study. J Psychiatry Neurosci 2011;36:127–34.
42. Ziermans T, Schothorst P, Sprong M, et al. Reduced prepulse inhibition as an early vulnerability marker of the psychosis prodrome in adolescence. Schizophr Res 2012;134:10–5.
43. Cadenhead KS. Startle reactivity and prepulse inhibition in prodromal and early psychosis: effects of age, antipsychotics, tobacco and cannabis in a vulnerable population. Psychiatry Res 2011;188:208–16.
44. Brockhaus-Dumke A, Schultze-Lutter F, Mueller R, et al. Sensory gating in schizophrenia: P50 and N100 gating in antipsychotic-free subjects at risk, first-episode, and chronic patients. Biol Psychiatry 2008;64:376–84.
45. Cadenhead KS, Light GA, Shafer KM, et al. P50 suppression in individuals at risk for schizophrenia: convergence of clinical, familial, and vulnerability marker risk assessment. Biol Psychiatry 2005;57:1504–9.
46. Nieman D, Becker H, van de Fliert R, et al. Antisaccade task performance in patients at ultra-high-risk for developing psychosis. Schizophr Res 2007;95:54–60.
47. Atkinson RJ, Michie PT, Schall U. Duration mismatch negativity and P300a in first-episode psychosis and individuals at ultra-high risk. Biol Psychiatry 2012;71:98–104.
48. Brockhaus-Dumke A, Tendolkar I, Pukrop R, et al. Impaired mismatch negativity generation in prodromal subjects and patients with schizophrenia. Schizophr Res 2005;73:297–310.
49. Bodatsch M, Ruhrmann S, Wagner M, et al. Prediction of psychosis by mismatch negativity. Biol Psychiatry 2011;69:959–66.
50. van Tricht MJ, Nieman DH, Koelman JH, et al. Auditory ERP components before and after transition to a first psychotic episode. Biol Psychol 2011;87:350–7.
51. Fusar-Poli P, Crossley N, Woolley J, et al. White matter alterations related to P300 abnormalities in individuals at high risk for psychosis: an MRI-EEG study. J Psychiatry Neurosci 2011;36:239–48.
52. Uchida H, Takeuchi H, Graff-Guerrero A, et al. Dopamine D2 receptor occupancy and clinical effects. J Clin Psychopharmacol 2011;31:497–502.
53. Miyake N, Thompson J, Skinbjerg M, et al. Presynaptic dopamine in schizophrenia. CNS Neurosci Ther 2011;17:104–9.
54. Bauer M, Praschak-Rieder N, Kasper S, et al. Is dopamine neurotransmission altered in prodromal schizophrenia? A review of the evidence. Curr Pharm Des 2012;18:1568–79.
55. Howes OD, Bose SK, Turkheimer F, et al. Dopamine synthesis capacity before onset of psychosis: prospective [18F]-DOPA PET imaging study. Am J Psychiatry 2011;168:1311–7.

56. Allen P, Luigjes J, Howes OD, et al. Transition to psychosis associated with pre-frontal and subcortical dysfunction in ultra-high-risk individuals. Schizophr Bull 2012;38(6):1268–76.
57. Kantrowitz JT, Javitt DC. N-methyl-D-aspartate receptor dysfunction or dysregu-lation: the final common pathway on the road to schizophrenia? Brain Res Bull 2010;83:108–21.
58. de la Fuente-Sandoval C, Leon-Ortiz P, Favila R, et al. Higher levels of glutamate in the associative-striatum of subjects with prodromal symptoms of schizo-phrenia and patients with first-episode psychosis. Neuropsychopharmacology 2011;36:1781–91.
59. Correll CU, Hauser M, Auther AM, et al. Research in people with psychosis risk syndrome: a review of current evidence, future directions. J Child Psychol Psy-chiatry 2010;51:390–431.
60. Egerton A, Fusar-Poli P, Stone JM. Glutamate and psychosis risk. Curr Pharm Des 2012;18:466–78.
61. Stone JM, Morrison PD, Pilowsky LS. Glutamate and dopamine dysregulation in schizophrenia–a synthesis and selective review. J Psychopharmacol 2007;21:440–52.
62. Stone JM, Howes OD, Egerton A. Altered relationship between hippocampal glutamate levels and striatal dopamine function in subjects at ultra high risk of psychosis. Biol Psychiatry 2010;68:599–602.
63. Sugranyes G, Thompson JL, Corcoran CM. HPA-axis function, symptoms, and medication exposure in youths at clinical high risk for psychosis. J Psychiatr Res 2012;46:1389–93.
64. Walker EF, Brennan PA, Esterberg ML, et al. Longitudinal changes in cortisol secretion and conversion to psychosis in at-risk youth. J Abnorm Psychol 2010;119:401–8.
65. Garner B, Pariente C, Wood S, et al. Pituitary volume predicts future transition to psychosis in individuals at ultra-high risk of developing psychosis. Biol Psychi-atry 2005;58:417–23.
66. Mizrahi R, Addington J, Rusjan PM, et al. Increased stress-induced dopamine release in psychosis. Biol Psychiatry 2012;71(6):561–7.
67. Carpenter WT, van Os J. Should attenuated psychosis syndrome be a DSM-5 diagnosis? Am J Psychiatry 2011;168:460–3.
68. Yung AR, Woods SW, Ruhrmann S, et al. Whither the attenuated psychosis syn-drome? Schizophr Bull 2012;38:1130–4.
69. Salokangas RK, Ruhrmann S, von Reventlow HG, et al. Axis I diagnoses and transition to psychosis in clinical high-risk patients EPOS project: prospective follow-up of 245 clinical high-risk outpatients in four countries. Schizophr Res 2012;138:192–7.
70. Cadenhead KS, Addington J, Cannon T, et al. Treatment history in the psychosis prodrome: characteristics of the North American Prodrome Longitudinal Study cohort. Early Interv Psychiatry 2010;4:220–6.
71. Fusar-Poli P, Borgwardt S, Bechdolf A, et al. The psychosis high-risk state: a comprehensive state-of-the-art review. Arch Gen Psychiatry 2012;19:1–14.

Affective Disorders and Psychosis in Youth

Gabrielle A. Carlson, MD

KEYWORDS

• Mania • Depression • Bipolar psychosis • Mood congruent/incongruent

KEY POINTS

• Studies in both adults and youth of mood disorders with psychosis have been compli-cated by misunderstanding the state versus trait aspect of the psychosis and, in the case of bipolar disorder, failing to distinguish whether psychosis is occurring during mania, depression, or both.

• It is important to distinguish between psychosis and nonspecific odd beliefs and transitory hallucinations.

• Psychosis seems to be associated with severity but people can have equally severe mood episodes and not be psychotic.

• Rates of lifetime psychosis in children with mood disorders vary widely from study to study; current psychosis is less common in mania. Hallucinations are more common in young children; delusions are more common in adolescents and adults.

HISTORY

Although manic depression was considered a psychosis in Diagnostic and Statistical Manual of Mental Disorders (DSM)–I and DSM-II, severe psychosis was mostly asso-ciated with schizophrenia rather than mood disorder in both adults and youth until the 1980s. Three related events increased the importance of psychosis in depression and mania. First, there was a growing realization in the 1960s that psychiatric diagnoses were unreliable. A cross-national study of the diagnosis of mental disorders among hospital patients in New York and London established that, although the symptoms of patients admitted to psychiatric hospitals in the United States and United Kingdom were similar, the proportion of patients given a diagnosis of schizophrenia was nearly twice as high in the United States as in the United Kingdom.[1] The US concept of schizophrenia was broad and encompassed patients who, in the United Kingdom, were regarded as suffering from depression, mania (sometimes with psychosis), or

Disclosures: The author has received research funding from NIMH, Glaxo-Smith-Kline, Bristol Myers Squibb/Otsuka, Pfizer, and Merck.
Child and Adolescent Psychiatry, Stony Brook University School of Medicine, Putnam Hall, South Campus, Stony Brook, NY 11794-8790, USA
E-mail address: gabrielle.carlson@stonybrook.edu

personality disorder. Shortly after this, the International Pilot Study of Schizophrenia confirmed that psychiatrists in the United States (and also in Moscow) had a broader concept of the disorder than psychiatrists in other countries.[2]

A second relevant contribution came from Washington University of St. Louis's Department of Psychiatry where research operationalizing psychiatric diagnostic criteria and using standardized interviews had been taking place. Two important publications, the 1973 Feighner Criteria[3] and a book on *Manic-depressive Illness* by Winokur and colleagues,[4] delineated the phenomenology of manic depression. The goal to revolutionize psychiatric diagnosis, which led to DSM-III, emerged from this renewed interest in phenomenology, and, among other things, schizophrenia became more narrowly defined and symptoms of mania and depression with psychosis were explained more clearly.

The other important influence resulted from the approval of lithium carbonate for the acute and prophylactic treatment of mania in 1970, which made the task of recognizing manic depression and differentiating it from schizophrenia of great clinical importance.[5] Several studies were published highlighting that there could be periods during an affective psychosis in which symptoms were indistinguishable from schizophrenia,[6,7] and that proper diagnosis of what is now called bipolar disorder could be life changing for patients.[5]

Child and adolescent psychiatrists eventually acknowledged that mood disorders were common, at least in adolescents, and that distinguishing schizophrenia from serious cases of mood disorders could be avoided by obtaining more systematic information on patient history, phenomenology, and family history.[8,9] In addition, there was the observation that adolescents with mania, and sometimes depression, could be psychotic and more likely misdiagnosed with schizophrenia than adults.[9–11] This possibility had not been a problem in prepubertal children, given the diagnosis of bipolar disorder in which psychotic symptoms are said to be present but are not as dramatic as they are in teens.

ISSUES COMPLICATING THE STUDY OF AFFECTIVE PSYCHOSIS

Several issues complicate interpretation of studies of affective psychosis. The first is that, at least with mood disorders, psychosis is a state, not a trait. By definition, psychosis can occur only within a mood episode. Mood episodes are often recurrent. Thus, patients can be psychotic within one episode and not another.[12] They can have one manic episode with psychosis and another without; or a mania with psychosis and a depression without. In a county-wide sample of patients with a first hospitalization for psychosis,[13] 37% of the sample had subsequent mood episodes but no further psychosis over the next 48 months (unpublished data). Thus it is important to understand whether a study was done on a patient with a lifetime psychosis (which has since remitted) or a current psychosis.

The significance of psychosis also is not clear.[14] In some cases it is a severity marker,[15] although, when that interpretation was examined specifically, another sample of patients with equally severe mood symptoms by other criteria were not psychotic.[16,17] Psychosis seems to be more common in mania than depression but bipolar depression with psychosis is not rare; a psychotic depression in an adolescent may be the harbinger of a future bipolar course (for review see Refs.[18,19]).

Also at issue is the term bipolar psychosis, or bipolar disorder with psychosis. This diagnosis does not identify whether the patient was psychotic within their mania or depression or both. It is possible that makes a difference but this cannot be determined unless the study breaks out the information that way. Some studies indicate that psychosis during mania worsens prognosis, including more frequent relapse, greater chronicity, and less complete remission between episodes, although other studies have found no difference in outcome.[13] In the Collaborative Depression Study, psychotic features that accompanied depression strongly predicted the number of weeks with psychosis during follow-up, particularly among individuals whose episodes at intake were less acute.[20] Although, at least in young people, a first episode of psychotic depression may portend a bipolar course, psychotic symptoms in a non-bipolar depression may portend a schizophrenic course.[21]

In addition, there is a spectrum of psychosis that includes nondiagnostic phenomena (eg, brief hallucinations) that occur in up to 10% of the general population[22] and are even more common in children, with 17% of patients between 9 and 12 years-old and 7.5% of patients between 13 and 18 ears old reporting symptoms.[23] Common psychotic-like experiences may potentially be distinguished from prodromal symptoms by self-report when factors such as symptom frequency, distress, and help seeking are taken into account. So-called emotional valence is also important. For hallucinations, it includes the negative content of voices, the degree of negative content, and the overall impairment conferred by these voices with negative content.[24]

In an emotionally disturbed sample, psychotic symptoms that are detailed and dramatic or in which content is associated with past traumatic experiences, or only present when the person is angry, or while negotiating for some particular need to be met are unstable and do not represent true psychosis.[25] These symptoms, even when they occur in the context of a depressive state, probably do not represent true affective psychosis.

RATES OF PSYCHOSIS IN CLINIC SAMPLES

Rates of psychosis in samples of youth with affective disorder depend on where the sample is obtained (research or clinic sample), the age of the child (child or adolescent), and the type interview used to elicit psychotic symptoms (eg, Refs.[26–31]). The largest clinic sample in which psychotic symptoms were described comes from Western Psychiatric Institute and Clinics using the Schedule for Affective Disorders and Schizophrenia for School Aged Children Present and Lifetime Version (KSADS-PL)[26] in a sample of 2031 youths aged 5 to 21 years.[32] Of these, 91 (4.5%) had definite psychotic symptoms, another 95 (4.7%) had probable psychotic symptoms, and 1845 (90.8%) did not have psychotic symptoms. Among those with definite psychosis, 44% had major depressive disorder (MDD), 22% had bipolar disorder (presumably mania but this was not specified), and the rest had assorted other disorders, conduct disorder (16.5%) being the largest residual category. Factor analysis of the psychotic symptoms indicated that hallucinations explained most of the variance (21%), followed by thought disorder (11%), delusions (6%), and manic thought disorder (6%). However, the factor analysis was for all psychotic symptoms, not specifically for mood-related psychosis.

Within mood disorders, bipolar disorder has been studied more frequently than non-bipolar major depression. Studies in this category can be divided into those that examine lifetime versus current psychosis. In bipolar disorder (presumably mania), lifetime psychotic symptoms vary considerably from a low of about 16%[33,34] to a high of 60%[35,36] and 75%. In the Course and Outcome of Bipolar Youth Study (COBY), Axelson and colleagues[37] found a rate of 34.5% in subjects with bipolar I disorder. In a factor analysis of manic symptoms derived from the KSADS-PL, a disorganized/psychotic factor emerged in the teens (but not the preadolescents).[38] Kowatch and colleagues[39] summed this up with a meta-analysis of studies, deriving a weighted rate of psychosis of 42% (95% confidence interval [CI] 24%–62%) but with statistically significant differences in rates among the samples. The range of psychosis in adults with bipolar disorder is higher, with a weighted mean of 62% and range from 47% to 90%.[40(p53)]

Rates of current manic symptoms are more difficult to glean from reported studies and are best obtained from drug studies in which it is clear both which mood episode is being measured, and that it is a current episode that is being rated. These rates are lower.[41] In studies of patients between 10 and 17 years old with acute or mixed manic symptoms, rates of psychosis ranged from 8.6% in the study of lithium and divalproex,[42] 5.2% in the aripiprazole versus placebo study,[43] 11% in the divalproex-ER study[44] and 27.3% in the study of patients between 13 and 17 years old with olanzapine.[45] This contrasts with adult drug studies in which rates of psychosis ranged from 27.7%[46] to 55.6%.[47]

In young people, comparisons of samples of bipolar patients with and without lifetime psychosis suggest that psychosis in probands predicted a greater likelihood of a family history of anxiety disorders and suicide attempts.[48,49] Samples with psychosis also had more psychiatric hospitalizations, higher rates of comorbidity, and worse cognitive functioning and worse global functioning than bipolar patients without psychosis.[49] Psychiatric hospitalization and thoughts of death were also associated with psychosis.[50]

Psychotic symptoms have been subtyped as mood congruent and mood incongruent. Mood-congruent delusions and hallucinations in depression contain themes of nihilism, guilt, deserved punishment, or personal failures that are consistent with depression. Those themes that involve inflated self-worth, extraordinary powers, knowledge, or relationship to a deity or famous person are consistent with mania. Persecutory delusions/paranoia may be mood congruent in the context of severe depression or mania (the patient is being persecuted because of terrible failings, or because of having some valuable power). Mood-incongruent delusions include Schneiderian symptoms as well as certain delusions of persecution or reference.

If psychosis is unstable across episodes, so is mood congruence. Although 66% of a cohort of bipolar patients had lifetime mood-incongruent psychosis, evaluating all 1539 episodes in the sample of 182 patients revealed that only one-third (32%) of the episodes showed mood incongruence. People had more episodes without than with mood-incongruent psychosis.[51] The contention has been that mood-incongruent psychosis carries a worse prognosis, although not all studies have found that. Furthermore, the type of mood incongruence may be important. Schneiderian symptoms were associated with lower global functioning and more time ill during follow-up, but paranoia was not associated with poor outcome (see Ref.[13] for review).

Mood incongruence has not been studied in young-onset patients.

PSYCHOTIC SYMPTOMS: DEFINITIONS AND PREVALENCE IN MANIA

Positive psychotic symptoms are most often associated with affective disorders, although they have to occur concurrently with the mood symptoms to be classified as part of the mood disorder.

A hallucination is "a sensory perception that has the compelling sense of reality of a true perception but that occurs without external stimulation of the relevant sensory organ."[52(p823)] Hallucinations may be auditory, visual, somatic, tactile, or gustatory. Auditory hallucinations, the most common type, may come from within or outside the head and range from a single word, uncertainly heard, to a few words, to words or phrases that subject think may just be their own thoughts or conscience. The patients' state of alertness, age/cognitive development, ability to express their internal state, and interviewer bias and conviction help determine whether to count a phenomenon as a true hallucination. In 91 youth with psychosis described by Ulloa and colleagues,[32] 73% had auditory hallucinations, 38.5% visual hallucinations, and 26.2% olfactory hallucinations.

Dunayvech and Keck[14] noted that, even in adults with mania, hallucinations tend to be "brief, fragmented and related to religious themes," although they can be more pronounced in severe, delirious states.[6] People who hear commands, commenting voices, or conversations between voices have crossed the threshold and have prominent hallucinations. Goodwin and Jamison[40] provide a weighted mean frequency of hallucinations in mania of 23% for a current episode. Child bipolar studies report hallucinations that range from 22% auditory and 18% visual[49] to 37.4% (pathologic hallucinations including visual).[36]

Delusions are false beliefs, not culturally accepted, and firmly held despite incontrovertible evidence to the contrary. Again, a spectrum exists between overvalued ideas and delusions.[52(p821)] Judgment is required in ascertaining the impact of development on cultural acceptance: convictions of a monster in the closet are not considered delusional in a young child, but would be considered delusional in a teen. In addition, the boundary between an obsession and a delusion is not always clear.

Grandiose delusions ("delusions of inflated worth, power, knowledge, identity or special relationship to a deity or famous person"[52]) are common in mania, but can also occur in schizophrenia. Grandiosity occurs often in mania (87%), but delusions occurred in about 31% of manic adults.[40] In children and adolescents, lifetime grandiosity occurred in more than 70% in 3 large studies of mania (86%,[36] 83%,[34] 75.5%[37]), although grandiose delusions were less common. The Washington University Kiddie Schedule for Affective Disorders and Schizophrenia (WASH-U KSADS) provided rates of 67% of respondents with grandiose delusions.[36] Geller and colleagues[35] described a grandiose child[22]: an 8-year-old girl, failing at school, met the mayor, she stated that she spent her evenings practicing for when she would be the first female president. She was also planning how to train her husband to be the First Gentleman. When asked how she could fail school and still be president, she said she just knew.

The following are examples of grandiose delusions in adolescents: a 13-year-old manic girl thought she was having labor pains from being pregnant and would give birth to Moses; a 14.5–year-old boy stated that he is the Messiah and that he feared he was going to die because he had seen God; a 16.5-year-old girl thought she was the reincarnation of Newton or Jesus.[8]

Persecutory/paranoid delusions include feelings of being attacked, harassed, cheated, persecuted, or conspired against. Almost 40% of adults with mania were paranoid,[40] but paranoia occurred in only 8.2% of one sample of children and adolescents.[36] In a different study,[8] examples of delusions in teens with psychosis were: "claims the staff and patients are purposely making toilets flush louder than normal, changing the water temperature in the shower, and pressurizing the room to wake her up." Another was: "I'm being watched by everyone – they have a special plan for me." Paranoia in young adults with mania was associated with a greater number of psychotic episodes over a 4-year follow-up but not with poorer function per se.[13]

Delusions of reference are defined as the conviction that events, objects or other persons in one's immediate environment have a particular and unusual significance. Tillman reported rates of 5.8% in children, and 8% in teens.[36]

Mood-incongruent delusions are those of being controlled (feelings, impulses, thoughts, or actions being under the control of some external force), thought broadcasting (an individual's thoughts are being broadcast out loud so that they can be perceived by others), thought insertion (individuals' thoughts are not their own, but rather are inserted into their minds), and bizarre delusions (other delusions that are totally implausible).[52] Considered first-rank symptoms of schizophrenia as originally delineated by Schneider (see Ref.[53] for review), they can occasionally occur in other conditions including mania. Passivity delusions were 12% and Schneiderian symptoms, 17% in adults and were rare in the sample described by Tillman and colleagues.[36] Even when they occurred in manic episodes early in the course of illness, they portended a worse outcome, being associated with lower global functioning and more time ill.[13]

Somatic delusions (centering on appearance or abnormal things happening to the patient's body), and the delusion that someone is in love with the subject are also described.

Formal thought disorder, known in DSM-IV as disorganized speech, has been operationalized in the Scale for the Assessment of Positive Symptoms (SAPS),[54] as follows: "Positive formal thought disorder is fluent speech that tends to communicate poorly for a variety of reasons. The subject tends to skip from topic to topic without warning, to be distracted by events in the nearby environment, to join words together because they are semantically or phonologically alike, even though they make no sense, or to ignore the question and ask another. This type of speech may be rapid, and it frequently seems quite disjointed. Unlike alogia (negative formal thought disorder), a wealth of detail is provided, and the flow of speech tends to have an energetic, rather than an apathetic quality to it."[54]

In older studies, Abrams and Taylor[7] noted rates disorganized speech of 84%; Carlson and Strober[9] reported rates in hospitalized manic teens of 44%. Kowatch and colleagues'[39] meta-analysis reported rates of flight-of-ideas from 44% to 69% with a weighted percent of 56%. On the Young Mania Rating Scale (YMRS),[55] used in pharmacologic studies of antimanic drugs, one of the items is Language/Thought Disorder. Anchors are 0 = absent; 1 = circumstantial, mild distractibility, quick thoughts; 2 = distractible, loses goal of thought, changes topics frequently, racing thoughts; 3 = flight of ideas, tangentiality, difficult to follow, rhyming, echolalia; 4 = incoherent, communication impossible. Pooled item score from 457 youth (mean age 14.2 years) was 2.2 ± 0.7. The comparable score in 649 adults was 2.2 ± 1.0.[41] Although the difference between youths and adults was significant ($P = .002$) the difference was not large.

PSYCHOTIC SYMPTOMS IN DEPRESSION

Psychosis during depression is as frightening as it is in mania. In terms of prevalence, in a population study of almost 20,000 people aged 15 years and older, 16.5% of the sample reported at least 1 depressive symptom on a questionnaire. Of these, 12.5% had either delusions or hallucinations. The prevalence of a major depressive episode with psychotic features was 0.4% (95% CI 0.35%–0.54%), and without psychotic features was 2.0% (95% CI 1.9%–2.1%). In all, 18.5% of the subjects who fulfilled the criteria for a major depressive episode had psychotic features. Rates of treatment seeking were higher in depressed subjects with psychotic features than in depressed subjects with no psychotic features.[56]

Among Ulloa and colleagues'[32] sample from an outpatient depression/anxiety clinic, 44% of the 91 children and adolescents with psychotic symptoms had a major depressive episode. In one of the first comprehensive studies of prepubertal major depression with the KSADS,[57] 38% of 58 children with MDD had psychopathologically meaningful hallucinations, 36% of which were auditory (mostly command), and 16% nonauditory, mostly visual. This percentage was considerably higher than in teens (10%). Delusions were found in only 7% of the sample.

In an old study comparing prepubertal, adolescent, and adult patients with major depression,[58] depressive hallucinations seemed to decrease with age (22% hallucinations in children, 14.1% in adolescents, and 9% in adults). In contrast, depressive delusions increased with age (4.2% in children and adolescents, 9% in adults). Chambers and colleagues,[57] concluded that the psychopathologic meaning of psychotic symptoms in prepubertal children was unclear.

With the exception of these older studies, major depression with psychosis is understudied in youth outside its predictive relationship to the development of bipolar disorder[18,19] and is usually an exclusionary criterion for antidepressant studies. It occurs in 10% to 19% of community samples of adults with major depression[59] and in one large study,[60] among those with a psychotic depression, most have either a bipolar I (48.5%) or II (10.5%) disorder.

In a first admission for psychosis sample, diagnostic stability is less certain than in older samples later in the course. In the 104 subjects who had been assessed 4 times over 48 months (71% of the sample) only 31% had MDD with psychosis diagnosed at all 4 time points. Of those with inconsistent diagnoses, 8.9% switched to bipolar disorder, 16.4% were rediagnosed with schizophrenia or schizoaffective disorder, and 37% had other patterns of diagnostic change.[59] This finding may have implications for children and adolescents with psychotic depression because of their early age of onset.

ASSESSMENT OF PSYCHOSIS IN MOOD DISORDERS

A good history is vital to understanding mood disorder in general and affective disorder with psychosis in particular. Not only is it necessary to track onset and polarity of episodes, it is imperative to ascertain whether, and in which episode, psychosis occurred, and whether it occurred outside the mood symptoms, which would suggest a schizoaffective state.

Assessing for psychosis is part of all mental status examinations, and asking about whether they have been observed should be part of routine questions asked of parents or caretakers. However, deciding how to ask the question, making sure the child understands what you are talking about, and interpreting the response takes a great deal of experience. As noted earlier, hallucinatory phenomena are not rare in children. The question is whether the phenomena elicited mean anything diagnostically. Most structured interviews take the examiner through a list of questions that become increasingly specific.[26,27,29–31] They start with questions like, "Do you ever think your ears are playing tricks on you," and progress through "Do you hear sounds and realize there was probably nothing there," "Do you ever hear a voice that others do not seem to or cannot hear?" "Does it sound clear like the way I'm sounding?" "What is it saying?"

Mood-related hallucinations are most often auditory. If they are mood congruent, and depressive, the voices heard are telling the person that he or she is bad, ugly, evil, nasty, and so forth. The clinician should therefore ask whether the child or adolescent has described symptoms of depression, whether he or she has ever felt so down and depressed that their imagination started to play tricks on them? Did they hear something or someone saying insulting or bad things about them? During mania, clinicians should ask whether the person ever felt so good that they started to experience something really special, like hearing from God, or hearing beautiful music, or seeing mystical things.

Rating scales (eg, the Brief Psychiatric Rating Scale for Children [BPRS-C])[61] help anchor the severity of what is being elicited. In the case of auditory hallucinations, they are rated as not present, mild (hears name called), moderate-severe (definite voices, comment or command), or extremely severe (eg, constantly commanding voices).

If hallucinations are difficult to elicit, delusions are even more difficult. Three levels of misunderstanding can occur with ascertaining delusions in general and grandiosity in particular.[61] The first occurs because children may be unable to accurately self-evaluate and distinguish between pretend and reality. Another source of misunderstanding comes from misinterpreting the question. It is also possible that what an adult thinks is delusional is caused either by the child not interpreting things the way the parent wants or by them being true. A child told this author that he pitched the fastest ball on the east coast. It sounded grandiose. It turned out to be true. Parents often think their child is delusional when the child says he does not have to study for a test because he knows it all, or that she will get into the college of her choice even with grades that are failing.[62] Most of the time the children know that what they are saying is not true but they will not give the parent the satisfaction of admitting it. The examiner can usually ascertain this by asking, "Is this really true, or do you just wish it were true?"

Examples of items from the Structured Interview for Prodromal Symptoms (SIPS)[63] that address grandiosity, for instance, ask "Do you feel you have special gifts or talents? Do people ever tell you that your plans or goals are unrealistic? Do you ever think of yourself as a famous or important person? Or chosen by God for a special role?"

Questions eliciting paranoid feelings include, "Do you feel people around you are thinking of you in a negative way? Are you mistrustful or suspicious of other people? Do feel you have to pay close attention to what's going on to feel safe? Do you feel like you are being singled out or watched? Or that people might be intending to harm you?"

Examples of questions about depressive delusions from the KSADS-PL[26] include, "Was there ever a time you felt something was happening to your body? Did you believe it was rotting from the inside or that something was very wrong with it? Did you ever feel convinced that the world was coming to an end? Do you ever feel you did something terrible? Something you should be punished for?" In the case of young children, the KSADS gives an example of 3 children each of whom had done something trivial but wrong. The examiner asks whether the child would be most like one who apologizes and moves on, one who thinks about it constantly and cannot get it out of his/her mind, or one who feels guilty for things that are not even his/her fault?

The BPRS-C anchors delusions as follows: not present; mild, occasionally thinks strangers may be looking/talking or laughing at them; moderate-severe, frequent distortion of thinking, mistrust, suspicious; extremely severe, mistrusts everything, cannot distinguish from reality.

SUMMARY

- Studies in both adults and youth of mood disorders with psychosis have been complicated by misunderstanding the state versus trait aspect of the psychosis and, in the case of bipolar disorder, failing to distinguish whether psychosis is occurring during mania, depression, or both.
- Especially in children, it is important to distinguish between true psychosis and nonspecific odd beliefs and transitory hallucinations.

- Psychosis seems to be associated with severity but people can have equally severe mood episodes and not be psychotic. The meaning of psychotic symptoms in adults or children is not understood.
- Rates of lifetime psychosis in children with mood disorders vary widely from study to study; current psychosis is less common in mania. Hallucinations are more common in young children; delusions are more common in adolescents and adults.
- Ascertaining psychotic symptoms in youth requires experience. There are several structured assessments that help word the questions.

REFERENCES

1. Cooper JE, Kendall RE, Gurland BJ, et al. Psychiatric diagnosis in New York and London: A comparative study of mental hospital admissions. Maudsley Monograph 20. Oxford University Press; 1972.
2. World Health Organization. Report of the International Pilot Study of Schizophrenia. Geneva (Switzerland): WHO; 1973.
3. Feighner JP, Robins E, Guze SB, et al. Diagnostic criteria for use in psychiatric research. Arch Gen Psychiatry 1972;26(1):57–63.
4. Winokur G, Clayton P, Reich T. Manic depressive illness. St Louis (MO): CV Mosby; 1969.
5. Goodwin FK, Ghaemi SN. The impact of the discovery of lithium on psychiatric thought and practice in the USA and Europe. Aust N Z J Psychiatry 1999; 33(Suppl):S54–64.
6. Carlson GA, Goodwin FK. The stages of mania. A longitudinal analysis of the manic episode. Arch Gen Psychiatry 1973;28(2):221–8.
7. Abrams R, Taylor MA. Importance of schizophrenic symptoms in the diagnosis of mania. Am J Psychiatry 1981;138(5):658–61.
8. Carlson GA, Strober M. Manic-depressive illness in early adolescence. A study of clinical and diagnostic characteristics in six cases. J Am Acad Child Psychiatry 1978;17(1):138–53.
9. Carlson GA, Strober M. Affective disorder in adolescence: issues in misdiagnosis. J Clin Psychiatry 1978;39(1):59–66.
10. Joyce PR. Age of onset in bipolar affective disorder and misdiagnosis as schizophrenia. Psychol Med 1984;14(1):145–9.
11. Carlson GA, Fennig S, Bromet EJ. The confusion between bipolar disorder and schizophrenia in youth: where does it stand in the 1990s? J Am Acad Child Adolesc Psychiatry 1994;33(4):453–60.
12. Winokur G, Scharfetter C, Angst J. Stability of psychotic symptomatology (delusions, hallucinations), affective syndromes, and schizophrenic symptoms (thought disorder, incongruent affect) over episodes in remitting psychoses. Eur Arch Psychiatry Neurol Sci 1985;234(5):303–7.
13. Carlson GA, Kotov R, Chang SW, et al. Early determinants of four-year clinical outcomes in bipolar disorder with psychosis. Bipolar Disord 2012;14(1):19–30.
14. Dunayevich E, Keck PE Jr. Prevalence and description of psychotic features in bipolar mania. Curr Psychiatry Rep 2000;2(4):286–90.
15. Coryell W, Leon A, Winokur G, et al. Importance of psychotic features to long-term course in major depressive disorder. Am J Psychiatry 1996;153(4):483–9.
16. Coryell W, Leon AC, Turvey C, et al. The significance of psychotic features in manic episodes: a report from the NIMH collaborative study. J Affect Disord 2001;67(1–3):79–88.

17. Forty L, Jones L, Jones I, et al. Is depression severity the sole cause of psychotic symptoms during an episode of unipolar major depression? A study both between and within subjects. J Affect Disord 2009;114(1–3):103–9.

18. Strober M, Carlson G. Bipolar illness in adolescents with major depression: clinical, genetic, and psychopharmacologic predictors in a three- to four-year prospective follow-up investigation. Arch Gen Psychiatry 1982;39(5):549–55.

19. DelBello MP, Carlson GA, Tohen M, et al. Rates and predictors of developing a manic or hypomanic episode 1 to 2 years following a first hospitalization for major depression with psychotic features. J Child Adolesc Psychopharmacol 2003;13(2):173–85.

20. Coryell W, Winokur G, Shea T, et al. Long term stability of depressive subtypes. Am J Psychiatry 1994;151:199–204.

21. Bromet EJ, Kotov R, Fochtmann LJ, et al. Diagnostic shifts during the decade following first admission for psychosis. Am J Psychiatry 2011;168(11):1186–94.

22. van Os J, Linscott RJ, Myin-Germeys I, et al. A systematic review and meta-analysis of the psychosis continuum: evidence for a psychosis-proneness-persistence-impairment model of psychotic disorder. Psychol Med 2008;8:1–17.

23. Kelleher I, Cannon M. Psychotic-like experiences in the general population: characterizing a high-risk group for psychosis. Psychol Med 2011;41(1):1–6.

24. Daalman K, Boks MP, Diederen KM, et al. The same or different? A phenomenological comparison of auditory verbal hallucinations in healthy and psychotic individuals. J Clin Psychiatry 2011;72(3):320–5.

25. Hlastala SA, McClellan J. Phenomenology and diagnostic stability of youths with atypical psychotic symptoms. J Child Adolesc Psychopharmacol 2005;15: 497–509.

26. Kaufman J, Birmaher B, Brent D, et al. Schedule for Affective Disorders and Schizophrenia for School-age Children–Present and Lifetime Version (K-SADS-PL): initial reliability and validity data. J Am Acad Child Adolesc Psychiatry 1997;36:980–8.

27. Orvaschel H. Schedule for Affective Disorders and Schizophrenia for School-age Children-Epidemiologic Version. 5th edition. Fort Lauderdale (FL): Nova Southeastern University; 1994.

28. Geller B, Williams M, Zimerman B, et al. Washington University in St. Louis Kiddie Schedule for Affective Disorders and Schizophrenia (WASH-U-KSADS). St Louis (MO): Washington University; 1996.

29. Angold A, Cox A, Prendergast M, et al. The Child and Adolescent Psychiatric Assessment (CAPA). Durham (NC): Duke University; 1998.

30. Shaffer D, Fisher P, Lucas C, NIMH DISC Editorial Board, editors. Diagnostic Interview Schedule for Children (DISC-IV), Parent Version. New York: Columbia University/New York State Psychiatric Institute; 1998.

31. Spitzer RL, Williams J, Gibbon M, et al. The Structured Clinical Interview for DSM-III-R (SCID). I: history, rationale, and description. Arch Gen Psychiatry 1992;49:624–9.

32. Ulloa RE, Birmaher B, Axelson D, et al. Psychosis in a pediatric mood and anxiety disorders clinic: phenomenology and correlates. J Am Acad Child Adolesc Psychiatry 2000;39(3):337–45.

33. Wozniak J, Biederman J, Kiely K, et al. Mania-like symptoms suggestive of childhood-onset bipolar disorder in clinically referred children. J Am Acad Child Adolesc Psychiatry 1995;34:867–76.

34. Findling RL, Gracious BL, McNamara NK, et al. Rapid, continuous cycling and psychiatric co-morbidity in pediatric bipolar I disorder. Bipolar Disord 2001;3: 202–10.

35. Geller B, Zimerman B, Williams M, et al. Phenomenology of prepubertal and early adolescent bipolar disorder: examples of elated mood, grandiose behaviors, decreased need for sleep, racing thoughts and hypersexuality. J Child Adolesc Psychopharmacol 2002;12(1):3–9.
36. Tillman R, Geller B, Klages T, et al. Psychotic phenomena in 257 young children and adolescents with bipolar I disorder: delusions and hallucinations (benign and pathological). Bipolar Disord 2008;10(1):45–55.
37. Axelson D, Birmaher B, Strober M, et al. Phenomenology of children and adolescents with bipolar spectrum disorders. Arch Gen Psychiatry 2006;63(10): 1139–48.
38. Topor DR, Swenson L, Hunt JI, et al. Manic symptoms in youth with bipolar disorder: factor analysis by age of symptom onset and current age. J Affect Disord 2013;145(3):409–12.
39. Kowatch RA, Youngstrom EA, Danielyan A, et al. Review and meta-analysis of the phenomenology and clinical characteristics of mania in children and adolescents. Bipolar Disord 2005;7(6):483–96.
40. Goodwin FK, Jamison KR. Manic-depressive illness: bipolar disorders and recurrent depression. New York: Oxford University Press; 2007.
41. Safer DJ, Zito JM, Safer AM. Age-grouped differences in bipolar mania. Compr Psychiatry 2012;53(8):1110–7.
42. Findling RL, McNamara NK, Youngstrom EA, et al. Double-blind 18-month trial of lithium versus divalproex maintenance treatment in pediatric bipolar disorder. J Am Acad Child Adolesc Psychiatry 2005;44(5):409–17.
43. Mankoski R, Zhao J, Carson WH, et al. Young mania rating scale line item analysis in pediatric subjects with bipolar I disorder treated with aripiprazole in a short-term, double-blind, randomized study. J Child Adolesc Psychopharmacol 2011;21:359–64.
44. Wagner KD, Redden L, Kowatch RA, et al. A double-blind, placebo-controlled trial of divalproex extended release in the treatment of bipolar disorder in children and adolescents. J Am Acad Child Adolesc Psychiatry 2009;48:519–32.
45. Tohen M, Krzyhanovskaya L, Carlson G, et al. Olanzapine versus placebo in the treatment of adolescents with bipolar mania. Am J Psychiatry 2007;164: 1547–56.
46. Tohen M, Sanger TM, McElroy SL, et al. Olanzapine versus placebo in the treatment of acute mania. Am J Psychiatry 1999;156:702–9.
47. Bowden CL, Mosolov S, Hranov L, et al. Efficacy of valproate versus lithium in mania or mixed mania: a randomized, open 12-week trial. Int Clin Psychopharmacol 2010;28:60–7.
48. Rende R, Birmaher B, Axelson D, et al. Psychotic symptoms in pediatric bipolar disorder and family history of psychiatric illness. J Affect Disord 2006;96(1–2): 127–31.
49. Hua LL, Wilens TE, Martelon M, et al. Psychosocial functioning, familiality, and psychiatric comorbidity in bipolar youth with and without psychotic features. J Clin Psychiatry 2011;72(3):397–405.
50. Caetano SC, Olvera RL, Hunter K, et al. Association of psychosis with suicidality in pediatric bipolar I, II and bipolar NOS patients. J Affect Disord 2006;91(1): 33–7.
51. Marneros A, Röttig S, Röttig D, et al. Bipolar I disorder with mood-incongruent psychotic symptoms: a comparative longitudinal study. Eur Arch Psychiatry Clin Neurosci 2009;259(3):131–6.
52. DSM-IV TR.

53. Tanenberg-Karant M, Fennig S, Ram R, et al. Bizarre delusions and first-rank symptoms in a first-admission sample: a preliminary analysis of prevalence and correlates. Compr Psychiatry 1995;36(6):428–34.
54. Andreasen NC. Scale for the Assessment of Positive Symptoms (SAPS); Scale for the Assessment of Negative Symptoms (SANS). Iowa City (IA): University of Iowa; 1984.
55. Young RC, Biggs JT, Ziegler VE, et al. A rating scale for mania: reliability, validity and sensitivity. Br J Psychiatry 1978;133:429–35.
56. Ohayon MM, Schatzberg AF. Prevalence of depressive episodes with psychotic features in the general population. Am J Psychiatry 2002;159(11):1855–61.
57. Chambers WJ, Puig-Antich J, Tabrizi MA, et al. Psychotic symptoms in prepubertal major depressive disorder. Arch Gen Psychiatry 1982;39(8):921–7.
58. Carlson GA, Kashani JH. Phenomenology of major depression from childhood through adulthood: analysis of three studies. Am J Psychiatry 1988;145(10): 1222–5.
59. Ruggero CJ, Kotov R, Carlson GA, et al. Diagnostic consistency of major depression with psychosis across 10 years. J Clin Psychiatry 2011;72(9): 1207–13. PubMed PMID: 21903033.
60. Souery D, Zaninotto L, Calati R, et al. Phenomenology of psychotic mood disorders: lifetime and major depressive episode features. J Affect Disord 2011; 135(1–3):241–50.
61. Hughes CW, Rintelmann J, Emslie GJ, et al. A revised anchored version of the BPRS-C for childhood psychiatric disorders. J Child Adolesc Psychopharmacol 2001;11(1):77–93.
62. Carlson GA, Meyer SE. Phenomenology and diagnosis of bipolar disorder in children, adolescents, and adults: complexities and developmental issues. Dev Psychopathol 2006;18(4):939–69.
63. Miller TJ, McGlashan TH, Rosen JL, et al. Prospective diagnosis of the initial prodrome for schizophrenia based on the Structured Interview for Prodromal Syndromes: preliminary evidence of interrater reliability and predictive validity. Am J Psychiatry 2002;159(5):863–5.

Congenital and Acquired Disorders Presenting as Psychosis in Children and Young Adults

Sheldon Benjamin, MD[a],*, Margo D. Lauterbach, MD[d,e],
Aimee L. Stanislawski, MD[b,c]

KEYWORDS

- Psychosis • Congenital disorders • Inherited disorders • Genetic disorders
- Differential diagnosis

KEY POINTS

FOR EVALUATING CHILDREN AND ADOLESCENTS WITH PSYCHOTIC SYMPTOMS

- Perform a standard medical and laboratory evaluation, then examine for the presence of dysmorphic features, major neurologic signs, and major organ system problems.
- In a child without dysmorphic features, intellectual disability, or family history of psychotic disorder, perform a comprehensive neurologic and medical evaluation.
- Become familiar with the 7 more common, easily missed, congenital disorders that can include psychosis (acute intermittent porphyria, Asperger disorder, Gilbert syndrome, glucose-6-phosphate dehydrogenase deficiency, Huntington disease, neurofibromatosis type 1, XXX karyotype).

INTRODUCTION

Psychiatrists, neurologists, and pediatricians are often called on to evaluate youth with psychotic symptoms for possible medical, neurologic, or neurodevelopmental causes. The diagnosis of acquired neurologic disorders, although not always straightforward, is most familiar to general psychiatric practitioners and is briefly reviewed. In contrast, a bewildering array of rare congenital neuropsychiatric conditions that

None of the authors have any conflicts of interest to disclose relevant to this paper.
[a] Departments of Psychiatry and Neurology, University of Massachusetts Medical School, 55 Lake Avenue North, Worcester, MA 01655, USA; [b] Behavioral Health, VA Western NY Healthcare System, 3495 Bailey Avenue, Buffalo, NY 14215, USA; [c] Department of Psychiatry, School of Medicine and Biomedical Sciences, State University of New York at Buffalo, Buffalo, NY 14215, USA; [d] Department of Psychiatry, University of Maryland School of Medicine, Baltimore, MD, USA; [e] Neuropsychiatry Program, Sheppard Pratt Health System, 6501 North Charles Street, PO Box 6815, Baltimore, MD 21285-6815, USA
* Corresponding author.
E-mail address: sheldon.benjamin@umassmed.edu

Child Adolesc Psychiatric Clin N Am 22 (2013) 581–608
http://dx.doi.org/10.1016/j.chc.2013.04.004
1056-4993/13/$ – see front matter © 2013 Elsevier Inc. All rights reserved.

include psychosis has been described. Although some reviews of congenital disorders that include psychosis have been published,[1-5] clear guidance on the neuropsychiatric evaluation and differential diagnosis of these conditions can be difficult to find.

To address this dearth of information, in a previous publication,[6] we described the congenital disorders that may include psychosis, and proposed a straightforward neuropsychiatric approach to their differential diagnosis based on major associated signs and relative prevalence of the disorders. In this article, we update the diagnostic guide using similar methodology, searching PubMed using the term psychosis paired with the terms metabolic, genetic, congenital, or neurodevelopmental. Disorders were included if they were heritable or congenital, typically present by young adulthood, included at least 3 case reports, and contained adequate description of psychotic symptoms. Descriptors of psychotic symptoms included such terms as hallucinations, delusions, schizophrenialike, and schizophreniform, as well as known psychotic syndromes such as Capgras. Standard neurology textbooks were consulted for additional information.[7-11] Disorders were categorized by the presence of 1 or more of 20 prominent groups of associated signs with an emphasis on those of neurologic significance that occur most commonly in each disorder. Epidemiologic information gathered via OMIM (Online Mendelian Inheritance in Man),[12] GeneTests,[13] and orphanet[14] was used to classify disorders into more common (prevalence greater than 1/10,000), rare (prevalence 1/10,000 to 1/50,000), and extremely rare (prevalence less than 1/50,000) groups. Guidance on laboratory and neurodiagnostic evaluation is offered for each disorder, along with a list of known genetic loci.

CLINICAL APPROACH

The evaluation of children and adolescents with new-onset psychosis begins with a thorough personal, psychosocial, medication (prescription and over-the-counter), and family history, followed by physical and neurologic examination. Although secondary psychotic symptoms can occur in any child, the absence of dysmorphic features, intellectual disability, or family history of psychosis should increase suspicion of an acquired medical or neurologic cause. The list of acquired disorders reported to present with psychosis is extensive.[15,16] There is no gold standard laboratory evaluation, but a screening examination including complete blood count, hepatic and renal function tests, serum electrolytes and glucose, vitamin B_{12} and folate, thyroid-stimulating hormone, erythrocyte sedimentation rate, and antinuclear antibody, along with urinalysis, is typically recommended, with testing for the human immunodeficiency virus if risk factors are present, serum ceruloplasmin in the presence of a movement disorder, and serum or urine toxicology if ingestion or drug abuse was possible. A history of seizures or brief stereotyped behavioral episodes is evaluated with a sleep-deprived electroencephalogram. Focal findings or a history of traumatic brain injury are followed up with cranial magnetic resonance imaging (MRI). Evidence of delirium, seizures, or catatonia indicates expansion of laboratory evaluation to include toxicologic screening, cerebrospinal fluid (CSF) analysis, and anti-N-methyl-D-aspartate (NMDA) receptor antibodies, the most frequent causes of such presentations being infection-related, drug-induced, traumatic, autoimmune, and metabolic.[17] The subacute development of psychosis, variable memory impairment, followed by either delirium or variable consciousness, seizures, catatonia, involuntary movement disorder, or autonomic instability may indicate the presence of autoimmune limbic encephalitis. This constellation is an indication for MRI (to seek evidence of limbic hyperintensities on fluid-attenuated inversion recovery images), CSF examination (to look for pleocytosis, oligoclonal bands, anti-NMDA NR-1 subunit antibodies), and electroencephalography (for disorganized, encephalopathic, or epileptiform pattern). Serum is also sent for autoantibody titers. Ultrasonography or MRI examination for ovarian teratoma is performed in females, with tumors responsible in 58% of women older than 18 years and only 15% of girls 14 years and younger.[18,19] Anti-NMDA receptor autoimmune limbic encephalitis is 4 times more common in females.

Having carefully evaluated and excluded the possibility of acquired medical or neurologic causes of psychosis, the clinician is faced with an increasing number of congenital and inherited disorders that can present with psychotic symptoms. In an attempt to rationalize the differential diagnosis of these disorders, 60 congenital disorders that may present from childhood to young adulthood with symptoms of psychosis were identified (**Table 1**). Prominent associated neurologic and physical signs are listed in **Box 1**. In brief:

- 43 disorders (72%) have prominent associated neurologic features that facilitate differential diagnosis.
- 18 disorders (30%) have readily recognizable unique phenotypes.
- 43 disorders (72%) may present without intellectual disability.
- 5 disorders (8%) are caused by chromosomal nondisjunction.
- 16 disorders (27%) have an estimated prevalence of 1/10,000 or greater (**Box 2**).

A diagnostic approach that takes relative prevalence into account is suggested to simplify a differential diagnosis that includes a large number of rare disorders. Although most of these disorders are unlikely to present to psychiatrists, neurologists, or pediatricians more than occasionally, the failure of physicians to recognize them may lead to unnecessary delay in diagnosis, misdiagnosis, or missed opportunities to offer genetic counseling. Many of these disorders have prominent unique phenotypes that are readily recognizable at a distance, which we have called doorway diagnoses, listed in **Box 3**. Fifty-two percent of the disorders we identified have subtypes that present without intellectual disability or easily recognized phenotype and are thus easily missed (**Box 4**). Seven of these easily missed disorders are common (acute intermittent porphyria, Asperger disorder, Gilbert syndrome, glucose-6-phosphate dehydrogenase deficiency, Huntington disease, neurofibromatosis type 1, XXX karyotype). Chromosomal microarray testing has been shown to detect more abnormalities than standard karyotype and fragile X studies in autism spectrum disorders,[20] but its role in routine evaluation of children with psychosis or autistic features is not yet established. If other members of a patient's family seem to share the patient's phenotype, the family should be referred to an academic genetics laboratory for more comprehensive testing.

LIMITATIONS OF THIS APPROACH

Although we have tried to exclude inherited disorders of which too few cases of psychosis have been described, or of which the descriptions are inadequate, there are several potential problems with relying on case report literature. It is difficult to determine whether the psychotic symptoms are caused directly by the disorder, are a common behavioral response to environmental or medical stress, or are merely coincidental. Despite the inclusion of misleading terms such as schizophreniform, schizophrenialike, or manic in many reports, the histories of many of the reported disorders do not seem to be consistent with disorders such as schizophrenia, schizoaffective disorder, bipolar mania, or major depression with psychotic features, despite

Table 1
Congenital diseases that may include psychosis. Prevalence code: 1 ≥1/10,000; 2 = 1/50,000–1/10,000; 3 ≤1/50,000. Diagnostic codes from Box 1, bold capitals denote neurologic signs

Prevalence	Diagnostic Code	Diagnosis	Workup	Gene(s)	References
1	**P** **Z** c r	Acute intermittent porphyria	U: ↑ porphobilinogen & δ-aminolevulinic acid	11q23.3 hydroxymethylbilane synthase (HMBS)	24–28
2	**D P T X Z** e n s u	Adrenoleukodystrophy	B: ↑ VLCFA (very long chain fatty acids)	Xq28 adenosine triphosphate-binding cassette, subfamily D, member 1 (ABCD1)	29–31
3	**L** a b k n y	Albright hereditary osteodystrophy	X: brachydactyly, subcutaneous ossifications, lumbar stenosis	20q13.2 GNAS complex locus (AHO)	32–35
3	**X** b y h **L** r	α-Mannosidosis	B: ↑ acid α-mannosidase activity	19p13.2-p13.11 Lysosomal α-mannosidase (MAN2B1)	36,37
1	None	Asperger disorder	N/A	N/A	38–40
1	**L** y	Autism	N/A	2,3,6,7,13,15,17	41,42
2	**D L T X Z** b c e r k s	Cerebrotendinous xanthomatosis	B: ↑ cholestanol	2q33-qter sterol 27-hydroxylase (CYP27A1)	43,44
3	**M Z** r n u	Citrullinemia, type 2	B/U: ↑ citrulline	7q21.3 solute carrier family 25 (mitochondrial carrier, citrin), member 13 (SLC25A13)	45,46
2	**M L** a b c h y	Coffin-Lowry syndrome	X: XR distal tufting of fingertip bones	Xp22.2-p22.1 ribosomal protein S6 kinase (RPS6KA3)	47–49
3	**L Z** k	Darier disease	T: skin biopsy	12q23-q24.1 ATPase, Ca²⁺-dependent, slow-twitch, cardiac muscle-2 (ATP2A2)	50–52
3	**D M L X Z**	Dentatorubral-pallidoluysian atrophy (DRPLA)	G: CAG repeats	12p13.31 atrophin 1 (DRPLA)	53,54
1	**D L** a c g h r k o y	Down syndrome	G: trisomy 21	N/A	55
2	**P** c e r k u	Fabry disease	B: ↓ α-galactosidase A	Xq22 galactosidase, α (GLA)	56–58

3	D M X Z s u	Fahr disease	X: BG calcification	14q basal ganglia calcification, idiopathic (IBGC1)	59-62
2	X e h r s	Familial hemiplegic migraine	G: CACNA1A gene mutation	19p13 calcium channel, voltage-dependent, P/Q type, α 1A subunit (CACNA1A)	63,64
1	L b c u y	Fragile X syndrome	G: CGG repeats	Xq27.3 fragile X MR gene (FXMR1)	65,66
3	None	Gaucher disease, type 1	B: ↓ β-glucosylceramidase	1q21 glucosidase, acid β (GBA)	67,68
1	g	Gilbert syndrome	B: fluctuating ↑ indirect bilirubin	2q37 UDP-glycosyltransferase 1 family (UGT1A1)	69
1	e g r n o	Glucose-6-phosphate dehydrogenase deficiency	B: red blood cell glucose-6-phosphate dehydrogenase test/fluorescent spot test	Xq28 glucose-6-phosphate dehydrogenase (G6PD)	70,71
3	Z c r k p	Hereditary coproporphyria	U/S: ↑ coproporphyrin	3q12 coproporphyrinogen oxidase (CPO)	28
3	D P T	hereditary spastic paraparesis SPG4	G: SPG4 gene mutation	2p22.p21 spastin (SPG4)	72
3	D P L T e s	Hereditary spastic paraparesis, SPG15-Kjellin syndrome	G: SPG15 gene mutation	14q22-q24 (SPG15)	72
3	L a b c e	Homocystinuria	B/U: ↑ methionine and homocysteine	MANY	73-79
1	D M	Huntington disease	G: CAG repeats	4p16.3 Huntington (HD)	60,80,81
2	c r	Kartagener syndrome	T: mucosal biopsy	9p21-p13 dynein, axonemal, intermediate chain 1 (DNAI1); 7p21 dynein, axonemal, heavy chain-11 (DNAH11); 5p15-p14 dynein, axonemal, heavy chain 5 (DNAH5)	82,83

(continued on next page)

Table 1
(continued)

Prevalence	Diagnostic Code	Diagnosis	Workup	Gene(s)	References
1	n	Klinefelter syndrome XXY	G: XXY	N/A	84–87
3	D M T X e s	Late-Onset Tay-Sachs disease	B: ↓ hexosaminidase A activity	15q23-q24 hexosaminidase A, α polypeptide (HEXA)	88–96
3	L T a e u y	Laurence-Moon/Biedl-Bardet	N/A	MANY	97–100
3	L T a s y	Lujan-Fryns syndrome	NA	Xq13 mediator of RNA polymerase II transcription subunit 12 (MED12)	101–104
1	a b c e y	Marfan syndrome	NA	15q21.1 fibrillin 1 (FBN1)	105,106
3	M L T X u	MR with psychosis pyramidal signs and macroorchidism (PPM-X)	G: mutation analysis	Xq28 methyl-CpG-binding protein 2 (MECP2)	107,108
2	D M P T	Metachromatic leukodystrophy	B: ↓ arylsulfatase A	22q13.31-qter arylsulfatase A (ARSA)	109–113
3	D M Z c r	Mitochondrial encephalopathy, lactic acidosis, and strokelike episodes (MELAS)	B: ↑ lactate, ↓ pyruvate	MANY	114–118
3	D M Z b	Nasu-Hakola	X: polycystic osseous lesions	19q13.1 tyrosine kinase-binding protein (TYROBP); 6p21.2 triggering receptor expressed on myeloid cells 2 (TREM2)	119–125
3	D M X Z e g s	Neimann-Pick disease type C	T: skin biopsy (fibroblasts)	18q11-q12 NPC1 gene (NPC1); 14q24.3 epididymal secretory protein HE1 (NPC2)	126–130
3	D M P Z e s	Neurooacanthocytosis	B: acanthocytosis; X: MRI caudate nuclei atrophy	9q21 vacuolar protein sorting 13A (chorein) (VPS13A)	131–134

3	L Z k	Neurocutaneous melanosis	X: MRI melanin deposits	MANY	135,136
3	D M e s	Neurodegeneration with brain iron accumulation (NBIA)	X: MRI T2 central pallidal hyperintensity with hypointense surround (eye of the tiger sign)	20p13-p12.3 pantothenate kinase 2 (PANK2)	137
1	b e k y	Neurofibromatosis, type 1	NA	17q11.2 neurofibromin (NF1)	138-140
2	D M X Z	Neuronal ceroid lipofuscinosis	T: increased dolichol levels in brain, muscle, or skin biopsy U: increased dolichol levels	Unknown (CLN4)	141
3	L e h	Norrie disease	G: mutation analysis	Xp11.4 Norrin (NDP)	142,143
1	e k o	Oculocutaneous albinism	G: mutation analysis	OCA1:11q14-q21 tyrosinase (TYR); OCA2:15q11.2-q12 pink-eye dilution, murine, homologue of (OCA2) and 16q24.3 melanocortin 1 receptor (MC1R)	144-147
3	c e r u y	Patau syndrome	G: trisomy 13	NA	148
3	D M X s	Pelizeus-Merzbacher disease	X: MRI white matter disease	Xq22 proteolipid protein 1 (PLP1)	149
1	L T Z s	Phenylketonuria	B: ↑ phenylalanine	12q24.1 phenylalanine hydroxylase (PAH)	150-154
2	k p	Porphyria variegata	U: ↑ porphobilinogen and δ-aminolevulinic acid	1q22 protoporphyrinogen oxidase (PPOX); 6p21.3 hemochromatosis gene (HFE)	
2	a n u	Prader-Willi syndrome	G: DNA methylation analysis	15q11-q13 necdin (NDN); 15q12 small nuclear ribonucleoprotein polypeptide N (SNRPN)	155-162
3	M s	Spinocerebellar atrophy	G: CAG repeats	Multiple gene loci	163-167

(continued on next page)

Table 1
(continued)

Prevalence	Diagnostic Code	Diagnosis	Workup	Gene(s)	References
2	Z e	Sturge-Weber syndrome	X: MRI and CT angiomatosis/gyral calcifications	N/A	168–170
3	M L X Z	Succinic semialdehyde dehydrogenase (SSADH) deficiency	U: ↑ γ-hydroxybutyric acid	6p22 succinic semialdehyde dehydrogenase (SSADH)	171,172
2	M	Gilles de la Tourette syndrome	N/A	13q31 SLIT-like and NTRK-like family, member 1(SLITRK1); 11q23 Gilles de la Tourette syndrome (GTS)	173,174
2	Z	Tuberous sclerosis	X: MRI and CT calcified nodules	9q34 hamartin (TSC1); 16p 13.3 tuberin (TSC2)	175–179
1	a c n y	Turner syndrome	G: XO	N/A	180,181
2	e h	Usher syndrome	O: ERG and ENG	11q13.5 myosin VIIA (MYO7A)	182–187
1	L Z c y	Velocardiofacial syndrome	G: FISH	22q11.2 T-box 1 (VCFS)	160,188,189
3	a c e k n y	Werner syndrome	N/A	8p12-p11.2 DNA helicase, RecQ-like 2 (WRN)	190–192
2	D M g	Wilson disease	B: ↓ ceruloplasmin and ↑ copper	13q14.3-q21.1 ATPase, Cu^{2+} transporting, β polypeptide (ATP7B)	60,110,193,194
3	e h n u	Wolfram syndrome	N/A	4p16.1 wolframin (WFS1); 4q22-q24 Wolfram syndrome 2 (WFS2)	195–197
1	*None*	XXX karyotype	G: XXX	N/A	198
2	*None*	XYY karyotype	G: XYY	N/A	199–201

Abbreviations: ATPase, adenosine triphosphatase; CT, computed tomography; N/A, not applicable.

Box 1
Disorders by major associated signs (letters in parentheses are codes used in Table 1; major neurologic signs are indicated in bold capitals)

ABNORMAL BODY SIZE (a)

- Albright hereditary osteodystrophy (short stature, obesity)
- Coffin-Lowry syndrome (short stature)
- Down syndrome (short stature)
- Homocystinuria (marfanoid habitus)
- Laurence-Moon/Bardet-Biedl (obese, small hands/feet, syndactyly, brachydactyly or polydactyly)
- Lujan-Fryns syndrome (marfanoid habitus)
- Marfan syndrome (marfanoid habitus)
- Prader-Willi syndrome (childhood-onset obesity, short stature, small hands/feet)
- Turner syndrome (short stature)
- Werner syndrome (short stature, slender limbs)

ATAXIA (**X**)

- Adrenoleukodystrophy
- α-Mannosidosis
- Cerebrotendinous xanthomatosis
- Dentatorubral-pallidoluysian atrophy
- Fahr disease
- Familial hemiplegic migraine
- Neuronal ceroid lipofuscinosis
- Late-onset Tay-Sachs
- Psychosis pyramidal signs and macroorchidism (PPM-X)
- Neimann-Pick type C
- Pelizaeus-Merzbacher disease
- Succinic semialdehyde dehydrogenase (SSADH) deficiency

BONE/CONNECTIVE TISSUE ABNORMALITIES (b)

- Albright hereditary osteodystrophy (brachydactyly)
- α-Mannosidosis (dysostosis multiplex, scoliosis, deformation of sternum)
- Cerebrotendinous xanthomatosis (osteoporosis)
- Coffin-Lowry syndrome (cervical lordosis, kyphoscoliosis, spinal stenosis)
- Fragile X syndrome (joint instability)
- Homocystinuria (osteoporosis)
- Marfan syndrome (weakened connective tissue)
- Nasu-Hakola (bone cysts, pathologic fractures)
- Neurofibromatosis, type 1 (osseous lesions, scoliosis)

(continued on next page)

Box 1
Disorders by major associated signs (letters in parentheses are codes used in Table 1; major neurologic signs are indicated in bold capitals)
(*continued*)

CARDIOVASCULAR ABNORMALITIES (c)

- Acute intermittent porphyria (hypertension, tachycardia)
- Cerebrotendinous xanthomatosis (atherosclerosis)
- Coffin-Lowry syndrome (mitral regurgitation, congestive heart failure)
- Down syndrome (atrioventricular septal defects)
- Fabry disease (peripheral vasculopathy and edema, arrhythmia, hypertrophic cardiomyopathy, stroke)
- Fragile X syndrome (mitral valve prolapse)
- Hereditary coproporphyria (hypertension)
- Homocystinuria (thromboembolic events)
- Kartagener syndrome (situs inversus)
- Marfan syndrome (mitral valve prolapse, mitral regurgitation, dilatation of the aortic root, and aortic regurgitation)
- MELAS (mitochondrial encephalopathy, lactic acidosis, and strokelike episodes)
- Patau syndrome (cardiac malformations)
- Turner syndrome (cardiac malformations, hypertension)
- Velocardiofacial syndrome (ventriculoseptal defect [VSD], tetralogy of Fallot, aortic arch defects)
- Werner syndrome (atherosclerosis)

COGNITIVE IMPAIRMENT-DEMENTIA (**D**)

- Adrenoleukodystrophy
- Cerebrotendinous xanthomatosis
- Dentatorubral-pallidoluysian atrophy
- Down syndrome
- Fahr disease
- Hereditary spastic paraparesis (SPG 4)
- Hereditary spastic paraparesis (SPG15-Kjellin syndrome)
- Huntington disease
- Neuronal ceroid lipofuscinosis
- Late-onset Tay-Sachs
- Metachromatic leukodystrophy
- MELAS
- Nasu-Hakola
- Neimann-Pick type C
- Neuroacanthocytosis
- NBIA

(*continued on next page*)

Box 1
Disorders by major associated signs (letters in parentheses are codes used in Table 1; major neurologic signs are indicated in bold capitals)
(*continued*)

- Pelizaeus-Merzbacher disease
- Wilson disease

DERMATOLOGIC ABNORMALITIES (k)

- Albright hereditary osteodystrophy (subcutaneous ossifications)
- Cerebrotendinous xanthomatosis (xanthomas)
- Darier disease (warty papules/plaques, palmoplantar pits, nail abnormalities)
- Down syndrome (abnormal dermatoglyphics)
- Fabry disease (angiokeratosis, hypohydrosis)
- Hereditary coproporphyria (photosensitivity)
- Neurocutaneous melanosis (large or multiple congenital melanocytic nevi)
- Neurofibromatosis, type 1 (café au lait spots, axillary freckling, neurofibromas)
- Oculocutaneous albinism (skin and hair hypopigmentation)
- Porphyria variegata
- Sturge-Weber syndrome (facial port wine stain hemangioma)
- Tuberous sclerosis (adenomata sebaceum)
- Werner syndrome (sclerodermalike skin changes, premature facial aging)

DYSMORPHIC FEATURES (y)

- Albright hereditary osteodystrophy
- α-Mannosidosis
- Coffin-Lowry syndrome
- Down syndrome
- Fragile X syndrome
- Laurence-Moon/Bardet-Biedl
- Lujan-Fryns syndrome
- Marfan syndrome
- Neurofibromatosis, type 1
- Patau syndrome
- Turner syndrome
- Velocardiofacial syndrome
- Werner syndrome

ENDOCRINE ABNORMALITIES (n)

- Adrenoleukodystrophy (adrenal insufficiency)
- Albright hereditary osteodystrophy (pseudohypoparathyroidism, hypothyroidism)
- Citrullinemia, type 2 (delayed menarche)

(continued on next page)

> **Box 1**
> **Disorders by major associated signs (letters in parentheses are codes used in Table 1; major neurologic signs are indicated in bold capitals)**
> (*continued*)

- Glucose-6-phosphate dehydrogenase deficiency (diabetes mellitus)
- Klinefelter syndrome (infertility)
- Prader-Willi syndrome (diabetes mellitus)
- Turner syndrome (hypothyroidism, infertility, type II diabetes)
- Werner syndrome (hypogonadism)
- Wolfram syndrome (diabetes mellitus, diabetes insipidus)

HEARING PROBLEM (h)

- α-Mannosidosis
- Coffin-Lowry syndrome (hearing deficit)
- Down syndrome (hearing loss)
- Familial hemiplegic migraine (deafness)
- Norrie disease (hearing loss)
- Usher syndrome (deafness)
- Wolfram syndrome (deafness)

HEMATOLOGIC ABNORMALITIES (o)

- Down syndrome (transient myeloproliferative disorder, megakaryoblastic leukemia)
- Glucose-6-phosphate dehydrogenase deficiency (hemolytic anemia)
- Oculocutaneous albinism (bleeding)

INTELLECTUAL DISABILITY (**L**)

- α-Mannosidosis
- Autism
- Cerebrotendinous xanthomatosis
- Coffin-Lowry syndrome
- Dentatorubral-pallidoluysian atrophy
- Down syndrome
- Fragile X syndrome
- Hereditary spastic paraparesis–SPG15-Kjellin syndrome
- Homocystinuria
- Laurence-Moon/Bardet-Biedl syndrome
- Lujan-Fryns syndrome
- PPM-X
- Neurocutaneous melanosis
- Norrie disease
- Patau syndrome

(continued on next page)

Box 1
Disorders by major associated signs (letters in parentheses are codes used in Table 1; major neurologic signs are indicated in bold capitals)
(continued)

- Phenylketonuria
- SSADH deficiency
- Velocardiofacial syndrome

MOVEMENT DISORDER (M)

- Citrullinemia, type 2 (tremor)
- Coffin-Lowry syndrome (cataplexy)
- Dentatorubral-pallidoluysian atrophy (choreoathetosis)
- Fahr disease (choreoathetosis, parkinsonism)
- Gilles de la Tourette syndrome (tics)
- Huntington disease (chorea, dystonia, parkinsonism)
- Neuronal ceroid lipofuscinosis (movement disorder and facial dyskinesia)
- Late-onset Tay-Sachs (dystonia, poor coordination)
- PPM-X (tremor, shuffling gait, bradykinesia)
- Metachromatic leukodystrophy (dystonia)
- MELAS (dystonia)
- Nasu-Hakola (choreoathetosis)
- Neimann-Pick type C (chorea, dystonia, myoclonus)
- Neuroacanthocytosis (chorea, dystonia, parkinsonism, motor or vocal tics)
- NBIA (choreoathetosis, dystonia)
- Pelizaeus-Merzbacher disease (choreoathetosis, nystagmus, tremor)
- Wilson disease (chorea, dystonia, tremor)

PERIPHERAL NEUROPATHY (P)

- Acute intermittent porphyria
- Adrenoleukodystrophy
- Fabry disease
- Hereditary coproporphyria
- Hereditary spastic paraparesis, SPG 4
- Hereditary spastic paraparesis, SPG15-Kjellin syndrome
- Metachromatic leukodystrophy
- Neuroacanthocytosis
- Porphyria variegata

RENAL OR GENITOURINARY ABNORMALITIES (u)

- Adrenoleukodystrophy (impotence)
- Citrullinemia, type 2 (enuresis)
- Fabry disease (renal insufficiency)

(continued on next page)

> **Box 1**
> **Disorders by major associated signs (letters in parentheses are codes used in Table 1; major neurologic signs are indicated in bold capitals)**
> (*continued*)

- Fahr disease (urinary incontinence)
- Fragile X syndrome (macroorchidism)
- Laurence-Moon/Bardet-Biedl (hypogonadism, hypogenitalism in males, structural or functional impairment of kidneys)
- PPM-X (macroorchidism)
- Patau syndrome (kidney malformations)
- Prader-Willi syndrome (hypogonadism)
- Wolfram syndrome (urinary tract abnormalities, neurogenic bladder)

SEIZURES (Z)

- Acute intermittent porphyria
- Adrenoleukodystrophy
- Cerebrotendinous xanthomatosis
- Citrullinemia, type 2
- Darier disease
- Dentatorubral-pallidoluysian atrophy
- Hereditary coproporphyria
- Neuronal ceroid lipofuscinosis
- Metachromatic leukodystrophy
- MELAS
- Nasu-Hakola
- Neimann-Pick type C
- Neuroacanthocytosis
- Neurocutaneous melanosis
- Phenylketonuria
- Sturge-Weber syndrome
- SSADH deficiency
- Tuberous sclerosis
- Velocardiofacial syndrome

SPASTICITY (T)

- Adrenoleukodystrophy
- Cerebrotendinous xanthomatosis (paraparesis/quadraparesis)
- Hereditary spastic paraparesis, SPG 4
- Hereditary spastic paraparesis, SPG15-Kjellin syndrome
- Late-onset Tay-Sachs
- Laurence-Moon

(continued on next page)

Box 1
Disorders by major associated signs (letters in parentheses are codes used in Table 1; major neurologic signs are indicated in bold capitals)
(continued)

- Lujan-Fryns syndrome
- PPM-X
- Metachromatic leukodystrophy
- Phenylketonuria

SPEECH PROBLEMS (s)

- Adrenoleukodystrophy (dysarthria)
- Fahr disease (dysarthria)
- Familial hemiplegic migraine (dysphasia)
- Hereditary spastic paraparesis, SPG15-Kjellin syndrome (dysarthria)
- Late-onset Tay-Sachs (dysarthria)
- Lujan-Fryns syndrome (hypernasal voice)
- Neimann-Pick type C (dysarthria)
- Neuroacanthocytosis (dysarthria from tongue/oral dystonia)
- NBIA (dysarthria)
- Pelizaeus-Merzbacher disease (slow speech)
- Spinocerebellar ataxias (ataxic speech)

SPLENIC OR HEPATIC ABNORMALITIES (g)

- Down syndrome (biliary tract malformations)
- Gilbert disease (hyperbilirubinemia, jaundice)
- Glucose-6-phosphate dehydrogenase deficiency (cholelithiasis, jaundice)
- Neimann-Pick type C (hepatic disease or splenomegaly)
- Wilson disease (cirrhosis, hepatitis, liver failure)

VISUAL SYSTEM ABNORMALITY (e)

- Adrenoleukodystrophy (Balint syndrome)
- Cerebrotendinous xanthomatosis (cataract)
- Fabry disease (corneal and lenticular opacities)
- Familial hemiplegic migraine (hemianopsia, blurred vision, retinal degeneration)
- Glucose-6-phosphate dehydrogenase deficiency (cataract)
- Hereditary spastic paraparesis, SPG15-Kjellin syndrome (macular pigmentation)
- Homocystinuria (ectopia lentis)
- Late-onset Tay-Sachs (coarse saccades)
- Laurence-Moon/Bardet-Biedl (retinitis pigmentosa, retinal dystrophy)
- Marfan syndrome (myopia, ectopia lentis)
- Neimann-Pick type C (vertical supranuclear gaze palsy)

(continued on next page)

> **Box 1**
> **Disorders by major associated signs (letters in parentheses are codes used in Table 1; major neurologic signs are indicated in bold capitals)**
> (*continued*)
>
> - Neuroacanthocytosis (supranuclear gaze palsy)
> - NBIA (retinitis pigmentosa, leading to blindness)
> - Neurofibromatosis, type 1 (Lisch nodules, iris hamartoma)
> - Norrie disease (bilateral blindness)
> - Oculocutaneous albinism (nystagmus, photophobia, decreased acuity)
> - Patau syndrome (microphthalmia)
> - Sturge-Weber syndrome (glaucoma)
> - Usher syndrome (retinitis pigmentosa)
> - Werner syndrome (cataracts)
> - Wolfram syndrome (optic atrophy)
>
> MISCELLANEOUS (r)
> - Acute intermittent porphyria (abdominal pain, constipation, vomiting)
> - α-Mannosidosis (upper airway infections)
> - Cerebrotendinous xanthomatosis (diarrhea)
> - Citrullinemia, type 2 (insomnia, sleep reversal, night sweats/terrors, diarrhea, vomiting)
> - Down syndrome (gastrointestinal malformations)
> - Fabry disease (febrile crises, dyspnea, gastrointestinal disturbance)
> - Familial hemiplegic migraine (headache, unilateral paresthesia, hemiparesis)
> - Glucose-6-phosphate dehydrogenase deficiency (back pain)
> - Hereditary coproporphyria (abdominal pain, constipation, vomiting)
> - Kartagener syndrome (rhinitis, bronchitis, bronchiectasis, sinusitis, infertility)
> - MELAS (vomiting, headaches)

phenotypic similarity at the time of presentation. Few congenital disorders have been described that closely resemble schizophrenia. Metachromatic leukodystrophy is 1 such disorder that has both negative and positive signs and symptoms and may begin within the typical age range of schizophrenia onset. 22q11.2 deletion syndrome, or velocardiofacial syndrome, which typically progresses from mood disorder to schizophrenialike disorder and may account for up to 6% of childhood-onset schizophrenia, is another. Anti-NMDA receptor encephalitis is emerging as another potentially important cause of acquired psychosis in childhood, or late-onset autism, with fewer cases presenting as paraneoplastic in youth than in later life and reports of serum NMDA receptor autoantibodies in first-break psychosis without clear signs of an encephalitic process.[19,21–23]

Another potential limitation of this review arises from reliance on the most common presentations to determine the major associated neuropsychiatric signs. For example, although neurofibromatosis type 1 certainly may be a cause of seizures, seizures are estimated to occur only in 7% of affected individuals; therefore, neurofibromatosis type 1 was not included in the seizure group.

Box 2
Disorders with prevalence of at least 1/10,000

Acute intermittent porphyria

Asperger disorder

Autism

Down syndrome

Fragile X syndrome

Gilbert syndrome

Glucose-6-phosphate dehydrogenase deficiency

Huntington disease

Klinefelter syndrome XXY

Marfan syndrome

Neurofibromatosis, type 1

Oculocutaneous albinism

Phenylketonuria

Turner syndrome

Velocardiofacial syndrome

XXX karyotype

Box 3
Doorway diagnoses (easily recognized phenotypes)

α-Mannosidosis

Coffin-Lowry syndrome

Down syndrome

Fragile X syndrome

Klinefelter syndrome XXY

Laurence-Moon/Biedl-Bardet

Lujan-Fryns syndrome

Marfan syndrome

Norrie disease

Oculocutaneous albinism

Phenylketonuria

Prader-Willi syndrome

Sturge-Weber syndrome

Tuberous sclerosis

Turner syndrome

Usher syndrome

Werner syndrome

Wolfram syndrome

Box 4
Diagnoses easily missed (may present as nonintellectually disabled without easily recognized phenotype)

Acute intermittent porphyria

Adrenoleukodystrophy

Albright hereditary osteodystrophy

Asperger disorder

Citrullinemia, type 2

Darier disease

Dentatorubral-pallidoluysian atrophy

Fabry disease

Fahr disease

Familial hemiplegic migraine

Gaucher disease, type 1

Gilbert syndrome

Glucose-6-phosphate dehydrogenase deficiency

Hereditary coproporphyria

Hereditary spastic paraparesis

Huntington disease

Late-onset Tay-Sachs

Metachromatic leukodystrophy, adult onset

Mitochondrial encephalopathy, lactic acidosis, and strokelike episodes (MELAS)

Nasu-Hakola

Neimann-Pick disease type C

Neuroacanthocytosis

Neurodegeneration with brain iron accumulation

Neurofibromatosis, type 1

Neuronal ceroid lipofuscinosis

Pelizeus-Merzbacher disease

Porphyria variegata

Spinocerebellar degenerations

Wilson disease

XXX karyotype

XYY karyotype

SUMMARY

It would be cost prohibitive to conduct a comprehensive laboratory and neurodiagnostic evaluation to rule out all possible causes of psychosis in all youth presenting for evaluation, even if such an evaluation were reserved only for those cases with a natural history atypical for major psychotic disorders. A coherent neuropsychiatric approach, such as the one presented here, improves cost-effectiveness by providing a probability-guided, examination-based approach to direct the diagnostic workup.

ACKNOWLEDGMENTS

The authors gratefully acknowledge the assistance of Len Levin, Head of Educational and Clinical Services, the Lamar Soutter Library, University of Massachusetts Medical School, for his assistance and advice with our literature search strategies.

REFERENCES

1. Davison K. Schizophrenia-like psychoses associated with organic cerebral disorders: a review. Psychiatr Dev 1983;1(1):1–33.
2. Walterfang M, Wood SJ, Velakoulis D, et al. Diseases of white matter and schizophrenia-like psychosis. Aust N Z J Psychiatry 2005;39(9):746–56.
3. Gray RG, Preece MA, Green SH, et al. Inborn errors of metabolism as a cause of neurological disease in adults: an approach to investigation. J Neurol Neurosurg Psychiatr 2000;69(1):5–12.
4. Anglin RE, Garside SL, Tarnopolsky MA, et al. The psychiatric manifestations of mitochondrial disorders: a case and review of the literature. J Clin Psychiatry 2012;73(4):506–12.
5. Staretz-Chacham O, Choi JH, Wakabayashi K, et al. Psychiatric and behavioral manifestations of lysosomal storage disorders. Am J Med Genet B Neuropsychiatr Genet 2010;153B(7):1253–65.
6. Lauterbach MD, Stanislawski-Zygaj AL, Benjamin S. The differential diagnosis of childhood- and young adult-onset disorders that include psychosis. J Neuropsychiatry Clin Neurosci 2008;20(4):409–18.
7. Menkes J, Sarnat H, Maria B. Child neurology. 7th edition. Philadelphia: Lippincott Williams & Wilkins; 2006.
8. Rowland LP, Pedley TA. Merritt's neurology. 12th edition. Philadelphia: Lippincott Williams & Wilkins, Wolters Kluwer; 2010.
9. Ropper AH, Samuels MA, Adams RD, et al. Adams and Victor's principles of neurology. 9th edition. New York: McGraw-Hill; 2009.
10. Nyhan WL, Barshop BA, Al-Aqueel AI. Atlas of inherited metabolic diseases. 3rd edition. London: Hodder Arnold; 2012.
11. Rosenberg RN, DiMauro S, Paulson HL, et al. The molecular and genetic basis of neurologic and psychiatric disease. Philadelphia: Wolters Kluwer Health/Lippincott Williams & Wilkins; 2008.
12. Online Mendelian Inheritance in Man, OMIM®. 2012. Available at: http://omim.org. Accessed December 1, 2012.
13. GeneTests Medical Genetics Information Resource (database online). 2012. Available at: http://www.genetests.org/. Accessed December 1, 2012.
14. Orphanet encyclopedia. 2012. Available at: http://www.orpha.net/. Accessed December 1, 2012.
15. Algon S, Yi J, Calkins ME, et al. Evaluation and treatment of children and adolescents with psychotic symptoms. Curr Psychiatry Rep 2012;14(2):101–10.
16. Freudenreich O, Holt DJ, Cather C, et al. The evaluation and management of patients with first-episode schizophrenia: a selective, clinical review of diagnosis, treatment, and prognosis. Harv Rev Psychiatry 2007;15(5):189–211.
17. Hatherill S, Flisher AJ. Delirium in children and adolescents: a systematic review of the literature. J Psychosom Res 2010;68(4):337–44.

18. Dalmau J, Lancaster E, Martinez-Hernandez E, et al. Clinical experience and laboratory investigations in patients with anti-NMDAR encephalitis. Lancet Neurol 2011;10(1):63–74.
19. Lennox BR, Coles AJ, Vincent A. Antibody-mediated encephalitis: a treatable cause of schizophrenia. Br J Psychiatry 2012;200(2):92–4.
20. Shen Y, Dies KA, Holm IA, et al. Clinical genetic testing for patients with autism spectrum disorders. Pediatrics 2010;125(4):e727–35.
21. Gabilondo I, Saiz A, Galan L, et al. Analysis of relapses in anti-NMDAR encephalitis. Neurology 2011;77(10):996–9.
22. Hung TY, Foo NH, Lai MC. Anti-N-methyl-d-aspartate receptor encephalitis. Pediatr Neonatol 2011;52(6):361–4.
23. Wandinger KP, Saschenbrecker S, Stoecker W, et al. Anti-NMDA-receptor encephalitis: a severe, multistage, treatable disorder presenting with psychosis. J Neuroimmunol 2011;231(1–2):86–91.
24. Chinnery PF, Cartlidge NE, Burn DJ, et al. Management of parkinsonism and psychotic depression in a case of acute intermittent porphyria. J Neurol Neurosurg Psychiatr 1997;62(5):542.
25. Croarkin P. From King George to neuroglobin: the psychiatric aspects of acute intermittent porphyria. J Psychiatr Pract 2002;8(6):398–405.
26. Ellencweig N, Schoenfeld N, Zemishlany Z. Acute intermittent porphyria: psychosis as the only clinical manifestation. Isr J Psychiatry Relat Sci 2006;43(1):52–6.
27. Massey EW. Neuropsychiatric manifestations of porphyria. J Clin Psychiatry 1980;41(6):208–13.
28. Strauss J, DiMartini A. Use of olanzapine in hereditary coproporphyria. Psychosomatics 1999;40(5):444–5.
29. Garside S, Rosebush PI, Levinson AJ, et al. Late-onset adrenoleukodystrophy associated with long-standing psychiatric symptoms. J Clin Psychiatry 1999; 60(7):460–8.
30. Kopala LC, Tan S, Shea C, et al. Adrenoleukodystrophy associated with psychosis. Schizophr Res 2000;45(3):263–5.
31. Rosebush PI, Garside S, Levinson AJ, et al. The neuropsychiatry of adult-onset adrenoleukodystrophy. J Neuropsychiatry Clin Neurosci 1999;11(3):315–27.
32. Hay GG, Jolley DJ, Jones RG. A case of the Capgras syndrome in association with pseudo-hypoparathyroidism. Acta Psychiatr Scand 1974;50(1):73–7.
33. Levine MA. Clinical spectrum and pathogenesis of pseudohypoparathyroidism. Rev Endocr Metab Disord 2000;1(4):265–74.
34. Nakamura Y, Matsumoto T, Tamakoshi A, et al. Prevalence of idiopathic hypoparathyroidism and pseudohypoparathyroidism in Japan. J Epidemiol 2000; 10(1):29–33.
35. Preskorn SH, Reveley A. Pseudohypoparathyroidism and Capgras syndrome. Br J Psychiatry 1978;133:34–7.
36. Backman ML, Aberg LE, Aronen ET, et al. New antidepressive and antipsychotic drugs in juvenile neuronal ceroid lipofuscinoses–a pilot study. Eur J Paediatr Neurol 2001;5(Suppl A):163–6.
37. Malm D, Nilssen O. Alpha-mannosidosis. Orphanet J Rare Dis 2008;3:21.
38. Fombonne E. What is the prevalence of Asperger disorder? J Autism Dev Disord 2001;31(3):363–4.
39. Raja M, Azzoni A. Asperger's disorder in the emergency psychiatric setting. Gen Hosp Psychiatry 2001;23(5):285–93.
40. Ryan RM. Treatment-resistant chronic mental illness: is it Asperger's syndrome? Hosp Community Psychiatry 1992;43(8):807–11.

41. Dhossche DM. Autism as early expression of catatonia. Med Sci Monit 2004; 10(3):RA31–9.
42. Simashkova NV. Psychotic forms of atypical autism in children. Zh Nevrol Psikhiatr Im S S Korsakova 2006;106(10):17–26.
43. Berginer VM, Foster NL, Sadowsky M, et al. Psychiatric disorders in patients with cerebrotendinous xanthomatosis. Am J Psychiatry 1988;145(3):354–7.
44. Gallus GN, Dotti MT, Federico A. Clinical and molecular diagnosis of cerebrotendinous xanthomatosis with a review of the mutations in the CYP27A1 gene. Neurol Sci 2006;27(2):143–9.
45. Maruyama H, Ogawa M, Nishio T, et al. Citrullinemia type II in a 64-year-old man with fluctuating serum citrulline levels. J Neurol Sci 2001;182(2):167–70.
46. Saheki T, Kobayashi K. Mitochondrial aspartate glutamate carrier (citrin) deficiency as the cause of adult-onset type II citrullinemia (CTLN2) and idiopathic neonatal hepatitis (NICCD). J Hum Genet 2002;47(7):333–41.
47. Collacott RA, Warrington JS, Young ID. Coffin-Lowry syndrome and schizophrenia: a family report. J Ment Defic Res 1987;31(Pt 2):199–207.
48. Haspeslagh M, Fryns JP, Beusen L, et al. The Coffin-Lowry syndrome. A study of two new index patients and their families. Eur J Pediatr 1984;143(2):82–6.
49. Sivagamasundari U, Fernando H, Jardine P, et al. The association between Coffin-Lowry syndrome and psychosis: a family study. J Intellect Disabil Res 1994;38(Pt 5):469–73.
50. Hellwig B, Hesslinger B, Walden J. Darier's disease and psychosis. Psychiatry Res 1996;64(3):205–7.
51. Wojas-Pelc A, Setkowicz M, Pelc J. Familial Darier disease and mental retardation in mother and her two sons. Przegl Lek 2002;59(11):946–9.
52. Lange CL. Psychosis only skin deep. Am J Psychiatry 2000;157(12):2055.
53. Adachi N, Arima K, Asada T, et al. Dentatorubral-pallidoluysian atrophy (DRPLA) presenting with psychosis. J Neuropsychiatry Clin Neurosci 2001;13(2):258–60.
54. Potter NT, Meyer MA, Zimmerman AW, et al. Molecular and clinical findings in a family with dentatorubral-pallidoluysian atrophy. Ann Neurol 1995;37(2):273–7.
55. Hurley AD. The misdiagnosis of hallucinations and delusions in persons with mental retardation: a neurodevelopmental perspective. Semin Clin Neuropsychiatry 1996;1(2):122–33.
56. Liston EH, Levine MD, Philippart M. Psychosis in Fabry disease and treatment with phenoxybenzamine. Arch Gen Psychiatry 1973;29(3):402–3.
57. MacDermot KD, Holmes A, Miners AH. Anderson-Fabry disease: clinical manifestations and impact of disease in a cohort of 98 hemizygous males. J Med Genet 2001;38(11):750–60.
58. Shen YC, Haw-Ming L, Lin CC, et al. Psychosis in a patient with Fabry's disease and treatment with aripiprazole. Prog Neuropsychopharmacol Biol Psychiatry 2007;31(3):779–80.
59. Geschwind DH, Loginov M, Stern JM. Identification of a locus on chromosome 14q for idiopathic basal ganglia calcification (Fahr disease). Am J Hum Genet 1999;65(3):764–72.
60. Lauterbach EC, Cummings JL, Duffy J, et al. Neuropsychiatric correlates and treatment of lenticulostriatal diseases: a review of the literature and overview of research opportunities in Huntington's, Wilson's, and Fahr's diseases. A report of the ANPA Committee on Research. American Neuropsychiatric Association. J Neuropsychiatry Clin Neurosci 1998;10(3):249–66.
61. Oliveira JR, Spiteri E, Sobrido MJ, et al. Genetic heterogeneity in familial idiopathic basal ganglia calcification (Fahr disease). Neurology 2004;63(11):2165–7.

62. Shouyama M, Kitabata Y, Kaku T, et al. Evaluation of regional cerebral blood flow in Fahr disease with schizophrenia-like psychosis: a case report. AJNR Am J Neuroradiol 2005;26(10):2527–9.

63. Feely MP, O'Hare J, Veale D, et al. Episodes of acute confusion or psychosis in familial hemiplegic migraine. Acta Neurol Scand 1982;65(4):369–75.

64. Spranger M, Spranger S, Schwab S, et al. Familial hemiplegic migraine with cerebellar ataxia and paroxysmal psychosis. Eur Neurol 1999;41(3):150–2.

65. Al-Semaan Y, Malla AK, Lazosky A. Schizoaffective disorder in a fragile-X carrier. Aust N Z J Psychiatry 1999;33(3):436–40.

66. Khin NA, Tarleton J, Raghu B, et al. Clinical description of an adult male with psychosis who showed FMR1 gene methylation mosaicism. Am J Med Genet 1998;81(3):222–4.

67. Herrlin KM, Hillborg PO. Neurological signs in a juvenile form of Gaucher's disease. Acta Paediatr 1962;51:137–54.

68. Neil JF, Glew RH, Peters SP. Familial psychosis and diverse neurologic abnormalities in adult-onset Gaucher's disease. Arch Neurol 1979;36(2):95–9.

69. Molina Ramos R, Villanueva Curto S, Molina Ramos JM. Gilbert's syndrome and schizophrenia. Actas Esp Psiquiatr 2006;34(3):206–8.

70. Bocchetta A. Psychotic mania in glucose-6-phosphate-dehydrogenase-deficient subjects. Ann Gen Hosp Psychiatry 2003;2(1):6.

71. Nasr SJ. Glucose-6-phosphate dehydrogenase deficiency with psychosis. Arch Gen Psychiatry 1976;33(10):1202–3.

72. McMonagle P, Hutchinson M, Lawlor B. Hereditary spastic paraparesis and psychosis. Eur J Neurol 2006;13(8):874–9.

73. Bracken P, Coll P. Homocystinuria and schizophrenia. Literature review and case report. J Nerv Ment Dis 1985;173(1):51–5.

74. Freeman JM, Finkelstein JD, Mudd SH. Folate-responsive homocystinuria and "schizophrenia". A defect in methylation due to deficient 5,10-methylenetetrahydrofolate reductase activity. N Engl J Med 1975;292(10):491–6.

75. Ryan MM, Sidhu RK, Alexander J, et al. Homocystinuria presenting as psychosis in an adolescent. J Child Neurol 2002;17(11):859–60.

76. Hill KP, Lukonis CJ, Korson MS, et al. Neuropsychiatric illness in a patient with cobalamin G disease, an inherited disorder of vitamin B12 metabolism. Harv Rev Psychiatry 2004;12(2):116–22.

77. Hutto BR. Folate and cobalamin in psychiatric illness. Compr Psychiatry 1997; 38(6):305–14.

78. Lindenbaum J, Healton EB, Savage DG, et al. Neuropsychiatric disorders caused by cobalamin deficiency in the absence of anemia or macrocytosis. N Engl J Med 1988;318(26):1720–8.

79. Roze E, Gervais D, Demeret S, et al. Neuropsychiatric disturbances in presumed late-onset cobalamin C disease. Arch Neurol 2003;60(10):1457–62.

80. Correa BB, Xavier M, Guimaraes J. Association of Huntington's disease and schizophrenia-like psychosis in a Huntington's disease pedigree. Clin Pract Epidemiol Ment Health 2006;2:1.

81. Jardri R, Medjkane F, Cuisset JM, et al. Huntington's disease presenting as a depressive disorder with psychotic features. J Am Acad Child Adolesc Psychiatry 2007;46(3):307–8.

82. Glick ID, Graubert DN. Kartagener's syndrome and schizophrenia: a report of a case with chromosomal studies. Am J Psychiatry 1964;121:603–5.

83. Quast TM, Sippert JD, Sauve WM, et al. Comorbid presentation of Kartagener's syndrome and schizophrenia: support of an etiologic hypothesis of

anomalous development of cerebral asymmetry? Schizophr Res 2005; 74(2–3):283–5.

84. DeLisi LE, Maurizio AM, Svetina C, et al. Klinefelter's syndrome (XXY) as a genetic model for psychotic disorders. Am J Med Genet B Neuropsychiatr Genet 2005;135(1):15–23.

85. Kebers F, Janvier S, Colin A, et al. What is the interest of Klinefelter's syndrome for (child) psychiatrists? Encephale 2002;28(3 Pt 1):260–5.

86. Visootsak J, Graham JM Jr. Klinefelter syndrome and other sex chromosomal aneuploidies. Orphanet J Rare Dis 2006;1:42.

87. DeLisi LE, Friedrich U, Wahlstrom J, et al. Schizophrenia and sex chromosome anomalies. Schizophr Bull 1994;20(3):495–505.

88. MacQueen GM, Rosebush PI, Mazurek MF. Neuropsychiatric aspects of the adult variant of Tay-Sachs disease. J Neuropsychiatry Clin Neurosci 1998; 10(1):10–9.

89. Neudorfer O, Pastores GM, Zeng BJ, et al. Late-onset Tay-Sachs disease: phenotypic characterization and genotypic correlations in 21 affected patients. Genet Med 2005;7(2):119–23.

90. Rosebush PI, MacQueen GM, Clarke JT, et al. Late-onset Tay-Sachs disease presenting as catatonic schizophrenia: diagnostic and treatment issues. J Clin Psychiatry 1995;56(8):347–53.

91. Zelnik N, Khazanov V, Sheinkman A, et al. Clinical manifestations of psychiatric patients who are carriers of Tay-Sachs disease. Possible role of psychotropic drugs. Neuropsychobiology 2000;41(3):127–31.

92. Federico A, Palmeri S, Malandrini A, et al. The clinical aspects of adult hexosaminidase deficiencies. Dev Neurosci 1991;13(4–5):280–7.

93. Hamner MB. Recurrent psychotic depression associated with GM2 gangliosidosis. Psychosomatics 1998;39(5):446–8.

94. Lichtenberg P, Navon R, Wertman E, et al. Post-partum psychosis in adult GM2 gangliosidosis. A case report. Br J Psychiatry 1988;153:387–9.

95. Zaroff CM, Neudorfer O, Morrison C, et al. Neuropsychological assessment of patients with late onset GM2 gangliosidosis. Neurology 2004;62(12):2283–6.

96. Navon R, Argov Z, Frisch A. Hexosaminidase A deficiency in adults. Am J Med Genet 1986;24(1):179–96.

97. Klein D, Ammann F. The syndrome of Laurence-Moon-Bardet-Biedl and allied diseases in Switzerland. Clinical, genetic and epidemiological studies. J Neurol Sci 1969;9(3):479–513.

98. Weiss M, Meshulam B, Wijsenbeek H. The possible relationship between Laurence-Moon-Biedl-Bardet syndrome and a schizophrenic-like psychosis. J Nerv Ment Dis 1981;169(4):259–60.

99. Iannello S, Bosco P, Cavaleri A, et al. A review of the literature of Bardet-Biedl disease and report of three cases associated with metabolic syndrome and diagnosed after the age of fifty. Obes Rev 2002;3(2):123–35.

100. Moore SJ, Green JS, Fan Y, et al. Clinical and genetic epidemiology of Bardet-Biedl syndrome in Newfoundland: a 22-year prospective, population-based, cohort study. Am J Med Genet A 2005;132(4):352–60.

101. De Hert M, Steemans D, Theys P, et al. Lujan-Fryns syndrome in the differential diagnosis of schizophrenia. Am J Med Genet 1996;67(2):212–4.

102. Purandare KN, Markar TN. Psychiatric symptomatology of Lujan-Fryns syndrome: an X-linked syndrome displaying Marfanoid symptoms with autistic features, hyperactivity, shyness and schizophreniform symptoms. Psychiatr Genet 2005;15(3):229–31.

103. Van Buggenhout G, Fryns JP. Lujan-Fryns syndrome (mental retardation, X-linked, marfanoid habitus). Orphanet J Rare Dis 2006;1:26.
104. Lalatta F, Livini E, Selicorni A, et al. X-linked mental retardation with marfanoid habitus: first report of four Italian patients. Am J Med Genet 1991;38(2–3): 228–32.
105. Leone JC, Swigar ME. Marfan's syndrome and neuropsychiatric symptoms: case report and literature review. Compr Psychiatry 1986;27(3):247–50.
106. Stramesi F, Politi P, Fusar-Poli P. Marfan syndrome and liability to psychosis. Med Hypotheses 2007;68(5):1173–4.
107. Klauck SM, Lindsay S, Beyer KS, et al. A mutation hot spot for nonspecific X-linked mental retardation in the MECP2 gene causes the PPM-X syndrome. Am J Hum Genet 2002;70(4):1034–7.
108. Lindsay S, Splitt M, Edney S, et al. PPM-X: a new X-linked mental retardation syndrome with psychosis, pyramidal signs, and macroorchidism maps to Xq28. Am J Hum Genet 1996;58(6):1120–6.
109. Black DN, Taber KH, Hurley RA. Metachromatic leukodystrophy: a model for the study of psychosis. J Neuropsychiatry Clin Neurosci 2003;15(3):289–93.
110. Estrov Y, Scaglia F, Bodamer OA. Psychiatric symptoms of inherited metabolic disease. J Inherit Metab Dis 2000;23(1):2–6.
111. Kothbauer P, Jellinger K, Gross H, et al. Adult metachromatic leukodystrophy manifested as schizophrenic psychosis (author's transl). Arch Psychiatr Nervenkr 1977;224(4):379–87.
112. Mihaljevic-Peles A, Jakovljevic M, Milicevic Z, et al. Low arylsulphatase A activity in the development of psychiatric disorders. Neuropsychobiology 2001; 43(2):75–8.
113. Kumperscak HG, Paschke E, Gradisnik P, et al. Adult metachromatic leukodystrophy: disorganized schizophrenia-like symptoms and postpartum depression in 2 sisters. J Psychiatry Neurosci 2005;30(1):33–6.
114. Apostolova LG, White M, Moore SA, et al. Deep white matter pathologic features in watershed regions: a novel pattern of central nervous system involvement in MELAS. Arch Neurol 2005;62(7):1154–6.
115. Thomeer EC, Verhoeven WM, van de Vlasakker CJ, et al. Psychiatric symptoms in MELAS; a case report. J Neurol Neurosurg Psychiatr 1998;64(5):692–3.
116. Kato T. The other, forgotten genome: mitochondrial DNA and mental disorders. Mol Psychiatry 2001;6(6):625–33.
117. Finsterer J. Central nervous system manifestations of mitochondrial disorders. Acta Neurol Scand 2006;114(4):217–38.
118. Suzuki T, Koizumi J, Shiraishi H, et al. Mitochondrial encephalomyopathy (MELAS) with mental disorder. CT, MRI and SPECT findings. Neuroradiology 1990;32(1):74–6.
119. Haruta K, Matsunaga S, Ito H, et al. Membranous lipodystrophy (Nasu-Hakola disease) presenting an unusually benign clinical course. Oncol Rep 2003; 10(4):1007–10.
120. Kobayashi K, Kobayashi E, Miyazu K, et al. Hypothalamic haemorrhage and thalamus degeneration in a case of Nasu-Hakola disease with hallucinatory symptoms and central hypothermia. Neuropathol Appl Neurobiol 2000;26(1): 98–101.
121. Verloes A, Maquet P, Sadzot B, et al. Nasu-Hakola syndrome: polycystic lipomembranous osteodysplasia with sclerosing leucoencephalopathy and presenile dementia. J Med Genet 1997;34(9):753–7.

122. Bianchin MM, Capella HM, Chaves DL, et al. Nasu-Hakola disease (polycystic lipomembranous osteodysplasia with sclerosing leukoencephalopathy–PLOSL): a dementia associated with bone cystic lesions. From clinical to genetic and molecular aspects. Cell Mol Neurobiol 2004;24(1):1–24.
123. Paloneva J, Autti T, Raininko R, et al. CNS manifestations of Nasu-Hakola disease: a frontal dementia with bone cysts. Neurology 2001;56(11):1552–8.
124. Paloneva J, Kestila M, Wu J, et al. Loss-of-function mutations in TYROBP (DAP12) result in a presenile dementia with bone cysts. Nat Genet 2000; 25(3):357–61.
125. Ueki Y, Kohara N, Oga T, et al. Membranous lipodystrophy presenting with pal-ilalia: a PET study of cerebral glucose metabolism. Acta Neurol Scand 2000; 102(1):60–4.
126. Campo JV, Stowe R, Slomka G, et al. Psychosis as a presentation of physical disease in adolescence: a case of Niemann-Pick disease, type C. Dev Med Child Neurol 1998;40(2):126–9.
127. Imrie J, Vijayaraghaven S, Whitehouse C, et al. Niemann-Pick disease type C in adults. J Inherit Metab Dis 2002;25(6):491–500.
128. Josephs KA, Van Gerpen MW, Van Gerpen JA. Adult onset Niemann-Pick disease type C presenting with psychosis. J Neurol Neurosurg Psychiatr 2003; 74(4):528–9.
129. Shulman LM, David NJ, Weiner WJ. Psychosis as the initial manifestation of adult-onset Niemann-Pick disease type C. Neurology 1995;45(9):1739–43.
130. Walterfang M, Fietz M, Fahey M, et al. The neuropsychiatry of Niemann-Pick type C disease in adulthood. J Neuropsychiatry Clin Neurosci 2006;18(2):158–70.
131. Bruneau MA, Lesperance P, Chouinard S. Schizophrenia-like presentation of neu-roacanthocytosis. J Neuropsychiatry Clin Neurosci 2003;15(3):378–80.
132. Destounis N, Dincmen K. Salutary effects of prochlorperazine on chronic psychotic choreo-athetosis. Dis Nerv Syst 1966;27(3):195–6.
133. Hardie RJ, Pullon HW, Harding AE, et al. Neuroacanthocytosis. A clinical, hae-matological and pathological study of 19 cases. Brain 1991;114(Pt 1A):13–49.
134. Takahashi Y, Kojima T, Atsumi Y, et al. Case of chorea-acanthocytosis with various psychotic symptoms. Seishin Shinkeigaku Zasshi 1983;85(8):457–72.
135. Azzoni A, Argentieri R, Raja M. Neurocutaneous melanosis and psychosis: a case report. Psychiatry Clin Neurosci 2001;55(2):93–5.
136. Thomas CS, Toone BK, Rose PE. Neurocutaneous melanosis and psychosis. Am J Psychiatry 1988;145(5):649–50.
137. Oner O, Oner P, Deda G, et al. Psychotic disorder in a case with Hallervorden-Spatz disease. Acta Psychiatr Scand 2003;108(5):394–7 [discussion: 7–8].
138. Gillberg C, Forsell C. Childhood psychosis and neurofibromatosis–more than a coincidence? J Autism Dev Disord 1984;14(1):1–8.
139. Mouridsen SE, Andersen LB, Sorensen SA, et al. Neurofibromatosis in infantile autism and other types of childhood psychoses. Acta Paedopsychiatr 1992; 55(1):15–8.
140. Mouridsen SE, Sorensen SA. Psychological aspects of von Recklinghausen neurofibromatosis (NF1). J Med Genet 1995;32(12):921–4.
141. Reif A, Schneider MF, Hoyer A, et al. Neuroleptic malignant syndrome in Kufs' disease. J Neurol Neurosurg Psychiatr 2003;74(3):385–7.
142. Bateman JB, Kojis TL, Cantor RM, et al. Linkage analysis of Norrie disease with an X-chromosomal ornithine aminotransferase locus. Trans Am Ophthalmol Soc 1993;91:299–307 [discussion: 8].

143. Warburg M. Norrie's disease. Birth Defects Orig Artic Ser 1971;7(3):117–24.
144. Baron M. Albinism and schizophreniform psychosis: a pedigree study. Am J Psychiatry 1976;133(9):1070–3.
145. Clarke DJ, Buckley ME. Familial association of albinism and schizophrenia. Br J Psychiatry 1989;155:551–3.
146. Jurius G, Moh P, Levy AB. Oculocutaneous albinism and schizophrenia-like psychosis. J Nerv Ment Dis 1989;177(2):112.
147. Yi Z, Garrison N, Cohen-Barak O, et al. A 122.5-kilobase deletion of the P gene underlies the high prevalence of oculocutaneous albinism type 2 in the Navajo population. Am J Hum Genet 2003;72(1):62–72.
148. Nanjiani A, Hossain A, Mahgoub N. Patau syndrome. J Neuropsychiatry Clin Neurosci 2007;19(2):201–2.
149. Sasaki A, Miyanaga K, Ototsuji M, et al. Two autopsy cases with Pelizaeus-Merzbacher disease phenotype of adult onset, without mutation of proteolipid protein gene. Acta Neuropathol 2000;99(1):7–13.
150. Letter: phenylketonuria and psychosis. N Engl J Med 1973;289(19):1040–1.
151. Lowe TL, Tanaka K, Seashore MR, et al. Detection of phenylketonuria in autistic and psychotic children. JAMA 1980;243(2):126–8.
152. Pitt D. The natural history of untreated phenylketonuria. Med J Aust 1971;1(7):378–83.
153. Seim AR, Reichelt KL. An enzyme/brain-barrier theory of psychiatric pathogenesis: unifying observations on phenylketonuria, autism, schizophrenia and postpartum psychosis. Med Hypotheses 1995;45(5):498–502.
154. Richardson MA, Read LL, Clelland JD, et al. Phenylalanine hydroxylase gene in psychiatric patients: screening and functional assay of mutations. Biol Psychiatry 2003;53(6):543–53.
155. Clarke D, Boer H, Webb T, et al. Prader-Willi syndrome and psychotic symptoms: 1. Case descriptions and genetic studies. J Intellect Disabil Res 1998; 42(Pt 6):440–50.
156. Descheemaeker MJ, Vogels A, Govers V, et al. Prader-Willi syndrome: new insights in the behavioural and psychiatric spectrum. J Intellect Disabil Res 2002;46(Pt 1):41–50.
157. Verhoeven WM, Curfs LM, Tuinier S. Prader-Willi syndrome and cycloid psychoses. J Intellect Disabil Res 1998;42(Pt 6):455–62.
158. Verhoeven WM, Tuinier S. Prader-Willi syndrome: atypical psychoses and motor dysfunctions. Int Rev Neurobiol 2006;72:119–30.
159. Verhoeven WM, Tuinier S, Curfs LM. Prader-Willi syndrome: the psychopathological phenotype in uniparental disomy. J Med Genet 2003;40(10):e112.
160. Verhoeven WM, Tuinier S, Curfs LM. Prader-Willi psychiatric syndrome and velo-cardio-facial psychiatric syndrome. Genet Couns (Geneva, Switzerland) 2000; 11(3):205–13.
161. Vogels A, De Hert M, Descheemaeker MJ, et al. Psychotic disorders in Prader-Willi syndrome. Am J Med Genet A 2004;127(3):238–43.
162. Soni S, Whittington J, Holland AJ, et al. The course and outcome of psychiatric illness in people with Prader-Willi syndrome: implications for management and treatment. J Intellect Disabil Res 2007;51(Pt 1):32–42.
163. Alekseeva N, Kablinger AS, Pinkston J, et al. Hereditary ataxia and behavior. Adv Neurol 2005;96:275–83.
164. Brandt J, Leroi I, O'Hearn E, et al. Cognitive impairments in cerebellar degeneration: a comparison with Huntington's disease. J Neuropsychiatry Clin Neurosci 2004;16(2):176–84.

165. Kanai K, Sakakibara R, Uchiyama T, et al. Sporadic case of spinocerebellar ataxia type 17: treatment observations for managing urinary and psychotic symptoms. Mov Disord 2007;22(3):441–3.
166. Leroi I, O'Hearn E, Marsh L, et al. Psychopathology in patients with degenerative cerebellar diseases: a comparison to Huntington's disease. Am J Psychiatry 2002;159(8):1306–14.
167. Liszewski CM, O'Hearn E, Leroi I, et al. Cognitive impairment and psychiatric symptoms in 133 patients with diseases associated with cerebellar degeneration. J Neuropsychiatry Clin Neurosci 2004;16(1):109–12.
168. Kalaitzi CK, Sakkas D. Brief psychotic disorder associated with Sturge-Weber syndrome. Eur Psychiatry 2005;20(4):356–7.
169. Lee S. Psychopathology in Sturge-Weber syndrome. Can J Psychiatry 1990; 35(8):674–8.
170. Madaan V, Dewan V, Ramaswamy S, et al. Behavioral manifestations of Sturge-Weber syndrome: a case report. Prim Care Companion J Clin Psychiatry 2006; 8(4):198–200.
171. Gibson KM, Gupta M, Pearl PL, et al. Significant behavioral disturbances in succinic semialdehyde dehydrogenase (SSADH) deficiency (gamma-hydroxybutyric aciduria). Biol Psychiatry 2003;54(7):763–8.
172. Philippe A, Deron J, Genevieve D, et al. Neurodevelopmental pattern of succinic semialdehyde dehydrogenase deficiency (gamma-hydroxybutyric aciduria). Dev Med Child Neurol 2004;46(8):564–8.
173. Kerbeshian J, Burd L. Are schizophreniform symptoms present in attenuated form in children with Tourette disorder and other developmental disorders. Can J Psychiatry 1987;32(2):123–35.
174. Lawlor BA, Most R, Tingle D, et al. Atypical psychosis in Tourette syndrome. Psychosomatics 1987;28(9):499–500.
175. Herkert EE, Wald A, Romero O. Tuberous sclerosis and schizophrenia. Diseases of the Nervous System 1972;33(7):439–45.
176. Holschneider DP, Szuba MP. Capgras' syndrome and psychosis in a patient with tuberous sclerosis. The Journal of Neuropsychiatry and Clinical Neurosciences 1992;4(3):352–3.
177. Raznahan A, Joinson C, O'Callaghan F, et al. Psychopathology in tuberous sclerosis: an overview and findings in a population-based sample of adults with tuberous sclerosis. Journal of Intellectual Disability Research JIDR 2006; 50(Pt 8):561–9.
178. Sedky K, Hughes T, Yusufzie K, et al. Tuberous sclerosis with psychosis. Psychosomatics 2003;44(6):521–2.
179. Zlotlow M, Kleiner S. Catatonic Schizophrenia Associated with Tuberous Sclerosis. Psychiatric Quarterly 1965;39:466–75.
180. Prior TI, Chue PS, Tibbo P. Investigation of Turner syndrome in schizophrenia. Am J Med Genet 2000;96(3):373–8.
181. Catinari S, Vass A, Heresco-Levy U. Psychiatric manifestations in Turner syndrome: a brief survey. Isr J Psychiatry Relat Sci 2006;43(4):293–5.
182. Hess-Rover J, Crichton J, Byrne K, et al. Diagnosis and treatment of a severe psychotic illness in a man with dual severe sensory impairments caused by the presence of Usher syndrome. J Intellect Disabil Res 1999;43(Pt 5):428–34.
183. Jumaian A, Fergusson K. Psychosis in a patient with Usher syndrome: a case report. East Mediterr Health J 2003;9(1–2):215–8.
184. Keats BJ, Corey DP. The Usher syndromes. Am J Med Genet 1999;89(3): 158–66.

185. Schaefer GB, Bodensteiner JB, Thompson JN Jr, et al. Volumetric neuroimaging in Usher syndrome: evidence of global involvement. Am J Med Genet 1998; 79(1):1–4.

186. Waldeck T, Wyszynski B, Medalia A. The relationship between Usher's syndrome and psychosis with Capgras syndrome. Psychiatry 2001;64(3):248–55.

187. Wu CY, Chiu CC. Usher syndrome with psychotic symptoms: two cases in the same family. Psychiatry Clin Neurosci 2006;60(5):626–8.

188. Ivanov D, Kirov G, Norton N, et al. Chromosome 22q11 deletions, velo-cardio-facial syndrome and early-onset psychosis. Molecular genetic study. Br J Psychiatry 2003;183:409–13.

189. Sachdev P. Schizophrenia-like illness in velo-cardio-facial syndrome: a genetic subsyndrome of schizophrenia? J Psychosom Res 2002;53(2):721–7.

190. Barak Y, Sirota P, Kimhi R, et al. Werner's syndrome (adult progeria): an affected mother and son presenting with resistant psychosis. Compr Psychiatry 2001; 42(6):508–10.

191. Hashimoto K, Ikegami K, Nakajima H, et al. Werner syndrome with psychosis. Psychiatry Clin Neurosci 2006;60(6):773.

192. Tannock TC, Cook RF. A case of a delusional psychotic syndrome in the setting of Werner's syndrome (adult progeria). Br J Psychiatry 1988;152:703–4.

193. Akil M, Schwartz JA, Dutchak D, et al. The psychiatric presentations of Wilson's disease. J Neuropsychiatry Clin Neurosci 1991;3(4):377–82.

194. Scheinberg IH, Sternlieb I. Wilson disease and idiopathic copper toxicosis. Am J Clin Nutr 1996;63(5):842S–5S.

195. Swift RG, Perkins DO, Chase CL, et al. Psychiatric disorders in 36 families with Wolfram syndrome. Am J Psychiatry 1991;148(6):775–9.

196. Swift RG, Sadler DB, Swift M. Psychiatric findings in Wolfram syndrome homozygotes. Lancet 1990;336(8716):667–9.

197. Torres R, Leroy E, Hu X, et al. Mutation screening of the Wolfram syndrome gene in psychiatric patients. Mol Psychiatry 2001;6(1):39–43.

198. Crow TJ. Sex chromosomes and psychosis. The case for a pseudoautosomal locus. Br J Psychiatry 1988;153:675–83.

199. Gillberg C, Winnergard I, Wahlstrom J. The sex chromosomes–one key to autism? An XYY case of infantile autism. Appl Res Ment Retard 1984;5(3): 353–60.

200. Mors O, Mortensen PB, Ewald H. No evidence of increased risk for schizophrenia or bipolar affective disorder in persons with aneuploidies of the sex chromosomes. Psychol Med 2001;31(3):425–30.

201. Sorensen K, Nielsen J. Reactive paranoid psychosis in a 47, XYY male. Acta Psychiatr Scand 1977;55(3):233–6.

"Autism-plus" Spectrum Disorders
Intersection with Psychosis and the Schizophrenia Spectrum

David M. Cochran, MD, PhD[a],*, Yael Dvir, MD[b], Jean A. Frazier, MD[a]

KEYWORDS

- Autism • Psychosis • Schizophrenia • Multiple complex developmental disorder
- Multidimensionally impaired

KEY POINTS

- The core social communication deficits and restricted, repetitive behaviors and interests in patients with autism spectrum disorders (ASDs) can be misinterpreted as possible hallmarks of a psychotic disorder because of the abnormal thought patterns associated with ASDs.
- Although comorbid schizophrenia spectrum disorder (SSD) is rare in ASDs, individuals with childhood-onset schizophrenia frequently have a history of premorbid ASD, and there is evidence of a connection between ASD and SSD that warrants a careful assessment for comorbidity when the presence of psychosis is suspected.
- There is a subset of individuals with the diagnosis of pervasive developmental disorder not otherwise specified who present with a complex neurodevelopmental pattern consisting of transient hallucinations, excessive mood lability and anxiety, social deficits, and excessive interest in fantasy. These patients have significant psychosocial impairments and are at risk for developing more significant psychiatric comorbidity in adolescence and young adulthood.

OVERVIEW
Nature of the Problem

Autism spectrum disorders (ASDs) are defined by impairments in 3 domains: social interaction; communication; and restricted repetitive and stereotyped patterns of behavior, interests and activities.[1] For the purposes of this article, these include the

Disclosure: Dr Cochran and Dr Dvir have no disclosures of conflict to report. Dr Frazier receives research support from GlaxoSmith Kline, Seaside Therapeutics, Pfizer, Inc, and Roche Pharmaceuticals.
[a] Division of Child and Adolescent Psychiatry, Department of Psychiatry, University of Massachusetts Medical School, Biotech One, Suite 100, 365 Plantation Street, Worcester, MA 01605, USA; [b] Division of Child and Adolescent Psychiatry, Department of Psychiatry, University of Massachusetts Medical School, 55 Lake Avenue North, Worcester, MA 01655, USA
* Corresponding author.
E-mail address: david.cochran@umassmemorial.org

Diagnostic and Statistical Manual of Mental Disorders (DSM), Fourth Edition, Text Revision (DSM-IV-TR) diagnoses of autistic disorder, Asperger disorder, and pervasive developmental disorder not otherwise specified (PDD-NOS). During the course of a clinical evaluation of an individual with ASD, the question often arises about the possibility of psychotic symptoms and/or a possible comorbid schizophrenia spectrum disorder (SSD: schizophrenia, schizophreniform disorder, schizoaffective disorder, schizotypal personality disorder). The problem is compounded if there is comorbid intellectual disability or if the communication impairment is severe enough to impair the assessment of thought process and content sufficiently. However, even in the verbal, higher-functioning individuals with ASDs, assessment of psychosis can be difficult in the face of the triad of core deficits in ASDs.

The difficulties with evaluating the presence of psychosis in individuals with ASDs can be organized in 3 concepts that lead to diagnostic dilemmas:

1. The social and communication deficits and restricted thinking that are core features of ASDs can be misinterpreted as psychosis.
2. There is epidemiologic, clinical, neurobiological, and genetic evidence for a connection between autism and schizophrenia, so there may be comorbidity with psychotic disorders.
3. There is a subset of individuals with complex neurodevelopmental disorders with symptoms ranging across multiple domains of functioning and who do not fit neatly into the current diagnostic criteria and who often have varying degrees of social communication deficits and thought disorder.

Misdiagnosis of autistic symptoms as psychosis

The first point to recognize is that the core features of ASDs (**Box 1**) can be misinterpreted as psychosis, which can lead to clinical uncertainty about the presence of

---

Box 1
Symptom domains, as adapted from DSM-IV-TR diagnostic criteria for autistic disorder

- Impairment in social interaction:
  - Impairment in the use of multiple nonverbal behaviors to regulate social interaction
  - Failure to develop appropriate peer relationships
  - Lack of spontaneous seeking to share enjoyment, interests, or achievements with other people
  - Lack of social or emotional reciprocity
- Impairment in communication:
  - Delay in the development of language
  - Marked impairment in the ability to initiate or sustain a conversation with others
  - Stereotyped and repetitive use of language or idiosyncratic language
  - Lack of appropriate varied, spontaneous make-believe play or social imitative play
- Restricted repetitive and stereotyped patterns of behavior, interests, and activities:
  - Preoccupation with 1 or more stereotyped and restricted patterns of interest
  - Inflexible adherence to specific, nonfunctional routines or rituals
  - Stereotyped and repetitive motor mannerisms
  - Persistent preoccupation with parts of objects

psychotic symptoms. **Fig. 1** shows the confusions that can arise when assessing clinical features of ASDs that may seem to be psychotic in origin. These difficulties were recognized early after the introduction of so-called pervasive developmental disorders into the DSM-III.[2] A review of DSM criteria noted that verbal individuals with autism would meet some criteria for schizophrenia because of illogical thinking, incoherence, poverty of speech and inappropriate or blunted affect.[3] Also, in a study of DSM-III criteria in 50 children clinically diagnosed with autism, parents of 20% of the children indicated that their child's inner life interfered with or took the place of reality, indicating the difficulty in distinguishing autistic preoccupation from delusional thinking.[4]

Konstantareas and Hewitt[5] evaluated 14 men with autism and 14 men with schizophrenia using the Structured Clinical Interview, Schedule for Positive Symptoms, and Schedule for Negative Symptoms to evaluate for a DSM-III, Revised Version (DSM-III-R), diagnosis of schizophrenia disregarding the criteria that diagnosis of schizophrenia can only be made in autistic disorder if prominent delusions and hallucinations are present. Fifty percent of the individuals with autism would have met criteria for schizophrenia, disorganized type, with 4 out of 7 showing bizarre behavior, 1 out of 7 showing formal thought disorder, and 6 out of 7 showing negative symptoms of schizophrenia. None of the individuals with autism had hallucinations or delusions. The investigators noted the importance of clinician experience and careful clinical observations, because perseverative and echolalic statements could be misinterpreted as hallucinations or delusions. Several studies have confirmed evidence of formal thought disorder in ASDs, with more evidence of poverty of speech and perseveration, and less evidence for illogicality and derailment of thought.[6,7] Ghaziuddin and colleagues[8] also found a trend toward a greater level of disorganized thinking in Asperger syndrome compared with autism, although the numbers were small in each group evaluated. Van der Gaag and colleagues[9] found high formal thought disorder scores in individuals with autism, with the severity inversely related to the verbal intelligence quotient scores, highlighting the impact of developmental effects and verbal abilities on the appearance of thought disorder. In addition, correlations between autistic symptoms or traits and schizotypal traits (referential thinking, paranoid thinking, constricted affect, social affect, odd speech, eccentric behavior) have been found in individuals with ASDs[10] as well as in subthreshold traits in nonclinical control populations.[11]

Because abnormal thought processes are common in individuals with ASDs, at least 1 month of prominent delusions or hallucinations is required before a diagnosis

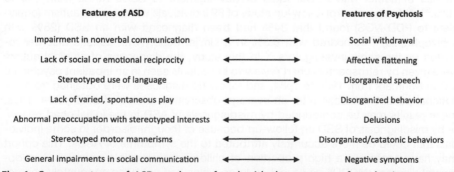

Features of ASD		Features of Psychosis
Impairment in nonverbal communication	←——————→	Social withdrawal
Lack of social or emotional reciprocity	←——————→	Affective flattening
Stereotyped use of language	←——————→	Disorganized speech
Lack of varied, spontaneous play	←——————→	Disorganized behavior
Abnormal preoccupation with stereotyped interests	←——————→	Delusions
Stereotyped motor mannerisms	←——————→	Disorganized/catatonic behaviors
General impairments in social communication	←——————→	Negative symptoms

Fig. 1. Core symptoms of ASD can be confused with the presence of psychotic symptoms. Developmental history and establishment of baseline thought process as well as change from baseline can be helpful in distinguishing between these presentations.

of schizophrenia is made.[1] In general, this requirement for prominent delusions or hallucinations is an important prerequisite before making any psychotic disorder diagnosis in individuals with ASDs. However, as noted in **Fig. 1**, the odd patterns of speech, rigidity of thinking, self-talk, and idiosyncratic thought processes seen in ASDs can also present a challenge to identifying delusions and hallucinations. An important key point is that the onset of psychotic disorder should coincide with the appearance of new symptoms and a decline in functioning from baseline in individuals on the autism spectrum. Thus, a careful developmental history with an elaboration of baseline presentation of core features of autism and any changes from the baseline presentation remain the essential standard for the evaluation of the presence of psychotic disorder in individuals with ASDs.

Comorbidity of ASD and psychotic disorder

Before the 1970s, autism was thought to be a manifestation of childhood schizophrenia, and there was no distinction between autistic disorder and psychosis or recognition of the broad spectrum of developmental disorders, which included autistic symptoms. The pioneering work of Kolvin and colleagues[12–17] made a distinction between psychosis that had its onset in infancy or early childhood (which would develop into the definition of ASD) and psychosis appearing in later childhood or adolescence (early-onset schizophrenia). Since that time, the connection between autism and schizophrenia has been continually debated and investigated, with mixed findings regarding the prevalence of SSDs in ASDs. Nevertheless, there is a subset of patients with comorbid ASDs and psychotic disorders, and a consideration of the evidence for a connection between the disorders is warranted.

Reports on the prevalence of SSD in ASD are variable. Volkmar and Cohen[18] studied 163 case records of individuals with autistic disorder, and only found 1 case that unequivocally met DSM-III-R criteria for schizophrenia, a frequency (0.6%) that was comparable with that of the general population. However, there are several case reports of individuals with autism who progress to a clear diagnosis of schizophrenia.[19–23] Some longitudinal studies, limited by the small number of patients followed (n <50), showed progression to schizophrenia in 3% to 10%.[24–26] In larger cohort studies of children and adolescents with ASDs, a diagnosis of any psychotic disorder is rare (1 out of 341 across 4 studies), although mood disorders, anxiety disorders, and disruptive behavior disorders were common.[27–30] Tantam[31] reported on 85 adults with Asperger disorder, and 21% had psychosis: most were associated with mood disorders, with only 3 diagnosed with schizophrenia. In larger cohort studies of adults with ASDs, rates of development of SSDs range from 0% to 16%.[32–36] A case-control follow-up study of 89 individuals with atypical autism (equivalent to PDD-NOS) found that 34% had been diagnosed with an SSD (28% with schizophrenia)[37] compared with 6.6% in a similar cohort with autistic disorder reported by the same investigators.[33] In this study, the diagnoses of atypical autism were given by retrospective chart review to individuals seen in an inpatient psychiatric unit in Denmark from 1960 to 1984, and follow-up diagnoses were obtained from the national patient database after an average observation period of 32.5 years. Thus, these results may be confounded by misdiagnosis of ASD in the initial chart review, or by misdiagnosis of SSD on follow-up because of thought disorder in some individuals that could be more accurately attributed to the symptoms of ASDs. This cohort may have contained a high proportion of children with multiple complex developmental disorder (MCDD), as described later, which had not been adequately characterized at the time of the study and may have a higher predisposition to development of SSD (discussed later).

Another confounding variable to take into account clinically is the relationship of psychotic symptoms to anxiety and mood disorders. Weisbrot and colleagues[38] examined anxiety and psychotic symptoms in children 6 to 12 years old with and without ASDs. Psychotic symptom severity was correlated with the level of anxiety in both groups, but children with ASDs had generally higher levels of both anxiety and psychotic symptoms. A history of psychotic symptoms that only present under conditions of extreme stress or anxiety may indicate the presence of a primary anxiety disorder driving the symptoms.[39] Mood disorders, both unipolar depression and bipolar mania and depression, can present with psychotic symptoms, and most of the epidemiologic studies noted earlier indicate an increased incidence of mood disorders, both with and without psychosis, in populations with ASDs.

In contrast with the moderate rates of SSD in individuals with ASDs, there is a marked preponderance of ASDs and atypical social development in individuals who develop childhood-onset schizophrenia (onset before the age of 12 years). Early small studies found an increased incidence of autism in childhood-onset schizophrenia (COS), and up to 65% of children with COS had language and/or motor development abnormalities.[40] A National Institute of Mental Health (NIMH) longitudinal study of COS confirmed these findings and found that 25% of the 75 children diagnosed with COS had a lifetime diagnosis of ASD, most of whom (16/19) were diagnosed with PDD-NOS, and these investigators later reported results confirming these proportions in a larger sample (N = 101).[41,42] Those individuals with and without ASD diagnosis in the NIMH sample did not differ on baseline or 2-year to 6-year outcome clinical measures (see article in this issue by Driver, Gogtay, and Rapoport: *Childhood Onset Schizophrenia and Early Onset Schizophrenia Spectrum Disorders*). Unenge-Hallerback and colleagues[43] carefully evaluated 32 adult patients with SSD cross-sectionally and 41% met criteria for ASDs based on parent interviews. Thus, clinically there does seem to be a substantial subset of patients with schizophrenia who have early neurodevelopmental histories consistent with ASDs, suggesting a connection between the disorders.

To summarize, consideration of comorbid ASD and SSD should be given whenever there is the concern for psychotic symptoms that are accompanied by a change from baseline presentation in individuals with ASDs. There is evidence for neurodevelopmental connections between these spectra of disorders, and a particularly high incidence of premorbid ASDs in individuals with COS. Particular attention should be paid to the evaluation for comorbid mood and anxiety disorders as well, which are more frequently seen with accompanying psychotic symptoms in children with ASDs.

Complex neurodevelopmental disorders with multiple domains of dysfunction

In addition to the diagnostic difficulty in assessing the thought process in individuals with ASDs, there is the added complexity of a subset of children who have a complex neurodevelopmental pattern of symptoms that cross diagnostic boundaries and include impairments in social functioning and reality testing. Many of these children are given diagnoses of ASD, particularly PDD-NOS, because of the severity of their social deficits. In the literature, these children have been described using various terms that also have overlapped with ASDs, including borderline syndrome of childhood[44] and schizoid personality in childhood.[45] Two constructs that have emerged have been developed to the point of having proposed diagnostic criteria and have been more rigorously studied: MCDD[46,47] and multidimensionally impaired (MDI) children.[48] These constructs are informative in the consideration of the overlap of autism and psychosis, particularly noting the similarities and differences in the development of these concepts.

The concept of MCDD grew out of studies at Yale Child Study Center designed to more accurately classify ASDs and particularly critiquing the DSM-III conceptualization and working toward the development of the PDD-NOS category that appeared in DSM-III-R and DSM-IV. Cohen and colleagues[46] described a subtype of children with ASDs who also displayed clinically significant disturbances in several areas of functioning, including affect and emotion regulation, severe anxieties, attachment relationships, and thought process. The thought disorder described in these children bordered on delusional thinking, with difficulty separating fantasy from reality. Criteria were developed (**Table 1**) to classify these children, and were later modified by Towbin and colleagues.[47] The descriptions of these children bring to mind clinical examples of individuals who seem to cross diagnostic boundaries of mood disorders, anxiety disorders, ASDs, and psychotic disorders. Children meeting these criteria have subsequently been studied by 2 clinical research groups in the Netherlands,[9,49–60] and

Table 1
Comparison of criteria for multiple complex developmental disorder[47] and multidimensionally impaired syndrome[66]

Multiple Complex Developmental Disorder	Multidimensionally Impaired Syndrome

• Impaired regulation of affective state and anxiety:
  ○ Intense anxiety, tension, irritability
  ○ Unusual fears and phobias
  ○ Recurrent panic episodes
  ○ Episodic behavioral disorganization or regression
  ○ Significant emotional variability
  ○ Idiosyncratic anxiety reactions
	Nearly daily periods of emotional lability disproportionate to precipitants

• Impaired social behavior and sensitivity:
  ○ Social disinterest, detachment, or avoidance
  ○ May appear friendly and cooperative but superficial
  ○ Inability to initiate or maintain peer relationships
  ○ High degree of ambivalent attachment to adults
  ○ Profound limitations in the capacity of empathy
	Impaired interpersonal skills despite desire to initiate social interactions with peers

• Impaired cognitive processing:
  ○ Thought problems including irrationality, intrusions on thought process, magical thinking, neologisms or nonsense words, illogical bizarre ideas
  ○ Confusion between reality and fantasy life
  ○ Perplexity and easy confusability
  ○ Fantasies of personal omnipotence, paranoid preoccupations, overengagement with fantasy figures, grandiose fantasies of special powers, and referential ideation
	Poor ability to distinguish fantasy from reality, as shown by ideas of reference and brief perceptual disturbances during stressful periods or while falling asleep

Data from Towbin KE, Dykens EM, Pearson GS, et al. Conceptualizing "borderline syndrome of childhood" and "childhood schizophrenia" as a developmental disorder. J Am Acad Child Adolesc Psychiatry 1993;32(4):775–82. http://dx.doi.org/10.1097/00004583-199307000-00011; and Kumra S, Jacobsen LK, Lenane M, et al. "Multidimensionally impaired disorder": is it a variant of very early-onset schizophrenia? J Am Acad Child Adolesc Psychiatry 1998;37(1):91–9.

1 each in the United States[61] and Sweden.[62] Sturm and colleagues[62] reviewed medical and psychiatric records of 101 children with ASDs and 8% met criteria for MCDD.

Several studies have compared children who meet criteria for both PDD-NOS and MCDD (PDD-NOS+MCDD) to those with autistic disorder (classic autism) and have suggested that MCDD may be more closely related to SSD. Compared with children with autistic disorder, children with PDD-NOS+MCDD had higher levels of psychotic thinking, anxiety, aggression, suspiciousness, and odd interactions, and lower levels of social communication deficits and stereotyped and rigid behaviors. There was also a marked fluctuation in functioning of children with PDD-NOS+MCDD compared with a more stable level in those with autistic disorder.[49] Children with PDD-NOS+MCDD also had a decreased stress response to a social stressor,[52] similar to a prior study in individuals with schizophrenia[63] and in contrast with an increased stress response seen in autistic disorder.[53] Likewise, in tracking of smooth pursuit eye movements, children with PDD-NOS+MCDD but not autistic disorder showed lower velocity gain compared with controls and similar to a group of adult patients with schizophrenia, although they did not have the same increased saccades as the group with schizophrenia.[56] Van Engeland and van der Gaag[64] reported follow-up studies of 43 adolescents and 12 adults who had been evaluated as children in an inpatient unit and who met criteria for MCDD. Twenty-two percent of the adolescents and 64% of the adults suffered from SSDs, primarily schizoid and schizotypal personality disorders. Two out of the 12 adults were diagnosed with schizophrenia. Sprong and colleagues[55] compared 32 adolescents with MCDD with 80 adolescents who were diagnosed with research criteria for at-risk mental state (ARMS), indicating a high risk for progression to psychosis. Seventy-eight percent of the individuals with MCDD also met criteria for ARMS, and the rate of first-degree relatives with psychotic disorder was comparable in the two groups. There were no differences between groups in schizotypal traits, but the MCDD group had more autistic traits, had been more impaired in early childhood, had significantly younger age at referral, and had earlier initiation of psychiatric treatment. These data indicate that children with PDD-NOS+MCDD may have a higher risk of developing psychotic disorders and may warrant more careful monitoring for emergence of psychosis.

The initial diagnostic criteria for MCDD were developed for a subset of patients who had already been identified as having ASD (specifically, PDD-NOS); however, other studies have identified patients who meet the explicit MCDD criteria, but not criteria for PDD-NOS.[59–61] For example, De Bruin and colleagues[59] reported that, out of 503 consecutive referrals of children aged 6 to 12 years to an outpatient treatment center, 5.9% met the research criteria for MCDD and 44% of these met criteria for PDD-NOS. Another 17.5% of referrals met criteria for PDD-NOS alone. Compared with children with PDD-NOS alone, children with MCDD had higher rates of obsessive-compulsive disorder, anxiety disorders, and disruptive behavior disorders, and higher rates of delusions and auditory hallucinations, although none had a diagnosis of schizophrenia. The children with MCDD, inclusive of those with PDD-NOS+MCDD, were less socially impaired than those with PDD-NOS alone. The study was not powered to compare those with MCDD alone or PDD-NOS alone with those with PDD-NOS+MCDD. One other study has compared children with PDD-NOS+MCDD with those with PDD-NOS without MCDD,[58] but it did not report on a comparison of social functioning between the groups. The PDD-NOS+MCDD group showed impairment in executive functioning with worse performance on a sustained attention task and more errors in an inhibition task.

In parallel with the development of the MCDD concept, researchers at the NIMH reported longitudinally on a group of children referred for an evaluation for COS.[48,65–74]

These children were determined not to have a diagnosis of schizophrenia, but instead displayed transient brief episodes of hallucinations during times of stress, difficulty distinguishing fantasy from reality, nearly daily periods of extreme emotional lability, impaired interpersonal skills despite the desire for social interaction, and attentional and information-processing deficits consistent with attention-deficit/hyperactivity disorder (ADHD) (see **Table 1**). They also had no evidence of formal thought disorder. These patients were initially labeled as having MDI syndrome,[48,65,66,73] although later reports identified their diagnosis as psychotic disorder not otherwise specified[67–72,74] (See article in this issue by Driver, Gogtay, and Rapoport: *Childhood Onset Schizophrenia and Early Onset Schizophrenia Spectrum Disorders*). Although the NIMH researchers did not consider these individuals to be associated with ASDs,[48] the surface resemblance of domains of dysfunction in MDI compared with MCDD is striking (see **Table 1**). Unlike the MCDD group, after 2 to 8 years of follow-up, none of the children with MDI had progressed to schizophrenia, and most had significant mood disorders or disruptive behavior disorders (38% bipolar disorder type I, 12% major depressive disorder, 3% schizoaffective disorder, 38% ADHD, 28% oppositional defiant disorder).

Taken together, these studies of MCDD and MDI indicate that there is a subset of children with complex neurodevelopmental disorders with symptoms that cut across various disorders but that are significantly impairing. It is counterintuitive that preliminary evidence suggests that those who have the most prominent psychotic symptoms in early childhood (the children with MDI, as shown by their referral to a research study for COS) have a propensity to develop significant mood disorders rather than SSD. In contrast, those who have been categorized as having MCDD, who have more prominent social impairments (given their association with PDD-NOS diagnosis), seem to have a higher propensity for development of SSD in adolescence and young adulthood. All of these associations should be regarded as preliminary given the small numbers of children who have been studied, especially in the MDI group, and understanding of these complex clinical presentations would be greatly enhanced by larger studies of children meeting these criteria, particularly with regard to long-term outcomes.

Symptom Criteria

Box 1 provides the symptom domains affected in ASDs, and **Table 1** compares the diagnostic criteria proposed for MCDD and MDI.

EVALUATION OF A PATIENT WITH ASD AND SUSPECTED PSYCHOSIS

Given the diagnostic dilemma raised by the presence of possible psychotic symptoms in an individual with ASD, it is helpful to have a framework for the evaluation with consideration for distinguishing between the misattribution of autistic core symptoms as psychotic, giving a diagnosis of comorbid psychotic disorder, or characterizing a complex neurodevelopmental disorder that is accompanied by dysfunction in several domains and a propensity toward the development of multiple possible comorbid psychiatric disorders. Much of the evaluation is centered on a careful developmental, behavioral, and psychiatric history, and the longitudinal assessment of mental status, because there are no current biological markers available for distinguishing between these various presentations.

Patient History

A careful developmental history is essential, with the focus on the time course and development of symptoms of concern. In addition, family history of psychotic disorders may be helpful in assessing an increased risk for progression to psychosis. **Box 2** shows elements within the patient history, specifically with regard to the suspected psychotic symptoms, that may weigh in favor of one of the 3 diagnostic possibilities outlined earlier.

Mental Status Examination Findings

Careful attention to the longitudinal evaluation of mental status can be helpful in clarifying the differential diagnosis of a possible psychotic disorder. For individuals in whom the core symptoms of ASDs are presenting in a way that raises the concern for psychosis, it is important to establish the child's baseline presentation. A stable historical pattern of rigid thinking, obsessive preoccupation with bizarre ideation, self-talk, or age-inappropriate fantastical beliefs or magical thinking may be more strongly indicative of the underlying abnormal thought patterns associated with ASD. However, new onset or acute progression of these symptoms is more consistent with the development of a psychotic process (ie, a distinct change from baseline). Also, formal thought disorder frequently is present in ASDs, and the conventional practice of requiring the presence of delusions or hallucinations to establish a psychotic disorder diagnosis is recommended in this population. In addition, transient psychotic episodes that are brief (often a few minutes) and infrequent (occurring only a few times a month, often in response to stress), accompanied by extreme mood lability and excessive anxiety, are more consistent with the patterns seen in individuals with MCDD/MDI. These individuals need to be monitored closely over time,

---

Box 2
Considerations in patient history to assess the question of psychotic symptoms in ASD

Core symptoms of ASD mistaken for psychosis

- Developmental history indicates presence of stable symptoms from early childhood
- Disorganized thought process without clear history of delusions or hallucinations
- Delusions consistent with abnormal preoccupation with stereotyped interests
- No decline in overall functioning from baseline

Comorbidity of SSD

- New onset of delusions and/or hallucinations lasting more than 1 month
- Disorganization of thought or behavior that is a clear change from baseline
- Degree of magical thinking or inability to distinguish fantasy from reality that is a clear change from baseline
- Also consider comorbidity of mood and/or anxiety disorder that coincides with onset of psychotic symptoms
- Significant decline in overall functioning

MCDD/MDI constructs (not DSM categories)

- Episodes of psychotic symptoms are transient and brief, and primarily occur in times of stress
- History also notable for extreme mood lability with daily severe mood changes
- Presence of unusually intense fears or phobias, or recurrent panic episodes
- Illogical thinking, magical thinking, and difficulty distinguishing fantasy from reality are present at baseline with no significant progression or worsening

because they have a propensity to develop significant mood disorders, disruptive behavior disorders, and possibly SSD as well.

Rating Scales and Standardized Assessments

Box 3 lists helpful diagnostic scales and standardized assessments that can be helpful in the evaluation of ASD and psychotic disorders.

Imaging

There have been interesting research findings regarding the various diagnostic entities under consideration; however, there are no clinically indicated imaging tests for the evaluation of possible psychosis in ASD unless the patient presents with focal neurologic signs that call for imaging as part of the standard clinical work-up. In general, imaging findings in autistic disorder and COS are different. In autistic disorder, the most consistent finding is increased head size and total brain volume in the first 3 years of life.[75,76] At later ages, the findings are inconsistent.[77] In COS, there is a striking loss of cortical gray matter in early childhood that progresses through adolescence,[78,79] which eventually develops into the adult schizophrenia pattern of prefrontal and superior temporal cortical gray matter loss.[80] Some have suggested a connection in these findings in that both represent an acceleration of the natural developmental maturation process.[42] Gogtay and colleagues[67] presented evidence that patients with COS had different cortical development trajectories than individuals with MDI, who did not differ from healthy controls. However, a subset of patients with COS who also had comorbid ASD had a faster gray matter loss through early adolescence than patients with COS without ASD.[41]

Box 3
Helpful diagnostic rating scales and standardized assessments

Evaluation of ASD

- Autism Diagnostic Observation Schedule[118]: standardized behavioral observation and coding; requires training for reliability as a diagnostic tool; administration time 40 to 60 minutes; second edition allows for assessment from 12 months of age to adulthood

- Autism Diagnostic Interview, Revised[119]: standardized caregiver interview and response coding; requires training for reliability as a diagnostic tool; administration time 1.5 to 2.5 hours

- Social Communication Questionnaire[120]: parent questionnaire with 40 Yes/No items; current and lifetime forms available; administration time less than 10 minutes; effective screening tool with total score cutoff; positive screen requires careful diagnostic interview/observation for confirmation of diagnosis

- Social Responsiveness Scale[121]: parent and/or teacher rating scale for ages 2.5 to 18 years; identifies presence and severity of social impairment within the autism spectrum and differentiates it from impairment that occurs in other disorders; administration time 15 to 20 minutes; useful for assessment of severity of impairment and assessment of various subdomains: social awareness, social cognition, social communication, social motivation, restricted interests, and repetitive behavior

Evaluation of psychotic disorder

- Positive and Negative Syndrome Scale[122]: clinician-completed rating scale based on observed and elicited symptoms during a clinical interview; administration time 30 to 40 minutes; in evaluation of individuals with comorbid ASD, must be combined with clinical judgment to determine whether symptoms indicate psychosis or underlying ASD

Genetics

There is compelling evidence for shared genetic factors linking ASDs and schizophrenia. Several common genes and chromosomal regions have been implicated in both disorders. Patients with deletions in chromosomal region 22q11.2, associated with velocardiofacial syndrome, have high rates of both ASDs and psychosis. In one study, 50% of patients with a 22q11.2 deletion met criteria for ASDs and 26.7% of patients with a 22q11.2 deletion had psychotic symptoms, with 11.7% being given a psychotic disorder diagnosis.[81] Eight percent of the patients had comorbid psychotic disorder and ASD, but the study did not report on the co-occurrence of ASDs and psychotic symptoms. Both microdeletions and microduplications of chromosome region 16p11.2 have been associated with autism (approximately 1% of patients),[82] and microduplications of this region have been associated with schizophrenia.[83] In terms of single genes implicated in these disorders, multiple genes involved in synaptogenesis and synapse maturation have copy number variants (CNVs) that are associated with both ASD and schizophrenia.[84] Deletions, mutations, and CNVs in the neurexin family,[85–87] which is involved in forming connections between neurons at synapses, have been reported in autism[88–97] and schizophrenia.[93,98–103] Likewise, mutations and single nucleotide polymorphisms in the genes for oxytocin, a hormone increasingly recognized to be a regulator of social interactions, and the oxytocin receptor have been found in cases of autism[104–108] and schizophrenia.[109–112] These findings are potentially clinically relevant, because preliminary studies of administration of intranasal oxytocin have shown some improvement in social impairments in autism[113,114] as well as enhanced antipsychotic effects on both positive and negative symptoms in individuals with schizophrenia.[115,116]

In terms of genetics testing, there is evidence that the initial diagnostic work-up for ASDs should include karyotyping and fragile X testing, and the Autism Consortium Clinical Genetics/DNA Diagnostics Collaboration recommended the consideration of chromosomal microarray to test for submicroscopic genomic deletions and duplications.[117] This may be particularly helpful if there is concern for comorbid psychosis, because it may identify genetic changes that are associated with both ASDs and schizophrenia, such as 22q11.2 deletions and 16p11.2 deletions and duplications. No other specific genetic testing has been studied for potential clinical usefulness in children with ASDs (See article in this issue by Benjamin, Stanislawski, and Lauterbach for discussion of medical and genetic evaluations of psychotic symptoms in childhood: *Congenital and Acquired Disorders Presenting as Psychosis in Children and Young Adults*).

SUMMARY

The concern for comorbid psychosis in patients with ASDs is a frequently encountered diagnostic dilemma. A careful assessment of the patient with particular regard to developmental history is important to determine whether symptoms are more consistent with a manifestation of the patient's core autistic symptoms than a true psychotic process. Nevertheless, there is growing evidence, as outlined earlier, for connections between ASDs and SSDs, and comorbid psychotic disorder must be on the differential diagnosis. In addition, as in the general population, psychotic symptoms in children and adolescents are more often associated with mood disorders, anxiety disorders, and disruptive behavior disorders than psychotic disorders, so a complete psychiatric assessment is needed. The diagnostic conundrum is further complicated by the presence of a subset of children with a complex neurodevelopmental disorder with symptoms that cross diagnostic boundaries. These children can present with psychotic symptoms but are notable for their excessive anxiety, mood lability, and information-processing deficits. This article summarizes the available literature on these complex individuals, particularly as elucidated in the MCDD/MDI constructs. Current research indicates a wide variety of diagnostic and clinical outcomes for these individuals, and more research is needed to better understand the predictors of outcome and development of appropriate interventions for these children.

REFERENCES

1. American Psychiatric Association. Diagnostic and statistical manual of mental disorders. 4th edition, Text Revision. Washington, DC: American Psychiatric Association; 2000.
2. American Psychiatric Association. Diagnostic and statistical manual of mental disorders. 3rd edition. Washington, DC: American Psychiatric Association; 1980.
3. Cohen DJ, Volkmar FR, Paul R. Issues in the classification of pervasive developmental disorders: history and current status of nosology. J Am Acad Child Psychiatry 1986;25(2):158–61.
4. Volkmar FR, Cohen DJ, Paul R. An evaluation of DSM-III criteria for infantile autism. J Am Acad Child Psychiatry 1986;25(2):190–7.
5. Konstantareas MM, Hewitt T. Autistic disorder and schizophrenia: diagnostic overlaps. J Autism Dev Disord 2001;31(1):19–28.
6. Dykens E, Volkmar F, Glick M. Thought disorder in high-functioning autistic adults. J Autism Dev Disord 1991;21(3):291–301.
7. Rumsey JM, Andreasen NC, Rapoport JL. Thought, language, communication, and affective flattening in autistic adults. Arch Gen Psychiatry 1986;43(8):771–7.
8. Ghaziuddin M, Leininger L, Tsai L. Brief report: thought disorder in Asperger syndrome: comparison with high-functioning autism. J Autism Dev Disord 1995;25(3):311–7.
9. van der Gaag R, Caplan R, van Engeland H, et al. A controlled study of formal thought disorder in children with autism and multiple complex developmental disorders. J Child Adolesc Psychopharmacol 2005;15(3):465–76.
10. Barneveld PS, Pieterse J, de Sonneville L, et al. Overlap of autistic and schizotypal traits in adolescents with autism spectrum disorders. Schizophr Res 2011; 126(1–3):231–6. http://dx.doi.org/10.1016/j.schres.2010.09.004.
11. Hurst RM, Nelson-Gray RO, Mitchell JT, et al. The relationship of Asperger's characteristics and schizotypal personality traits in a non-clinical adult sample. J Autism Dev Disord 2007;37(9):1711–20. http://dx.doi.org/10.1007/s10803-006-0302-z.
12. Kolvin I. Studies in the childhood psychoses. I. Diagnostic criteria and classification. Br J Psychiatry 1971;118(545):381–4.
13. Kolvin I, Ounsted C, Humphrey M, et al. Studies in the childhood psychoses. II. The phenomenology of childhood psychoses. Br J Psychiatry 1971;118(545):385–95.
14. Kolvin I, Ounsted C, Richardson LM, et al. Studies in the childhood psychoses. 3. The family and social background in childhood psychoses. Br J Psychiatry 1971;118(545):396–402.
15. Kolvin I, Garside RF, Kidd JS. Studies in the childhood psychoses. IV. Parental personality and attitude and childhood psychoses. Br J Psychiatry 1971; 118(545):403–6.
16. Kolvin I, Ounsted C, Roth M. Studies in the childhood psychoses. V. Cerebral dysfunction and childhood psychoses. Br J Psychiatry 1971;118(545):407–14.

17. Kolvin I, Humphrey M, McNay A. Studies in the childhood psychoses. VI. Cognitive factors in childhood psychoses. Br J Psychiatry 1971;118(545):415–9.
18. Volkmar FR, Cohen DJ. Comorbid association of autism and schizophrenia. Am J Psychiatry 1991;148(12):1705–7.
19. Petty LK, Ornitz EM, Michelman JD, et al. Autistic children who become schizophrenic. Arch Gen Psychiatry 1984;41(2):129–35.
20. Gillberg C. Asperger's syndrome and recurrent psychosis–a case study. J Autism Dev Disord 1985;15(4):389–97.
21. Trave Rodriguez AL, Barreiro Marin P, Galvez Borrero IM, et al. Association between autism and schizophrenia. J Nerv Ment Dis 1994;182(8):478–9.
22. Sverd J, Montero G, Gurevich N. Brief report: cases for an association between Tourette syndrome, autistic disorder, and schizophrenia-like disorder. J Autism Dev Disord 1993;23(2):407–13.
23. Clarke DJ, LittleJohns CS, Corbett JA, et al. Pervasive developmental disorders and psychoses in adult life. Br J Psychiatry 1989;155:692–9.
24. Larsen FW, Mouridsen SE. The outcome in children with childhood autism and Asperger syndrome originally diagnosed as psychotic. A 30-year follow-up study of subjects hospitalized as children. Eur Child Adolesc Psychiatry 1997; 6(4):181–90.
25. Wing L. Asperger's syndrome: a clinical account. Psychol Med 1981;11(1): 115–29.
26. Wolff S, Chick J. Schizoid personality in childhood: a controlled follow-up study. Psychol Med 1980;10(1):85–100.
27. Bradley E, Bolton P. Episodic psychiatric disorders in teenagers with learning disabilities with and without autism. Br J Psychiatry 2006;189: 361–6. http://dx.doi.org/10.1192/bjp.bp.105.018127.
28. Simonoff E, Pickles A, Charman T, et al. Psychiatric disorders in children with autism spectrum disorders: prevalence, comorbidity, and associated factors in a population-derived sample. J Am Acad Child Adolesc Psychiatry 2008; 47(8):921–9. http://dx.doi.org/10.1097/CHI.0b013e318179964f.
29. Ghaziuddin M, Weidmer-Mikhail E, Ghaziuddin N. Comorbidity of Asperger syndrome: a preliminary report. J Intellect Disabil Res 1998;42(Pt 4):279–83.
30. Leyfer OT, Folstein SE, Bacalman S, et al. Comorbid psychiatric disorders in children with autism: interview development and rates of disorders. J Autism Dev Disord 2006;36(7):849–61. http://dx.doi.org/10.1007/s10803-006-0123-0.
31. Tantam D. Asperger syndrome in adulthood. In: Frith U, editor. Autism and Asperger syndrome. Cambridge (United Kingdom): Cambridge University Press; 1991. p. 147–83.
32. Hutton J, Goode S, Murphy M, et al. New-onset psychiatric disorders in individuals with autism. Autism 2008;12(4):373–90. http://dx.doi.org/10.1177/1362361308091650.
33. Mouridsen SE, Rich B, Isager T, et al. Psychiatric disorders in individuals diagnosed with infantile autism as children: a case control study. J Psychiatr Pract 2008;14(1):5–12. http://dx.doi.org/10.1097/01.pra.0000308490.47262.e0.
34. Stahlberg O, Soderstrom H, Rastam M, et al. Bipolar disorder, schizophrenia, and other psychotic disorders in adults with childhood onset AD/HD and/or autism spectrum disorders. J Neural Transm 2004;111(7):891–902. http://dx.doi.org/10.1007/s00702-004-0115-1.
35. Tsakanikos E, Costello H, Holt G, et al. Psychopathology in adults with autism and intellectual disability. J Autism Dev Disord 2006;36(8):1123–9. http://dx.doi.org/10.1007/s10803-006-0149-3.

36. Hofvander B, Delorme R, Chaste P, et al. Psychiatric and psychosocial problems in adults with normal-intelligence autism spectrum disorders. BMC Psychiatry 2009;9:35. http://dx.doi.org/10.1186/1471-244X-9-35.

37. Mouridsen SE, Rich B, Isager T. Psychiatric disorders in adults diagnosed as children with atypical autism. A case control study. J Neural Transm 2008; 115(1):135–8. http://dx.doi.org/10.1007/s00702-007-0798-1.

38. Weisbrot DM, Gadow KD, DeVincent CJ, et al. The presentation of anxiety in children with pervasive developmental disorders. J Child Adolesc Psychopharmacol 2005;15(3):477–96. http://dx.doi.org/10.1089/cap.2005.15.477.

39. Biederman J, Petty C, Faraone SV, et al. Phenomenology of childhood psychosis: findings from a large sample of psychiatrically referred youth. J Nerv Ment Dis 2004;192(9):607–14.

40. Watkins JM, Asarnow RF, Tanguay PE. Symptom development in childhood onset schizophrenia. J Child Psychol Psychiatry 1988;29(6):865–78.

41. Sporn A, Addington A, Gogtay N, et al. Pervasive developmental disorder and childhood-onset schizophrenia: comorbid disorder or a phenotypic variant of a very early onset illness? Biol Psychiatry 2004;55(10):989–94.

42. Rapoport J, Chavez A, Greenstein D, et al. Autism spectrum disorders and childhood-onset schizophrenia: clinical and biological contributions to a relation revisited. J Am Acad Child Adolesc Psychiatry 2009;48(1):10–8.

43. Unenge Hallerback M, Lugnegard T, Gillberg C. Is autism spectrum disorder common in schizophrenia? Psychiatry Res 2012;198(1):12–7. http://dx.doi.org/10.1016/j.psychres.2012.01.016.

44. Petti TA, Vela RM. Borderline disorders of childhood: an overview. J Am Acad Child Adolesc Psychiatry 1990;29(3):327–37.

45. Wolff S. 'Schizoid' personality in childhood and adult life. I: the vagaries of diagnostic labelling. Br J Psychiatry 1991;159:615–20, 634–5.

46. Cohen DJ, Paul R, Volkmar FR. Issues in the classification of pervasive and other developmental disorders: toward DSM-IV. J Am Acad Child Psychiatry 1986; 25(2):213–20.

47. Towbin KE, Dykens EM, Pearson GS, et al. Conceptualizing "borderline syndrome of childhood" and "childhood schizophrenia" as a developmental disorder. J Am Acad Child Adolesc Psychiatry 1993;32(4):775–82. http://dx.doi.org/10.1097/00004583-199307000-00011.

48. McKenna K, Gordon CT, Lenane M, et al. Looking for childhood-onset schizophrenia: the first 71 cases screened. J Am Acad Child Adolesc Psychiatry 1994;33(5):636–44. http://dx.doi.org/10.1097/00004583-199406000-00003.

49. Van der Gaag RJ, Buitelaar J, Van den Ban E, et al. A controlled multivariate chart review of multiple complex developmental disorder. J Am Acad Child Adolesc Psychiatry 1995;34(8):1096–106.

50. Buitelaar JK, van der Gaag RJ. Diagnostic rules for children with PDD-NOS and multiple complex developmental disorder. J Child Psychol Psychiatry 1998; 39(6):911–9.

51. Kemner C, van der Gaag RJ, Verbaten M, et al. ERP differences among subtypes of pervasive developmental disorders. Biol Psychiatry 1999;46(6):781–9.

52. Jansen LM, Gispen-de Wied CC, Van der Gaag RJ, et al. Unresponsiveness to psychosocial stress in a subgroup of autistic-like children, multiple complex developmental disorder. Psychoneuroendocrinology 2000;25(8):753–64.

53. Jansen LM, Gispen-de Wied CC, van der Gaag RJ, et al. Differentiation between autism and multiple complex developmental disorder in response

to psychosocial stress. Neuropsychopharmacology 2003;28(3):582–90. http://dx.doi.org/10.1038/sj.npp.1300046.

54. Lahuis BE, Durston S, Nederveen H, et al. MRI-based morphometry in children with multiple complex developmental disorder, a phenotypically defined subtype of pervasive developmental disorder not otherwise specified. Psychol Med 2008;38(9):1361–7. http://dx.doi.org/10.1017/S0033291707001481.

55. Sprong M, Becker HE, Schothorst PF, et al. Pathways to psychosis: a comparison of the pervasive developmental disorder subtype multiple complex developmental disorder and the "at risk mental state". Schizophr Res 2008;99(1–3): 38–47.

56. Lahuis BE, Van Engeland H, Cahn W, et al. Smooth pursuit eye movement (SPEM) in patients with multiple complex developmental disorder (MCDD), a subtype of the pervasive developmental disorder. World J Biol Psychiatry 2009;10(4 Pt 3):905–12. http://dx.doi.org/10.1080/15622970801901828.

57. Oranje B, Lahuis B, van Engeland H, et al. Sensory and sensorimotor gating in children with multiple complex developmental disorders (MCDD) and autism. Psychiatry Res 2012;206(2–3):287–92. http://dx.doi.org/10.1016/j.psychres. 2012.10.014.

58. van Rijn S, de Sonneville L, Lahuis B, et al. Executive function in MCDD and PDD-NOS: a study of inhibitory control, attention regulation and behavioral adaptivity. J Autism Dev Disord 2012. http://dx.doi.org/10.1007/s10803-012-1688-4.

59. de Bruin E, de Nijs PF, Verheij F, et al. Multiple complex developmental disorder delineated from PDD-NOS. J Autism Dev Disord 2007;37(6):1181–91.

60. Herba CM, de Bruin E, Althaus M, et al. Face and emotion recognition in MCDD versus PDD-NOS. J Autism Dev Disord 2008;38(4):706–18. http://dx.doi.org/10.1007/s10803-007-0438-5.

61. Lincoln AJ, Bloom D, Katz M, et al. Neuropsychological and neurophysiological indices of auditory processing impairment in children with multiple complex developmental disorder. J Am Acad Child Adolesc Psychiatry 1998;37(1): 100–12. http://dx.doi.org/10.1097/00004583-199801000-00023.

62. Sturm H, Fernell E, Gillberg C. Autism spectrum disorders in children with normal intellectual levels: associated impairments and subgroups. Dev Med Child Neurol 2004;46(7):444–7.

63. Jansen LM, Gispen-de Wied CC, Kahn RS. Selective impairments in the stress response in schizophrenic patients. Psychopharmacology (Berl) 2000;149(3): 319–25.

64. Van Engeland H, van der Gaag RJ. MCDD in childhood: a precursor of schizophrenic spectrum disorders. Schizophr Res 1994;11:197.

65. Kumra S, Wiggs E, Krasnewich D, et al. Brief report: association of sex chromosome anomalies with childhood-onset psychotic disorders. J Am Acad Child Adolesc Psychiatry 1998;37(3):292–6. http://dx.doi.org/10.1097/00004583-199803000-00014.

66. Kumra S, Jacobsen LK, Lenane M, et al. "Multidimensionally impaired disorder": is it a variant of very early-onset schizophrenia? J Am Acad Child Adolesc Psychiatry 1998;37(1):91–9.

67. Gogtay N, Sporn A, Clasen LS, et al. Comparison of progressive cortical gray matter loss in childhood-onset schizophrenia with that in childhood-onset atypical psychoses. Arch Gen Psychiatry 2004;61(1):17–22. http://dx.doi.org/10.1001/archpsyc.61.1.17.

68. Kumra S, Wiggs E, Bedwell J, et al. Neuropsychological deficits in pediatric patients with childhood-onset schizophrenia and psychotic disorder not otherwise specified. Schizophr Res 2000;42(2):135–44.

69. Kumra S, Giedd JN, Vaituzis AC, et al. Childhood-onset psychotic disorders: magnetic resonance imaging of volumetric differences in brain structure. Am J Psychiatry 2000;157(9):1467–74.

70. Kumra S, Sporn A, Hommer DW, et al. Smooth pursuit eye-tracking impairment in childhood-onset psychotic disorders. Am J Psychiatry 2001;158(8):1291–8.

71. Nicolson R, Lenane M, Brookner F, et al. Children and adolescents with psychotic disorder not otherwise specified: a 2- to 8-year follow-up study. Compr Psychiatry 2001;42(4):319–25. http://dx.doi.org/10.1053/comp.2001.24573.

72. Stayer C, Sporn A, Gogtay N, et al. Multidimensionally impaired: the good news. J Child Adolesc Psychopharmacol 2005;15(3):510–9. http://dx.doi.org/10.1089/cap.2005.15.510.

73. Gogtay N, Ordonez A, Herman DH, et al. Dynamic mapping of cortical development before and after the onset of pediatric bipolar illness. J Child Psychol Psychiatry 2007;48(9):852–62. http://dx.doi.org/10.1111/j.1469-7610.2007.01747.x.

74. Gogtay N, Weisinger B, Bakalar JL, et al. Psychotic symptoms and gray matter deficits in clinical pediatric populations. Schizophr Res 2012;140(1–3):149–54. http://dx.doi.org/10.1016/j.schres.2012.07.006.

75. Courchesne E, Carper R, Akshoomoff N. Evidence of brain overgrowth in the first year of life in autism. JAMA 2003;290(3):337–44. http://dx.doi.org/10.1001/jama.290.3.337.

76. Hazlett HC, Poe M, Gerig G, et al. Magnetic resonance imaging and head circumference study of brain size in autism: birth through age 2 years. Arch Gen Psychiatry 2005;62(12):1366–76. http://dx.doi.org/10.1001/archpsyc.62.12.1366.

77. Mosconi M, Zwaigenbaum L, Piven J. Structural MRI in autism: findings and future directions. Clin Neurosci Res 2006;6:135–44.

78. Thompson PM, Hayashi KM, Sowell ER, et al. Mapping cortical change in Alzheimer's disease, brain development, and schizophrenia. Neuroimage 2004;23(Suppl 1):S2–18. http://dx.doi.org/10.1016/j.neuroimage.2004.07.071.

79. Gogtay N, Giedd JN, Lusk L, et al. Dynamic mapping of human cortical development during childhood through early adulthood. Proc Natl Acad Sci U S A 2004;101(21):8174–9. http://dx.doi.org/10.1073/pnas.0402680101.

80. Greenstein D, Lerch J, Shaw P, et al. Childhood onset schizophrenia: cortical brain abnormalities as young adults. J Child Psychol Psychiatry 2006;47(10):1003–12. http://dx.doi.org/10.1111/j.1469-7610.2006.01658.x.

81. Vorstman JA, Morcus ME, Duijff S, et al. The 22q11.2 deletion in children: high rate of autistic disorders and early onset of psychotic symptoms. J Am Acad Child Adolesc Psychiatry 2006;45(9):1104–13.

82. Weiss LA, Shen Y, Korn JM, et al. Association between microdeletion and microduplication at 16p11.2 and autism. N Engl J Med 2008;358(7):667–75. http://dx.doi.org/10.1056/NEJMoa075974.

83. McCarthy SE, Makarov V, Kirov G, et al. Microduplications of 16p11.2 are associated with schizophrenia. Nat Genet 2009;41(11):1223–7. http://dx.doi.org/10.1038/ng.474.

84. Guilmatre A, Dubourg C, Mosca AL, et al. Recurrent rearrangements in synaptic and neurodevelopmental genes and shared biologic pathways in schizophrenia, autism, and mental retardation. Arch Gen Psychiatry 2009;66(9):947–56. http://dx.doi.org/10.1001/archgenpsychiatry.2009.80.

85. Carroll L, Owen M. Genetic overlap between autism, schizophrenia and bipolar disorder. Genome Med 2009;1(10):102.
86. Reichelt AC, Rodgers RJ, Clapcote SJ. The role of neurexins in schizophrenia and autistic spectrum disorder. Neuropharmacology 2012;62(3):1519–26. http://dx.doi.org/10.1016/j.neuropharm.2011.01.024.
87. Burbach JP, van der Zwaag B. Contact in the genetics of autism and schizophrenia. Trends Neurosci 2009;32(2):69–72. http://dx.doi.org/10.1016/j.tins.2008.11.002.
88. Marshall CR, Noor A, Vincent JB, et al. Structural variation of chromosomes in autism spectrum disorder. Am J Hum Genet 2008;82(2):477–88. http://dx.doi.org/10.1016/j.ajhg.2007.12.009.
89. Kim HG, Kishikawa S, Higgins AW, et al. Disruption of neurexin 1 associated with autism spectrum disorder. Am J Hum Genet 2008;82(1):199–207. http://dx.doi.org/10.1016/j.ajhg.2007.09.011.
90. Zahir FR, Baross A, Delaney AD, et al. A patient with vertebral, cognitive and behavioural abnormalities and a de novo deletion of NRXN1alpha. J Med Genet 2008;45(4):239–43. http://dx.doi.org/10.1136/jmg.2007.054437.
91. Autism Genome Project Consortium, Szatmari P, Paterson AD, Zwaigenbaum L, et al. Mapping autism risk loci using genetic linkage and chromosomal rearrangements. Nat Genet 2007;39(3):319–28. http://dx.doi.org/10.1038/ng1985.
92. Feng J, Schroer R, Yan J, et al. High frequency of neurexin 1beta signal peptide structural variants in patients with autism. Neurosci Lett 2006;409(1):10–3. http://dx.doi.org/10.1016/j.neulet.2006.08.017.
93. Gauthier J, Siddiqui TJ, Huashan P, et al. Truncating mutations in NRXN2 and NRXN1 in autism spectrum disorders and schizophrenia. Hum Genet 2011;130(4):563–73. http://dx.doi.org/10.1007/s00439-011-0975-z.
94. Alarcon M, Abrahams BS, Stone JL, et al. Linkage, association, and gene-expression analyses identify CNTNAP2 as an autism-susceptibility gene. Am J Hum Genet 2008;82(1):150–9. http://dx.doi.org/10.1016/j.ajhg.2007.09.005.
95. Arking DE, Cutler DJ, Brune CW, et al. A common genetic variant in the neurexin superfamily member CNTNAP2 increases familial risk of autism. Am J Hum Genet 2008;82(1):160–4. http://dx.doi.org/10.1016/j.ajhg.2007.09.015.
96. Bakkaloglu B, O'Roak BJ, Louvi A, et al. Molecular cytogenetic analysis and resequencing of contactin associated protein-like 2 in autism spectrum disorders. Am J Hum Genet 2008;82(1):165–73. http://dx.doi.org/10.1016/j.ajhg.2007.09.017.
97. Rossi E, Verri AP, Patricelli MG, et al. A 12Mb deletion at 7q33-q35 associated with autism spectrum disorders and primary amenorrhea. Eur J Med Genet 2008;51(6):631–8. http://dx.doi.org/10.1016/j.ejmg.2008.06.010.
98. Walsh T, McClellan J, McCarthy S, et al. Rare structural variants disrupt multiple genes in neurodevelopmental pathways in schizophrenia. Science 2008;320(5875):539–43.
99. Kirov G, Gumus D, Chen W, et al. Comparative genome hybridization suggests a role for NRXN1 and APBA2 in schizophrenia. Hum Mol Genet 2008;17(3):458–65. http://dx.doi.org/10.1093/hmg/ddm323.
100. Kirov G, Rujescu D, Ingason A, et al. Neurexin 1 (NRXN1) deletions in schizophrenia. Schizophr Bull 2009;35(5):851–4. http://dx.doi.org/10.1093/schbul/sbp079.
101. Rujescu D, Ingason A, Cichon S, et al. Disruption of the neurexin 1 gene is associated with schizophrenia. Hum Mol Genet 2009;18(5):988–96. http://dx.doi.org/10.1093/hmg/ddn351.

102. International Schizophrenia Consortium. Rare chromosomal deletions and duplications increase risk of schizophrenia. Nature 2008;455(7210):237–41. http://dx.doi.org/10.1038/nature07239.

103. Friedman JI, Vrijenhoek T, Markx S, et al. CNTNAP2 gene dosage variation is associated with schizophrenia and epilepsy. Mol Psychiatry 2008;13(3):261–6. http://dx.doi.org/10.1038/sj.mp.4002049.

104. Wu S, Jia M, Ruan Y, et al. Positive association of the oxytocin receptor gene (OXTR) with autism in the Chinese Han population. Biol Psychiatry 2005;58(1): 74–7. http://dx.doi.org/10.1016/j.biopsych.2005.03.013.

105. Jacob S, Brune CW, Carter CS, et al. Association of the oxytocin receptor gene (OXTR) in Caucasian children and adolescents with autism. Neurosci Lett 2007; 417(1):6–9. http://dx.doi.org/10.1016/j.neulet.2007.02.001.

106. Lerer E, Levi S, Salomon S, et al. Association between the oxytocin receptor (OXTR) gene and autism: relationship to Vineland Adaptive Behavior Scales and cognition. Mol Psychiatry 2008;13(10):980–8. http://dx.doi.org/10.1038/sj.mp.4002087.

107. Yrigollen CM, Han SS, Kochetkova A, et al. Genes controlling affiliative behavior as candidate genes for autism. Biol Psychiatry 2008;63(10):911–6. http://dx.doi.org/10.1016/j.biopsych.2007.11.015.

108. Campbell DB, Datta D, Jones ST, et al. Association of oxytocin receptor (OXTR) gene variants with multiple phenotype domains of autism spectrum disorder. J Neurodev Disord 2011;3(2):101–12. http://dx.doi.org/10.1007/s11689-010-9071-2.

109. Souza RP, de Luca V, Meltzer HY, et al. Schizophrenia severity and clozapine treatment outcome association with oxytocinergic genes. Int J Neuropsychopharmacol 2010;13(6):793–8. http://dx.doi.org/10.1017/S1461145710000167.

110. Souza RP, Ismail P, Meltzer HY, et al. Variants in the oxytocin gene and risk for schizophrenia. Schizophr Res 2010;121(1–3):279–80. http://dx.doi.org/10.1016/j.schres.2010.04.019.

111. Teltsh O, Kanyas-Sarner K, Rigbi A, et al. Oxytocin and vasopressin genes are significantly associated with schizophrenia in a large Arab-Israeli pedigree. Int J Neuropsychopharmacol 2011;1–11. http://dx.doi.org/10.1017/S1461145711001374.

112. Montag C, Brockmann EM, Bayerl M, et al. Oxytocin and oxytocin receptor gene polymorphisms and risk for schizophrenia: a case-control study. World J Biol Psychiatry 2012. http://dx.doi.org/10.3109/15622975.2012.677547.

113. Guastella AJ, Einfeld SL, Gray KM, et al. Intranasal oxytocin improves emotion recognition for youth with autism spectrum disorders. Biol Psychiatry 2010; 67(7):692–4. http://dx.doi.org/10.1016/j.biopsych.2009.09.020.

114. Andari E, Duhamel JR, Zalla T, et al. Promoting social behavior with oxytocin in high-functioning autism spectrum disorders. Proc Natl Acad Sci U S A 2010; 107(9):4389–94. http://dx.doi.org/10.1073/pnas.0910249107.

115. Feifel D, Macdonald K, Nguyen A, et al. Adjunctive intranasal oxytocin reduces symptoms in schizophrenia patients. Biol Psychiatry 2010;68(7):678–80. http://dx.doi.org/10.1016/j.biopsych.2010.04.039.

116. Pedersen CA, Gibson CM, Rau SW, et al. Intranasal oxytocin reduces psychotic symptoms and improves theory of mind and social perception in schizophrenia. Schizophr Res 2011;132(1):50–3. http://dx.doi.org/10.1016/j.schres.2011.07.027.

117. Shen Y, Dies K, Holm I, et al. Clinical genetic testing for patients with autism spectrum disorders. Pediatrics 2010;125(4):e727–35.

118. Lord C, Risi S, Lambrecht L, et al. The autism diagnostic observation schedule-generic: a standard measure of social and communication deficits associated with the spectrum of autism. J Autism Dev Disord 2000;30(3):205–23.
119. Lord C, Rutter M, Le Couteur A. Autism diagnostic interview-revised: a revised version of a diagnostic interview for caregivers of individuals with possible pervasive developmental disorders. J Autism Dev Disord 1994;24(5):659–85.
120. Rutter M, Bailey A, Lord C. Social Communication Questionnaire (SCQ). Los Angeles (CA): Western Psychological Services; 2003.
121. Constantino J, Gruber C. Social Responsiveness Scale (SRS). Los Angeles (CA): Western Psychological Services; 2005.
122. Kay SR, Fiszbein A, Opler LA. The Positive and Negative Syndrome Scale (PANSS) for schizophrenia. Schizophr Bull 1987;13(2):261–76.

Childhood Trauma and Psychosis

Yael Dvir, MD*, Brian Denietolis, PsyD, Jean A. Frazier, MD

KEYWORDS

- Childhood trauma • Childhood maltreatment • Childhood adversity • Child abuse
- Psychosis

KEY POINTS

- There is strong evidence that childhood adversity (defined as sexual abuse, physical abuse, emotional/psychological abuse, neglect, parental death, and bullying) is associated with increased risk for psychosis in adulthood.
- Particularly important to the clinician working with children and adolescents are the reported associations between peer victimization and bullying, and psychotic symptoms in childhood.
- There is a reported cumulative effect, showing an increased risk for psychosis with increase in number and types of childhood trauma, as well as hypothesized correlations between certain types of adversities and certain psychotic symptoms.
- There is consistent evidence that individuals with co-occurring psychosis and posttraumatic stress disorder can benefit from trauma-focused cognitive behavioral therapy interventions, despite recurrent and severe psychiatric symptoms, suicidal ideation, and psychosis.

INTRODUCTION

About one-fourth of children experience a traumatic event before the age of 18 years; these events may include physical or sexual abuse; domestic, community, or school violence; and/or the traumatic death of significant others. Neglect and placement in foster or institutional care are also among childhood adversities. Although most children are resilient after traumatic exposure, some develop significant and potentially long-lasting symptoms.[1] Over recent decades, child and adolescent psychiatry has moved away from explaining schizophrenia as being caused by parenting and abnormal communication styles in families, toward a more biological approach. However, current developmental psychopathology suggests reconsidering the interplay between environment and genetic vulnerabilities.[2]

Disclosures: Dr Frazier has received research support from Glaxo Smith Kline, Pfizer Inc., Seaside Therapeutics, and Roche pharmaceuticals. Drs Dvir and Denietollis have no disclosures.
Department of Psychiatry, University of Massachusetts Medical School, 55 Lake Avenue North, Worcester, MA 01655, USA
* Corresponding author.
E-mail address: yael.dvir@umassmed.edu

CHILDHOOD TRAUMA AND PSYCHOSIS

This article focuses on childhood maltreatment and its association with psychotic illness.

There are several potential links between childhood maltreatment and psychosis:

1. Childhood maltreatment has been associated with psychosis and suggested as a risk factor leading to psychosis and schizophrenia in adulthood.
2. Posttraumatic stress disorder (PTSD) has been suggested to have a psychotic subtype that includes secondary or comorbid psychotic features.
3. Psychotic symptoms themselves have been suggested to be traumatic, as have restraints and seclusion. As such, these experiences have been suggested to cause PTSD symptoms in youth with psychotic illnesses.

DO CHILDHOOD ADVERSITIES INCREASE THE RISK OF PSYCHOSIS?

Until recently, review articles attempting to synthesize findings of studies of the associations between childhood trauma and psychotic disorders have been narrative in nature, and reached inconsistent conclusions.[3–5] Of late, a meta-analysis of patient-control, prospective, and cross-sectional cohort studies by Varese and colleagues[6] published in *Schizophrenia Bulletin* (2012), reported strong evidence that childhood adversity (defined as sexual abuse, physical abuse, emotional/psychological abuse, neglect, parental death, and bullying) is associated with increased risk for psychosis in adulthood. This meta-analysis included 18 case-control studies (n = 2048 psychotic patients and 1856 nonpsychiatric controls), 10 prospective and quasiprospective studies (n = 41,803), and 8 population-based cross-sectional studies from 6 countries including the United States, the United Kingdom, and the Netherlands (n = 35,546). There were significant associations between adversity and psychosis across all research designs, suggesting that childhood adversity and trauma increase the risk of psychosis with an odds ratio (OR) of 2.8, and that patients with psychosis were 2.72 times more likely to have been exposed to childhood adversity than controls. Assuming causality, which has been supported by prospective studies, if childhood adversities were removed from the population as risk factors, the number of people with psychosis would be reduced by a third. The investigators also reported that 9 out of 10 of the studies that tested for dose-response effect found positive relationships. Those studies that controlled for parental mental illness found that parental mental illness does not attenuate associations between childhood adversity and psychosis.[4,7–10]

Because many of these studies used retrospective reports by patients, it is important to note that the reliability of retrospective reports of childhood abuse in patients with psychosis has been shown to be stable over a long period of time. It seems that severity of psychotic symptomatology at the time of report does not influence the likelihood of reporting childhood abuse, and that rates of childhood trauma are similar when obtained by different assessment instruments as well as by clinical notes.[11]

When addressing the associations between trauma and psychosis, studies that evaluate and attempt to separate the contributions of the genetics of parental mental illness from the environmental influences of exposure to traumatic events and parental mental illness are critical. To that end, a prospective study of 2230 Dutch youth, followed between the ages 10 and 16 years, evaluated the separate contributions of genetic (ie, familial) and environmental (ie, childhood trauma) factors to the development of subthreshold psychosis. There was no interaction between general and psychotic parental mental illness and childhood trauma. However, both parental mental illness and childhood trauma were correlated with persistent psychosis.[12] Husted and colleagues[10] (2010) investigated the history of prepsychosis childhood trauma in 184 members of 24 Canadian families in which multiple and multigenerational members had schizophrenia previously shown to be associated with a functional allele in the NOS1AP gene. In this sample, childhood trauma was more prevalent in those with narrowly defined schizophrenia (n = 79) than in their unaffected family members (n = 86) (OR = 4.17), even after adjusting for the NOS1AP risk phenotype, and for parental history of schizophrenia. This finding suggests that the association of schizophrenia with histories of childhood trauma is independent of familial and genetic risk.

Another aspect that may be particularly important to the clinician working with children and adolescents is the reported associations between peer victimization and bullying, and the development of psychotic symptoms in childhood. In a prospective cohort study, Schreier and colleagues[13] in the United Kingdom (2009) found that the risk of psychotic symptoms in early adolescence was twice as high in children who were victims of bullying at ages 8 to 10 years, independent of previously diagnosed psychiatric disorders, family psychosocial stressors, or the child's intelligence quotient (IQ). Chronic or severe bullying was associated with an even higher correlation. In another prospective study conducted in the United Kingdom, Arsenault and colleagues[9] (2011) followed 2232 twin children for traumatic experiences and psychotic symptoms between the ages of 5 and 12 years. Children who experienced maltreatment by an adult or bullying by peers were more likely than those who were not exposed to such events to report psychotic symptoms at age 12 years, regardless of when these events occurred. Again, this risk remained significant when controlling for prior internalizing or externalizing disorders, family adversity and socioeconomic status, IQ, and genetics, which was calculated for each pair of twins in accordance to zygosity and presence of psychosis. In a study of 6692 children in the United Kingdom interviewed at a mean age of 13 years, Fisher and colleagues[14] (2012) found that the association of bullying victimization and exposure to domestic violence with psychotic symptoms were only partially mediated by affective symptoms such as depression and anxiety. These findings highlight the need for clinicians working with children who report early symptoms of psychosis to inquire about traumatic events such as maltreatment and bullying.

ARE SPECIFIC TYPES OF TRAUMA ASSOCIATED WITH SPECIFIC PSYCHOTIC SYMPTOMS?

There is a reported cumulative effect, showing an increased risk for psychosis with increase in number and types of childhood trauma,[15,16] as well as hypothesized correlations between certain types of adversities and certain psychotic symptoms. Bentall and colleagues[17] (2012) examined the associations between different types of adversity (sexual trauma, physical abuse, bullying, and separation experiences) and reports of auditory hallucinations and paranoid beliefs in the 2006 to 2007 Adult Psychiatric Morbidity Survey in the United Kingdom. Childhood sexual abuse, especially rape, was associated with auditory verbal hallucinations, whereas victimization (physical abuse and bullying) predicted paranoia as well as auditory verbal hallucinations. Separation experiences (placements in foster care or institutions) were associated with paranoia. For each symptom, there was a dose-response relationship between the number of childhood traumatic events and the risk of the symptom.

A study by Hardy and colleagues[18] (2005) of the content of hallucinations in adults with nonaffective psychosis reported that 45% of patients who had experienced trauma (N = 40) had hallucinations with similar themes to their trauma, and 12.5%

had hallucinations with similar themes and content to their trauma. Traumas rated as intrusive were associated with intrusive hallucinations, and sexual abuse and bullying were most likely to be associated with hallucinations. Other studies have shown that psychotic symptoms with sexual content are related to history of previous sexual trauma[19]; and that although the association of trauma and paranoia may be explained by levels of anxiety, the association of trauma and hallucinations is not.[20]

Patients with psychotic illnesses and histories of childhood trauma may also have a different presentation at illness onset from those with psychotic illnesses and no exposure to childhood trauma. A chart review of 658 patients with first-episode psychosis showed that 34% had been exposed to sexual and physical abuse, and that these patients were more likely to have had PTSD and/or substance use disorders before psychosis onset, to have more history of suicide attempts, and poorer premorbid functioning.[21] Poor social adjustment predating the onset of psychosis has been shown in other studies.[22] It also seems that previous traumatic experiences are associated with more affective and positive symptoms in patients with first-episode psychosis.[23]

Although deficits in neurocognition have been described in association with psychosis, Aas and colleagues[24] showed worse deficits in cognitive performance in patients with first episode psychosis (FEP) who also experienced childhood trauma. They hypothesized that changes affected by stress through the hypothalamic-pituitary-adrenal axis lead to structural changes that explain this finding. The researchers used magnetic resonance imaging (MRI) to examine the association between childhood trauma, cognitive function, and amygdala and hippocampus volumes in 83 patients with first-episode psychosis (45% schizophrenia, 55% other psychosis) and 63 healthy controls (HCs). Mean amygdala volume was significantly smaller in patients compared with HCs, especially in those who experienced more significant childhood maltreatment, and seemed to have a mediating role between trauma exposure and cognitive impairment. Habets and colleagues[25] (2011) used MRI to measure cerebral cortical thickness in 88 patients with schizophrenia, 98 healthy siblings at higher than average genetic risk for schizophrenia, and 87 HCs. The researchers specifically assessed associations between cortical thickness and childhood trauma, and between cortical thickness and cannabis use. For both exposures, the schizophrenia group displayed stronger reduction of cortical thickness compared with the sibling group and to HCs. The opposite pattern was found in the sibling group, which displayed an increase in cortical thickness with higher levels of trauma.

In addition, the consideration of psychosis that is secondary to PTSD has been reported in adults only. Chronic PTSD with psychotic features has been described mostly in veterans with combat-related trauma, suggesting symptoms such as paranoid delusions, delusions of reference, hallucinations, and bizarre behavior that are distinct from PTSD-specific perceptual disturbances. The challenge remains in distinguishing whether such reports indicate poor symptom differentiation or increased risk and/or comorbidity. Intrusive recollections and flashbacks may mimic delusions and hallucination, whereas avoidance may mimic negative symptoms.[26] Braakman and colleagues[27] (2009) reviewed the evidence for a distinct diagnostic entity defined as PTSD with secondary psychosis (PTSD-SP) by reviewing 24 studies conducted in adults. PTSD-SP was defined as PTSD with later appearance of psychotic features not confined to episodes of reexperiencing. They reported distinct biological features differentiating PTSD-SP from both schizophrenia and PTSD: differences in smooth pursuit eye movement patterns, concentrations of corticotropin-releasing factor, and dopamine β-hydroxylase activity, suggesting that there is initial phenomenological and biological evidence for its validity as a diagnostic entity. However, the distinction of PTSD-SP with comorbid major depression versus PTSD with comorbid major depression with psychotic features was not clearly established.

MANIFESTATION OF CO-OCCURRING TRAUMA AND PSYCHOSIS IN ADOLESCENTS

Although the relationship between interpersonal trauma exposure and psychosis is well established within the literature, the exact psychological mechanisms by which trauma influences the development of psychosis are less clear. One theory that provides a cognitive explanation of the relationship between trauma and psychosis is Morrison's[28] integrative cognitive approach. This theory suggests that experiencing trauma at any age can alter a child's or adult's attributional style, fostering negative beliefs about the self, the world, and others.[29] In the wake of trauma, adolescents often consider themselves vulnerable, others as untrustworthy, and the world as dangerous and unsafe.[30] Kilcommons and Morrison[29] argued that these negative belief structures can alter attributional styles, making paranoid, distressing interpretations of ambiguous events more likely.

In a recent study, Kilcommons and Morrison[29] (2005) tested this theory by exploring the relationship between negative appraisals resulting from childhood and adult trauma exposure and the development of psychotic symptoms. Participants were between 18 and 60 years old (mean age 34.5 ± 9.96 years), and all met Diagnostic and Statistical Manual of Mental Disorders, Fourth Edition (DSM-IV) criteria for a range of schizophrenia spectrum disorders. Results of this study showed that the overall rate of childhood and adult trauma exposure in the population of individuals with symptoms of psychosis is larger than in the normative population, with 94% of this sample having been exposed to at least 1 traumatic event. Further, results suggest that the severity and recurrence of traumatic exposure in childhood and adulthood was strongly associated with the severity of psychotic symptoms that later developed. As postulated, correlational analysis revealed a relationship between negative attribution styles resulting from trauma and some psychotic symptoms, particularly hallucinations. There was a salient relationship between the content of the trauma previously experienced and the themes of delusions and hallucinations described by the subjects.[29] Thus, it seems as though experiencing interpersonal trauma may set in motion a deleterious developmental process whereby significant exposure to trauma alters the underlying schemata and cognitive appraisal systems of individuals, which may influence both the content of positive psychotic symptoms and the appraisal of internal and external experiences.

Clinical and Diagnostic Presentation

The scientific literature describing the clinical presentation of children and adolescents with co-occurring trauma and psychosis is nascent. However, research exploring this complex relationship within the adult population may provide insight into the diagnostic presentation of individuals experiencing trauma and psychosis. According to Braakman and colleagues,[27] adults presenting with PTSD and secondary psychosis often have more positive symptoms of psychosis than negative, and these positive symptoms are generally related to the traumatic events they have experienced. The delusional content is often paranoid and persecutory; the content of hallucinations is typically trauma related but accompanied by non–trauma-related content. Freeman and Fowler[20] (2009) conducted a study with adults showing that severe childhood sexual abuse was particularly associated with an increased risk for developing persecutory delusions and verbal hallucinations. In another study in adults between the ages of 18 and 60 years, physical abuse was associated with positive symptoms of psychosis in general, whereas sexual abuse was associated with verbal hallucinations in particular.[29]

Although the presence of bizarre behaviors is common in adults with co-occurring trauma and psychosis, disorganized thinking (eg, loose associations and flight of ideas) are almost never endorsed.[27] Instead, thinking is often linear and organized. Affect is observed as flat to blunted with depressed, irritable, and anxious content. Level of insight varies by individual; however, many individuals with co-occurring psychosis and trauma recognize and report their hallucinogenic experiences as nonreal and disturbing. In essence, these symptoms are often the most egodystonic features of their psychiatric condition. Many adults seem to develop posttraumatic stress disorder before developing psychosis. However, once developed, positive symptoms of psychosis are typically present even in the absence of acute reexperiencing symptoms, like flashbacks and intrusive recollections.[27] Thus, psychotic symptoms do not seem to occur only within the context of reexperiencing symptoms; instead, they seem pervasive and recurrent.

Diagnostic Comorbidities

Both posttraumatic stress disorder and psychosis are associated with a range of diagnostic comorbidities. In a seminal epidemiologic study, Kessler and colleagues[31] (1995) obtained a representative national sample of more than 5000 adults to clarify common comorbidities between psychiatric conditions. Results of the National Comorbidity Survey showed that 88% of men and 79% of women with PTSD had at least 1 comorbid diagnosis. Major depressive disorder was the most common comorbidity, occurring in slightly less than half of individuals with PTSD. Substance use disorders, disruptive behavior disorders, and other anxiety disorders were also common comorbid diagnoses for individuals with PTSD and for individuals with psychotic disorders.[31]

Evidence-based Assessment Procedures

Clinician-administered PTSD Scale for Children and Adolescents
There are a series of evidence-based assessments for evaluating the frequency and intensity of posttraumatic stress symptoms in children and adolescents (**Table 1**). One such measure is the Clinician-administered PTSD Scale for Children and Adolescents (CAPS-CA), a 33-item clinician-administered PTSD scale for youth between the ages of 8 and 18 years.[32] These carefully worded interview questions are designed to assess the frequency and intensity of 17 PTSD symptoms, as well as their effect on social, developmental, and academic functioning. Administration typically requires 45 minutes, depending on the severity of symptoms, and scoring requires 20 to 30 minutes. Given the strong psychometric properties of this instrument, it is considered the gold standard for posttraumatic stress research in youth. However, practitioners may find the instrument cumbersome given the time required for administration and scoring.

UCLA PTSD Index for Adolescents
The UCLA (University of California, Los Angeles) PTSD Index[33] is one of the most widely used instruments for the assessment of posttraumatic stress disorder in children and adolescents. There are 3 versions of this measure: Child Self-Report, Adolescent Self-Report, and Parent Report. The adolescent measure, designed for youth between the ages of 13 and 18 years, comprises 41 questions with the first 14 questions being designed to assess for exposure to a variety of traumatic events. Items 15 to 27 assess the adolescent's immediate response to any traumatic events endorsed (ie, shock; horror; peritraumatic dissociation). The remaining 14 items

Table 1
Evidence-based assessments for trauma and psychosis in adolescents

Name	Type of Instrument	Purpose	Age Range (y)	Time (min)	Cost ($)
CAPS-CA	Semistructured clinical interview	Designed to assess the frequency and intensity of 17 PTSD symptoms, as well as their effect on social, developmental, and academic functioning	8–18	Administration: 45 Scoring: 25–30	110.00
UCLA PTSD Index	Self-report screening tool	Designed to efficiently screen for symptoms of posttraumatic stress disorder	6–18	Administration: 15–25 Scoring: 5–10	Free
CPSS	Self-report screening tool	Designed to efficiently screen for symptoms of posttraumatic stress disorder	8–18	Administration: 10 Scoring: 5–10	Free
TSCC	Self-report diagnostic measure	Designed to assess symptoms of posttraumatic stress, as well as general anxiety, depression, anger, sexual concerns, and dissociation	8–17	Administration: 10–20 Scoring: 15–20	168.00
PANSS	Clinician-rated diagnostic measure	Designed to assess positive and negative symptoms of psychosis	18 and older	Administration: 30–40 Scoring: 20	275.00

Abbreviations: CPSS, Child PTSD Symptom Scale; PANSS, Positive and Negative Syndrome Scale; TSCC, Trauma Symptom Checklist for Children.

assess the frequency and severity of any symptoms of reexperiencing, avoidance, and hypervigilance/hyperarousal. All items correspond with the DSM-IV Text Revision (DSM-IV-TR) diagnostic criteria for PTSD. Completion of this self-report measure typically requires 15 to 25 minutes, depending on the age and ability of the adolescent, and scoring typically requires 5 to 10 minutes. Like the CAPS-CA, the UCLA PTSD Index has strong psychometric properties; however, it is more widely used within clinical settings because of the efficiency of the measure.

Child PTSD Symptom Scale

The Child PTSD Symptom Scale (CPSS) is a 24-item self-report measure designed to assess symptoms of PTSD in youth between the ages of 8 and 18 years.[34] The first 17 items are designed to assess reexperiencing, avoidance, and hyperarousal symptoms. In the remaining 7 items, respondents are asked about specific functional impairments resulting from symptoms of posttraumatic stress. All items correspond with the DSM-IV-TR diagnostic criteria for PTSD. Completion of this measure typically requires 10 minutes, and scoring typically requires 5 to 10 minutes. This measure, like those discussed earlier, has strong psychometric properties both in terms of internal consistency, test-retest reliability, and convergent validity.[34]

Trauma Symptom Checklist for Children

The Trauma Symptom Checklist for Children (TSCC)[35] is a 54-item self-report measure for youth ranging from 8 to 17 years, designed to assess symptoms of posttraumatic stress as well as related psychological sequelae associated with trauma exposure. The TSCC consists of 6 clinical scales and 2 validity scales. Validity scales measure both under-reporting and over-reporting, whereas the clinical scales measure general anxiety, depression, posttraumatic stress, sexual concerns, dissociation, and anger. Completion of this measure typically requires 10 to 20 minutes to complete, and scoring typically requires 10 to 15 minutes. Numerous research studies using the TSCC indicate strong psychometric properties in terms of convergent and predictive validity, as well as test-retest reliability.

The Positive and Negative Syndrome Scale

The Positive and Negative Syndrome Scale (PANSS)[36] is a 30-item screening tool designed to assess positive and negative symptoms of psychosis. Positive symptoms of psychosis assessed include hallucinatory behavior, persecution and suspiciousness, delusions, conceptual disorganization, excitement, and hostility. Negative symptoms of psychosis assessed include blunted affect, social withdrawal, emotional withdrawal, lack of flow and spontaneity of conversation, difficulty with abstract thinking, and stereotyped thinking. The psychometric properties of the PANSS have been well established within the adult literature, and it is considered one of the most widely used research measurement tools. It has also been included in large treatment studies with adolescents, like the Treatment of Early Onset Schizophrenia Study, which was funded by the National Institute of Mental Health. However, although some clinicians use this instrument to assess for psychosis in adolescents, this measure requires further scientific study to determine its validity, reliability, and developmental sensitivity for those within the adolescent population.

In clinical practice, these assessment tools can be used to help clinicians assess their clients' baseline functioning, select appropriate treatments, as well as evaluate clients' overall response to psychotherapeutic and pharmaceutical intervention. Data from these scales are most helpful when collected at the outset of treatment and then at regular intervals over the course of treatment.

When collected at regular intervals, data gleaned from these tools can assist clients and practitioners alike with making treatment decisions. For instance, a therapist-client dyad may choose to augment the treatment approach after discovering that, although the client's symptoms of PTSD have reduced over the past 12 weeks, symptoms of paranoia remain unchanged, thus warranting perhaps the addition of a low-dose atypical antipsychotic. Integrating clinical scales in this manner has been shown to increase both the efficiency and effectiveness of psychotherapeutic and psychopharmacologic treatment, because it encourages collaboration between practitioners and clients while also encouraging all parties to remain focused on a focal problem.

EVIDENCE-BASED TREATMENTS FOR TRAUMA AND PSYCHOSIS IN ADOLESCENTS
Cognitive Behavioral Interventions

The scientific literature exploring the efficacy of trauma-focused interventions for adolescents with co-occurring PTSD and psychosis is nascent. However, there is considerable evidence in the child and adolescent trauma literature indicating that cognitive behavior therapies (CBTs) are the most effective interventions for children and adolescents with PTSD.[37] In a recent meta-analysis, Silverman and colleagues[37] (2008) reviewed 21 scientifically rigorous treatment studies evaluating a variety of PTSD treatments for adolescents. Results from this meta-analysis showed that, overall, CBT interventions consistently produced statistically significant treatment effects compared with non-CBT interventions. Further, CBT interventions were more effective than non-CBT interventions at reducing secondary effects of trauma, including depression, anxiety, and externalizing behavior problems. In terms of specific therapeutic approaches, trauma-focused CBT was identified as the most effective and well-researched therapeutic intervention to date for adolescents with PTSD, having been evaluated through multiple randomized controlled trials using rigorous comparison conditions, assessment procedures, adequate sample sizes, and multisite clinical trials.[37]

Trauma-focused CBT is a 12-session to 16-session treatment model designed to address a range of psychological traumas experienced by children and adolescents.[30] Components of the treatment are reflected in the acronym PRACTICE: psychoeducation and parenting skills, relaxation skills, affect recognition and modulation, cognitive coping skills, trauma narrative, in-vivo exposure, conjoint parent-child sessions, cognitive restructuring, and enhancing future safety. As with many cognitive behavioral treatments for PTSD, this treatment model begins by normalizing symptoms of PTSD through psychoeducation, while also bolstering the adolescents' capacity for adaptive coping. Once sufficient safety and adaptive coping are established, the adolescent is gradually and systematically encouraged to complete a trauma narrative, or a detailed account of the specific trauma or traumas evoking symptoms of PTSD. Particular attention is paid to the adolescent's self-rated level of distress when reading the narrative, because this should decrease over time. The adolescent's cognitive appraisals of the traumatic events described are also closely monitored, because negative cognitions undergo cognitive restructuring once the narrative is complete. Treatment culminates with the adolescent sharing the trauma narrative with the caregivers, but only after preparation and support is provided to both parent and child.

In addition to exposure-based CBT modalities, non–exposure-based CBTs have also shown clinical efficacy, with adults presenting with co-occurring PTSD and psychosis. In a recent randomized controlled trial, Mueser and colleagues[38] (2008) evaluated a CBT for a PTSD program for 108 adults with a mean age of 44.2 years presenting with comorbid PTSD and either a major mood disorder with and without psychosis (85%) or schizophrenia/schizoaffective disorder (15%). The CBT for

PTSD program is a 12-session to 16-session therapeutic approach that focuses primarily on identifying and restructuring underlying maladaptive cognitions that contribute to and maintain posttraumatic stress responses. Compared with subjects assigned to the treatment-as-usual condition, participants in the CBT condition showed statistically significant reduction in symptoms of PTSD, depression, anxiety, and negative trauma-related beliefs. In a similar study, van der Gaag and colleagues[39] (2012) evaluated the efficacy of a CBT intervention designed to target maladaptive cognitive biases in adolescents deemed at ultrahigh risk for developing psychosis. When compared with treatment as usual, subjects within the CBT condition showed a statistically significant reduction in their risk for developing psychosis. Results also showed a reduction in subclinical psychotic symptoms. Although this study did not evaluate for histories of trauma in the youth at ultrahigh risk for developing psychosis, other investigators have found that many individuals at ultrahigh risk typically have increased rates of trauma exposure, with one study citing 83% of its sample experiencing physical abuse, 67% experiencing emotional abuse, and 27% experiencing sexual abuse.[40] Thus, findings from both of these studies highlight the efficacy of CBT interventions for comorbid serious mental illness and trauma exposure.

Rosenberg and colleagues[41] (2011) evaluated a similar non–exposure-based CBT program for adolescents with PTSD alone. This treatment modality, called CBT for PTSD in adolescents, is a program of 12 to 16 weeks that incorporates cognitive restructuring as the primary therapeutic agent. Treatment consists of psychoeducation regarding core and secondary symptoms associated with PTSD, relaxation training, identification of the common styles of thinking associated with trauma, and the 5 steps of cognitive restructuring. Results from this pilot study revealed that, from baseline to after treatment, subjects showed significant reductions in symptoms of PTSD and depression, and these treatment gains were maintained at a 3-month follow-up.

Findings from these studies provide consistent evidence that adults with co-occurring psychosis and PTSD can benefit from trauma-focused cognitive behavioral interventions, despite recurrent and severe psychiatric symptoms, suicidal ideation, and psychosis. To date, there is not a sufficient evidence basis for CBT intervention in adolescents who have both PTSD and psychosis. However, both cognitive restructuring and exposure therapy have strong empirical support for the treatment of PTSD in the adolescent population in general,[37] and there is emerging evidence that CBT is an effective intervention for youths at ultrahigh risk for psychosis. Future studies are warranted to evaluate CBT in the treatment of youth who have both PTSD and psychosis. Nonetheless, at this time, many trauma therapists advise proceeding judiciously when considering any exposure therapy for individuals suffering from psychosis, because individuals with psychotic disorders can be highly sensitive to stress.[42]

Although psychopharmacologic treatment of psychosis in youth is reviewed elsewhere is this issue by Kranzler and Cohen, the evidence basis for psychopharmacologic treatment of PTSD and trauma effects in youth is sparse. At present, the data do not support using selective serotonin reuptake inhibitor as first-line treatments for PTSD in children and adolescents. There is limited evidence, mainly case controls, to suggest that the brief use of antiadrenergic agents, second-generation antipsychotics, and several mood stabilizers may offer some relief from PTSD symptoms in youth.[43]

SUMMARY

This article highlights recent advances regarding the complex causal relationship between childhood trauma exposure and psychosis. According to a recent meta-analysis, there is strong evidence that childhood adversity and trauma significantly increase the risk for developing psychosis, and that those suffering from psychosis were 2.72 times more likely to have been exposed to childhood adversity than controls.[6] Several studies showed a dose-response relationship, showing that the risk for psychosis increases with the number and types of childhood traumas endorsed.[15,16] From the review of the literature, this article also discusses the relationship between specific adverse childhood experiences and specific symptoms of psychosis. According to Bentall and colleagues[17] (2012), child sexual abuse, especially rape, was associated with auditory verbal hallucination, physical abuse and bullying predicted paranoia and auditory verbal hallucinations, and separation experiences (ie, placement in foster care or institutions) were associated with increased rates of paranoia. The article culminates with a comprehensive review of evidence-based practices for assessing and treating co-occurring posttraumatic stress and psychosis in adolescents.

Although the relationship between trauma and psychosis has strong scientific support, the literature exploring exact underlying psychobiological and developmental mechanisms contributing to this complex relationship is inadequate. In addition, there is limited scientific evidence exploring the efficacy of evidence-based practices for adolescents with co-occurring PTSD and psychosis. At present, there are no randomized controlled trials or pilot studies that show the efficacy of specific therapeutic strategies for alleviating the psychological suffering of this unique population. Instead, practitioners are challenged to either apply interventions proved to be effective for adults with co-occurring PTSD and psychosis, or to use interventions that have shown efficacy with adolescents with PTSD in general. Further research is needed that comprehensively evaluates trauma-focused interventions for this population through the use of randomized controlled trials with rigorous comparison conditions and assessment procedures, and adequate sample sizes. In addition, the academe would benefit from research that focuses on elucidating the underlying psychobiological and developmental factors that contribute to the relationship between psychosis and trauma in adolescents. Expanding the scientific literature in these two areas will enhance the recovery process of numerous adolescents who, without support, would continue to suffer silently.

REFERENCES

1. Cohen JA, Bukstein O, Walter H, et al. Practice parameter for the assessment and treatment of children and adolescents with posttraumatic stress disorder. J Am Acad Child Adolesc Psychiatry 2010;49(4):414–30.
2. Rutter M, Sroufe LA. Developmental psychopathology: concepts and challenges. Dev Psychopathol 2000;12:265–96.
3. Read J, van Os J, Morrison AP, et al. Childhood trauma, psychosis and schizophrenia: a literature review with theoretical and clinical implications. Acta Psychiatr Scand 2005;112(5):330–50.
4. Morgan C, Fisher H. Environment and schizophrenia: environmental factors in schizophrenia: childhood trauma–a critical review. Schizophr Bull 2007;33(1):3–10.
5. Bendall S, Jackson HJ, Hulbert CA, et al. Childhood trauma and psychotic disorders: a systematic, critical review of the evidence. Schizophr Bull 2008;34(3):568–79.
6. Varese F, Smeets F, Drukker M, et al. Childhood adversities increase the risk of psychosis: a meta-analysis of patient-control, prospective- and cross-sectional cohort studies. Schizophr Bull 2012;38(4):661–71.
7. Janssen I, Krabbendam L, Bak M, et al. Childhood abuse as a risk factor for psychotic experiences. Acta Psychiatr Scand 2004;109(1):38–45.

8. Fisher HL, Jones PB, Fearon P, et al. The varying impact of type, timing and frequency of exposure to childhood adversity on its association with adult psychotic disorder. Psychol Med 2010;40(12):1967–78.

9. Arseneault L, Cannon M, Fisher HL, et al. Childhood trauma and children's emerging psychotic symptoms: a genetically sensitive longitudinal cohort study. Am J Psychiatry 2011;168(1):65–72.

10. Husted JA, Ahmed R, Chow EW, et al. Childhood trauma and genetic factors in familial schizophrenia associated with the NOS1AP gene. Schizophr Res 2010; 121(1–3):187–92.

11. Fisher HL, Craig TK, Fearon P, et al. Reliability and comparability of psychosis patients' retrospective reports of childhood abuse. Schizophr Bull 2011;37(3): 546–53.

12. Wigman JT, van Winkel R, Ormel J, et al. Early trauma and familial risk in the development of the extended psychosis phenotype in adolescence. Acta Psychiatr Scand 2012;126:266–73.

13. Schreier A, Wolke D, Thomas K, et al. Prospective study of peer victimization in childhood and psychotic symptoms in a nonclinical population at age 12 years. Arch Gen Psychiatry 2009;66(5):527–36.

14. Fisher HL, Schreier A, Zammit S, et al. Pathways between childhood victimization and psychosis-like symptoms in the ALSPAC birth cohort. Schizophr Bull 2012. [Epub ahead of print].

15. Shevlin M, Dorahy MJ, Adamson G. Trauma and psychosis: an analysis of the national comorbidity survey. Am J Psychiatry 2007;164(1):166–9.

16. Shevlin M, Houston JE, Dorahy MJ, et al. Cumulative traumas and psychosis: an analysis of the National Comorbidity Survey and the British Psychiatric Morbidity Survey. Schizophr Bull 2008;34(1):193–9.

17. Bentall RP, Wickham S, Shevlin M, et al. Do specific early-life adversities lead to specific symptoms of psychosis? A study from the 2007 The Adult Psychiatric Morbidity Survey. Schizophr Bull 2012;38(4):734–40.

18. Hardy A, Fowler D, Freeman D, et al. Trauma and hallucinatory experience in psychosis. J Nerv Ment Dis 2005;193(8):501–7.

19. Thompson A, Nelson B, McNab C, et al. Psychotic symptoms with sexual content in the "ultra high risk" for psychosis population: frequency and association with sexual trauma. Psychiatry Res 2010;177(1–2):84–91.

20. Freeman D, Fowler D. Routes to psychotic symptoms: trauma, anxiety and psychosis-like experiences. Psychiatry Res 2009;169(2):107–12.

21. Conus P, Cotton S, Schimmelmann BG, et al. Pretreatment and outcome correlates of sexual and physical trauma in an epidemiological cohort of first-episode psychosis patients. Schizophr Bull 2010;36(6):1105–14.

22. Tikka M, Luutonen S, Ilonen T, et al. Childhood trauma and premorbid adjustment among individuals at clinical high risk for psychosis and normal control subjects. Early Interv Psychiatry 2013;7(1):51–7.

23. Burns JK, Jhazbhay K, Esterhuizen T, et al. Exposure to trauma and the clinical presentation of first-episode psychosis in South Africa. J Psychiatr Res 2011; 45(2):179–84.

24. Aas M, Navari S, Gibbs A, et al. Is there a link between childhood trauma, cognition, and amygdala and hippocampus volume in first-episode psychosis? Schizophr Res 2012;137(1–3):73–9.

25. Habets P, Marcelis M, Gronenschild E, et al. Reduced cortical thickness as an outcome of differential sensitivity to environmental risks in schizophrenia. Biol Psychiatry 2011;69(5):487–94.

26. Seedat S, Stein MB, Oosthuizen PP, et al. Linking posttraumatic stress disorder and psychosis: a look at epidemiology, phenomenology, and treatment. J Nerv Ment Dis 2003;191(10):675–81.
27. Braakman MH, Kortmann FA, van den Brink W. Validity of 'post-traumatic stress disorder with secondary psychotic features': a review of the evidence. Acta Psychiatr Scand 2009;119(1):15–24.
28. Morrison AP. The interpretation of intrusions in psychosis: an integrative cognitive approach to hallucinations and delusions. Behavioral and Cognitive Psychotherapy 2001;29:257–76.
29. Kilcommons AM, Morrison AP. Relationships between trauma and psychosis: an exploration of cognitive and dissociative factors. Acta Psychiatr Scand 2005; 112(5):351–9.
30. Cohen JA, Mannarino AP, Deblinger E. Treating trauma and traumatic stress in children and adolescents. New York: The Guilford Press; 2006.
31. Kessler RC, Sonnega A, Bromet E, et al. Posttraumatic stress disorder in the National Comorbidity Survey. Arch Gen Psychiatry 1995;52(12):1048–60.
32. Nader K, Kriegler JA, Blake DD, et al. Clinician administered PTSD scale, child and adolescent version. White River Junction (VT): National Center for PTSD; 1996.
33. Steinberg AM, Brymer MJ, Decker KB, et al. The University of California at Los Angeles Post-traumatic Stress Disorder Reaction Index. Curr Psychiatry Rep 2004;6:96–100.
34. Foa EB, Johnson KM, Feeny NC, et al. The Child PTSD Symptom Scale: a preliminary examination of its psychometric properties. J Clin Child Psychol 2001;30(3): 376–84.
35. Briere J. Trauma Symptom Checklist for Children (TSCC) professional manual. Odessa (FL): Psychological Assessment Resources; 1996.
36. Kay SR, Fiszbein A, Opler LA. The positive and negative syndrome scale (PANSS) for schizophrenia. Schizophr Bull 1987;13(2):261–76.
37. Silverman WK, Ortiz CD, Viswesvaran C, et al. Evidence-based psychosocial treatments for children and adolescents exposed to traumatic events. J Clin Child Adolesc Psychol 2008;37(1):156–83.
38. Mueser KT, Rosenberg SD, Xie H, et al. A randomized controlled trial of cognitive-behavioral treatment for posttraumatic stress disorder in severe mental illness. J Consult Clin Psychol 2008;76(2):259–71.
39. van der Gaag M, Nieman DH, Rietdijk J, et al. Cognitive behavioral therapy for subjects at ultrahigh risk for developing psychosis: a randomized controlled clinical trial. Schizophr Bull 2012;38(6):1180–8.
40. Bechdolf A, Thompson A, Nelson B, et al. Experience of trauma and conversion to psychosis in an ultra-high-risk (prodromal) group. Acta Psychiatr Scand 2010; 121(5):377–84.
41. Rosenberg H, Jankowski M, Fortuna L, et al. A pilot study of a cognitive restructuring program for treating post-traumatic disorders in adolescents. Psychol Trauma 2011;3(1):94–9.
42. Butzlaff RL, Hooley JM. Expressed emotion and psychiatric relapse: a meta-analysis. Arch Gen Psychiatry 1998;55(6):547–52.
43. Strawn JR, Keeshin BR, DelBello MP, et al. Psychopharmacologic treatment of posttraumatic stress disorder in children and adolescents: a review. J Clin Psychiatry 2010;71(7):932–41.

Substance Abuse and Psychosis

Danielle Goerke, DO*, Sanjiv Kumra, MD

KEYWORDS

- Substance-induced psychosis • Adolescent psychosis • Dual diagnosis
- Cannabis and psychosis

KEY POINTS

- At initial presentation, substance-induced psychosis is almost indistinguishable from a primary psychotic disorder.
- All adolescents presenting with psychotic symptoms and co-occurring substance use should be considered at significant risk of developing a primary psychotic disorder.
- There is a paucity of data on the optimal treatment of patients with a psychotic disorder and co-occurring substance use, because most of these adolescents have been excluded from controlled treatment trials of antipsychotic medications.
- Cannabis use has been identified as a potential risk factor to the development of a primary psychotic illness in at-risk adolescents, and these data suggest that reduction or cessation of cannabis use should be recommended for all adolescents with psychotic symptoms to prevent further deterioration.
- Once psychotic symptoms have been stabilized with antipsychotic medications, developing a therapeutic alliance and ongoing psychoeducation are critical to keep these young people engaged in treatment and abstinent from substance use.

INTRODUCTION

Approximately one-third of people with a primary psychotic disorder experience their first psychotic episode before the age of 19 years. As part of healthy psychological development, adolescence is also a period in which individuals are emotionally separating from their parents. This developmental stage also represents a peak period of time for use and experimentation with alcohol, cannabis, and other illicit substances, which may reflect the influence of culture, media, and peer group in Western societies. Although the ability of illicit substances to induce psychotic symptoms has been well recognized, more recent epidemiologic studies have suggested that cannabis may represent a significant risk factor for the development of a psychotic illness in

Disclosures: Dr Goerke, None; Dr Kumra has received research support from the Minnesota Medical Foundation, the National Alliance for Research on Schizophrenia and, Depression, and AstraZeneca.
Division of Child and Adolescent Psychiatry, University of Minnesota Medical School, F256/2B West, 2450 Riverside Avenue, Minneapolis, MN 55454, USA
* Corresponding author.
E-mail address: morg0153@umn.edu

Child Adolesc Psychiatric Clin N Am 22 (2013) 643–654
http://dx.doi.org/10.1016/j.chc.2013.06.001
1056-4993/13/$ – see front matter © 2013 Elsevier Inc. All rights reserved.

childpsych.theclinics.com

at-risk individuals. In adolescents and young adults with a first episode of psychosis, co-occurring substance use has been reported as many as 74%,[1] and this comorbidity has been associated with less effective treatment responses, decreased medication adherence, and consequently a worsened course of illness.[2] By extension, these data suggest that identification and treatment of substance abuse are imperative to resolution of psychotic symptoms for adolescents with co-occurring disorders. This article selectively reviews the pertinent literature that provides guidance for clinicians with regard to the most pressing diagnostic and treatment challenges faced in working with this group of adolescents (aged 13–18 years).

The diagnosis of psychotic symptoms in adolescents is difficult, particularly if the adolescent is also abusing chemicals. A case vignette is presented later to highlight the problem of differentiating a substance-induced psychotic disorder (SIPD) from an early stage primary psychotic disorder (PPD) with co-occurring substance use. The vignette also helps to show the multimodal nature of treatment interventions required for this population in terms of psychoeducation, engagement of the patient and family in the treatment process, and use of antipsychotic medications. Recent data suggesting that cannabis may be a causal risk factor in psychotic illness are examined, because these data support clinical recommendations to reduce or cease cannabis use in this population. In addition, treatment strategies that have been found to be effective in adult patients that may be efficacious for youth to abstain from substances after the resolution of psychotic symptoms are presented.

CLINICAL VIGNETTE

Fifteen-year-old A.S. was brought to the emergency room by his parents after expressing concern that the TV was talking to him. Over the last several months, his parents had observed changes in their son's behavior: increasing social isolation, deteriorating school performance, and frequent episodes of being found passed out from alcohol intoxication. He admitted to daily marijuana use and several urine toxicology screens at various emergency department visits confirmed this misuse. At first, his family was turned away from inpatient care because emergency department physicians thought that he did not meet admission criteria because of a lack of behaviors that indicated danger to self or others. The patient started outpatient chemical dependency treatment, but he continued to use both alcohol and marijuana. Over the next several months, his symptoms expanded to include disorganized thought processes, paranoia, anxiety, and eventually refusing to leave his mother's side for several days. He was referred to a university psychiatric clinic where he was observed to have difficulty expressing his thoughts, decreased attention, poor motivation, social isolation, and a further decline in academic functioning. He was then referred for an inpatient evaluation for diagnostic clarification and stabilization of his symptoms. Quetiapine was started to address psychosis and anxiety, which resulted in a rapid cognitive clearing. However, once discharged from the hospital, he refused to take medication. He was insistent that his drug use was the source of his symptoms and that with sobriety all would be well. Weekly visits with his psychiatrist continued. Within 2 weeks, it was noted that he was laughing to himself in class, continuing to have failing grades, and refusing to interact with anyone but his family. He shared with his father his overwhelming fear that something horrible may happen to his family and that, if he took antipsychotic medication, it would not only damage his brain but his family would die. Despite denying all positive symptoms to his psychiatrist, he did express concern over his ongoing difficulty in concentration. With the support of his parents, a low dose of aripiprazole was initiated to help with focus and concentration. He refused to exceed a dose of 5 mg daily. However, thought process, academics, and social engagement with peers all improved. He relapsed on marijuana once, which resulted in a significant worsening of anxiety as noted by the patient. A new level of insight was achieved in that A.S. shared that he could no longer use marijuana because it was detrimental to his mental health. Despite observed improvement by his psychiatrist and family, medication compliance continued to be a daily struggle and, after 4 months, he requested that he be given a trial off medication. His parents agreed that he was looking better and so supported the discontinuation of medication against medical advice. Within 1 week, he was found heavily intoxicated with alcohol and returned to chemical dependency treatment. At continued monthly visits to his psychiatrist, his improvement in thought process and resolution of anxiety persisted, despite the discontinuation of his low-dose second-generation antipsychotic. Both the patient and his parents agreed to continue to follow with the psychiatrist, but did not want to resume antipsychotic medications at that time.

INITIAL EVALUATION

Adolescents are often concerned about confidentiality so separate interviews for the individual and family are optimal. The substances most commonly used by adolescents with schizophrenia are alcohol and cannabis. A detailed history and physical with a subsequent diagnosis is traditionally the primary goal at initial contact with an adolescent presenting to medical services. Based on this diagnosis, a treatment course is recommended. As illustrated in the vignette, the initial clinical presentation of SIPD and a PPD with co-occurring substance use is often indistinguishable. Clinicians rely on the definition of SIPD as stated in the Diagnostic and Statistical Manual of Mental Disorders, Fourth Edition (DSM-IV) (**Box 1**).

However, these criteria oversimplify the complexity of differentiating these diagnoses. Cannabis in particular has the potential to induce psychotic symptoms acutely and may play a causal role in primary psychotic illnesses. Therefore, it is possible for a young person to meet criteria for an SIPD and also be at high risk of developing a PPD over time.

Several studies have focused on differentiating a SIPD from a PPD with co-occurring substance use at initial presentation. The Psychiatric Research Interview for DSM-IV Substance and Mental Disorders (PRISM-IV) has proved reliable at this task. The length and the intensive training required to administer this structured

---

Box 1
DSM-IV Text Revision criteria for SIPD

a. Prominent hallucinations or delusions. Note: do not include hallucinations if the person has insight that they are substance induced.

b. There is evidence from the history, physical examination, or laboratory findings of either (1) or (2):

   1. The symptoms in criterion A developed during or within a month of substance intoxication or withdrawal

   2. Medication use is causally related to the disturbance

c. The disturbance is not better accounted for by a psychotic disorder that is not substance induced. Evidence that the symptoms are better accounted for by a psychotic disorder that is not substance induced might include the following: the symptoms precede the onset of the substance use (or medication use); the symptoms persist for a substantial period of time (eg, about a month) after the cessation of acute withdrawal or severe intoxication, or are substantially in excess of what would be expected given the type or amount of the substance used or the duration of use; or there is other evidence that suggests the existence of an independent non-SIPD (eg, a history of recurrent non–substance-related episodes).

d. The disturbance does not occur exclusively during the course of delirium.

Reprinted with permission from the Diagnostic and Statistical Manual of Mental Disorders, Fourth Edition, Text Revision. Copyright 2000 American Psychiatric Association.

interview hinder its usefulness in everyday practice; however, specific clinical markers with the potential to differentiate between these diagnoses were identified. For example, using the PRISM-IV, cannabis dependence, a history of trauma, and the absence of a family history of psychosis correctly identified 78.7% of patients with SIPD in a sample of young people experiencing their first episode of psychosis with concurrent substance use.[3] However, the consensus among longitudinal studies is that these initial diagnoses are not stable. A large number of those diagnosed with an SIPD, followed over time, eventually meet criteria for a PPD. A 3-year longitudinal study found that, out of a total of 238 patients, 44.5% of those diagnosed with cannabis-induced psychotic symptoms later developed a schizophrenia-spectrum disorder. This proportion increased with length of follow-up. Male gender and young age related to increased risk of conversion to a PPD. Compared with patients without a history of cannabis-induced psychosis, they developed schizophrenia at a significantly younger age. This effect was most marked for paranoid schizophrenia.[4–7]

A potential explanation for this high rate of conversion is that youth presenting for medical care of psychotic symptoms are in the early stages of the disease process. A well-defined period of decline with attenuated psychotic symptoms, often referred to as the prodromal period, can be identified in most patients presenting with a first episode of psychotic illness. Identification of those young people still in prodrome, deemed at ultrahigh risk to develop a psychotic illness, is now a top priority. A focus on this early stage of the illness has the potential to prevent cognitive decline and intervene while that patient maintains some insight into the symptoms. Often intervention in this earlier stage is better received by the adolescent and the treatment process has the potential to be more collaborative. Those presenting with attenuated psychotic symptoms are likely to present with co-occurring substance use given the average age of onset for both disorders. Therefore, a young person presenting in the prodrome or early stages of a psychotic illness with co-occurring substance use could be mistaken for SIPD.[5]

Given the high level of diagnostic instability, specifically the rate of conversion from an SIPD to a PPD with co-occurring substance use, differentiating between the two diagnoses may be arbitrary from a treatment perspective. Instead, recognizing that these individuals with early psychotic symptoms are on a spectrum at a substantially increased risk of developing PPD provides the framework necessary for an effective treatment plan.

TREATMENT CONSIDERATIONS

The treatment of adolescents is different from that of adult patients in that the families are typically more involved in the treatment process. It is common for parents to be scared and to be in shock and denial about the diagnosis. Adolescents frequently do not want to cooperate with the assessment or treatment process, regardless of diagnosis. With the lack of insight experienced in a psychotic illness, engaging them in treatment can be particularly challenging.

As in the case vignette, the treatment of dually diagnosed patients with mental illness and substance use disorders is often fragmented. It is common for mental health and substance use services to be provided separately. Practitioners may refer youth using substances to chemical dependency treatment programs. However, these programs are often not as helpful to the recovery process of those who are still actively psychotic. Staff and programming tend to be highly focused on chemical dependency with the mental illness as a secondary focus. This approach is helpful for other mental health diagnoses but is not suitable for actively psychotic youth. They may not be cognitively ready for the rigorous requirements of groups and their delusional state may make them vulnerable to peers. Paranoia and confusion may necessitate a locked unit. A multidisciplinary integrated approach that provides special attention to mental health concerns is optimal to promote retention in the treatment process.[8,9]

Some practitioners are reluctant to refer young people for psychiatric services because of fear of stigma or what they deem may be unnecessary antipsychotic medications because of the belief that substance-induced psychosis resolves spontaneously with cessation of the illicit substance. In our experience, there is a subgroup of adolescents who present with psychotic symptoms that persist beyond the period of intoxication and that result in a decline in adaptive function, dangerousness to self or others, and/or other types of deleterious consequences. In this context, antipsychotic medications may facilitate the treatment process by alleviating impairments in reality testing, reducing anxiety, promoting sleep, and stabilizing mood. Stabilization of psychotic symptoms may have other long-term benefits in terms of reducing the likelihood of future episodes of substance use and preventing the deterioration associated with untreated psychosis. In adults, substance use in combination with psychotic illness correlates with more frequent hospitalizations, suicide attempts, relapse of psychotic symptoms, homelessness, health problems, legal problems, violent behavior, and residential instability.[10-12]

Programs giving equal attention to substance use and mental health symptoms are preferable. Intervention should be multimodal and include individual and family therapy, medication, and referral to formal treatment programs for longer-term chemical dependency treatment. Some adolescents significantly decrease or discontinue substance use after their first episode of psychosis without specific substance abuse treatment. The experience of psychosis, education about the relationship of symptoms to use, treatment of psychosis, and interruption of social interactions are all postulated to contribute to discontinuation.[13-15] Integral to reduction of substance use is the treatment of psychotic symptoms. Youth engaged in a comprehensive mental health program with a primary focus on addressing psychotic symptoms display the lowest levels of chemical use with improved clinical outcomes.[1] Few patients begin using substances following entry into treatment.[1,16-20] However, in some instances, formal chemical dependency treatment may be helpful, particularly if the adolescent has little insight or motivation. In these programs, education by adult staff on the risks of use may be better received than that given by parents. Second, peers can hold adolescents accountable and peer accountability becomes the criterion for peer acceptance.

At present, specific guidelines regarding the use of antipsychotics in this patient population are lacking. To date, all of the clinical trials supporting the use of second-generation antipsychotic medications in adolescents with schizophrenia have excluded subjects actively using substances. In adult patients with schizophrenia, clozapine has been found to be the most effective medication in reducing cannabis and alcohol use. Because of the potential adverse effects of clozapine in youth, this is a second-line intervention reserved for treatment-refractory patients. The paucity of data regarding adolescents with schizophrenia and comorbid substance misuse makes it unclear whether any of the second-generation antipsychotic medications influence substance misuse or reduce drug cravings. To date, there have been no trials of anticraving agents (eg, naltrexone, topiramate) in these adolescents. Given that these youth are in their first episode of psychosis, lower doses of antipsychotic medications may be required to achieve remission of psychotic symptoms than what is typically recommended for adults with chronic schizophrenia. Frequent psychiatric appointments are essential, not only to build a therapeutic alliance but also to closely monitor side effects. Young people are more susceptible to side effects and tend to be resistant to taking medication in general. A collaborative effort by a mental health provider to reduce these side effects is likely to result in improved adherence. Recent studies have identified a high rate of relapse to psychotic symptoms after discontinuation of antipsychotic medications in those adequately treated for a first psychotic episode. However, if able to maintain sobriety and a quick resolution of psychotic symptoms is experienced, a brief period of antipsychotic medications may be enough. A high level of vigilance for the return of symptoms remains essential, including involvement of the patient's family, educators, and significant others who are often the first to observe reemergence of symptoms. Cannabis use is regarded as benign by most adolescents. Encouraging reduction and cessation of this substance in particular can be challenging. However, understanding of the role cannabis plays in psychotic illness is evolving.

CANNABIS

The role of cannabis in psychotic illness has been controversial. Experts have debated whether those who are psychosis prone are more likely to use cannabis or whether cannabis use independent of other risk factors can cause or precipitate psychotic symptoms.

Lifetime prevalence of cannabis use in grade 12 students in the United States was 49% in 2007.[21] In 2008, more than 15% of 12th graders reported using cannabis daily for at least a month.[22] This finding is particularly concerning given the increased risk of developing psychotic symptoms with increased frequency and dose used.[23–26] For example, transition to daily cannabis abuse in particular has been linked with an increased risk of psychotic symptoms up to 5 times that of nonusers.[23–31] Patients often report the onset of psychosis after the initiation of cannabis use and can recall that their first psychotic symptoms occurred while intoxicated.[31–33] This relationship indicates a causal role as opposed to use for self-medication.

Despite up to 15% of those who use the substance experiencing psychotic symptoms, only a minority go on to develop permanent impairments that include PPDs,[34] indicating that cannabis use alone is not sufficient to cause psychotic illness. Instead, it is likely that, in combination with predisposing risk factors (genetic vulnerability, environmental factors, obstetric insults, and social adversities), cannabis is an additive risk factor in those with increased vulnerability.[33,35,36] In those predisposed, cannabis use is associated with an earlier age of onset for a first episode of psychosis.[37–49] The higher rate of onset of schizophrenia in early cannabis users may reflect an interaction with the catechol O-methyltransferase (COMT) genotype.[50] In adults with schizophrenia, cannabis use was associated with greater brain volume loss over a 5-year period.[51]

Proposed theories focus on the role of the endocannabinoid system in the developing adolescent brain. The role of the endocannabinoids in the development of the infant brain has been shown. Of importance in adolescence, neurodevelopment continues to occur with the prefrontal cortex. During this critical time period (age 15–17 years), synaptic development and pruning, receptor distribution, volumetric growth, myelination, and programming of neurotrophic levels are particularly active.[52–55]

During this same time period, CB1 receptors have been found to increase greatly in the frontal cortex,[56] leading to the theory that the endocannabinoid system is integral to adolescent neurodevelopment as well.[57] Therefore, it is proposed that adolescence represents a critical time period in which the toxic effects of environmental factors, such as cannabis, have the potential to alter neurodevelopment. The prefrontal cortex has been implicated as a core region involved in PPDs. Overpruning of neuronal connections and decreased density of dendritic spines have been implicated in psychosis. Whether by direct toxic effects on neurons or through social deprivation essential to gaining life skills, heavy cannabis use in this critical time period poses a significant increased risk of developing a PPD that has not been observed in those who start using later in life.[58]

Practitioners must be vigilant in screening for cannabis use. Use of cannabis during adolescence is common and increasing in prevalence. With this increased use, it can be assumed that there will be an increase in the number of adolescents experiencing psychotic symptoms. Once identified as being at high risk, acutely stabilized, and educated on the likely contribution of cannabis to the symptoms, long-term engagement in treatment is essential to prevent relapse and potential future episodes.

TREATMENT ENGAGEMENT

Substance use is often cited as one of the strongest predictors of disengagement of treatment in specialized early psychosis programs.[59–62] Adolescents are particularly challenging to engage in treatment of any illness. Psychosis often presents with a low level of insight, making encouragement to take medications challenging. Antipsychotic medications have side effects, the most common being weight gain, fatigue, and sexual side effects, all of which negatively affect the social structure that is of utmost importance to adolescents. Adolescents with psychotic disorders frequently have neuropsychological deficits in attention and executive function. These deficits make psychoeducation and attendance of appointments particularly challenging. The social isolation that ensues with psychosis may alienate that person from those who would have been most helpful in managing day-to-day life.

First-episode programs have shown improved adherence and clinical outcomes, compared with treatment as usual. These programs focus on the lowest effective dose of medications, early engagement of family and caregivers, psychoeducation, group and individual psychotherapy, intensive case management services, and frequent interaction with mental health providers. Motivational interviewing and cognitive behavior therapy are emphasized to foster the therapeutic relationship and encourage participation. These programs have been shown to reduce substance use in patients with psychotic illness.[48,63]

Disengagement in treatment often results in relapse to substance use, which in turn leads to relapse of psychotic symptoms.[64] Even after patients are stabilized on antipsychotic medications, ongoing substance use can result in relapse of symptoms. Subsequent psychotic episodes not only tend to worsen in severity and duration, but may result in resistance to antipsychotic medications.

Early engagement of youth through showing genuine interest in their interests and opinions, including their opinion on what may be causing their symptoms, is imperative. Attention to their concerns (academic, social, and legal) shows desire to help them and to improve cohesiveness.[65]

Treatment recommendations for the combined treatment of psychosis and substance use include, first and foremost, treatment of the psychotic symptoms. A significant proportion of those who experience their first episode of psychosis stop using illicit substances with antipsychotic treatment and psychoeducation. Both of these treatment modalities require excellent engagement in a treatment plan to have efficacy.

SUMMARY

The diagnosis of adolescents with psychotic symptoms and co-occurring substance use disorders is a complex and dynamic process that must take developmental issues into account. Early interventions for adolescents presenting with psychotic symptoms are essential. In both SIPD and PPD, better premorbid adjustment, shorter duration of untreated psychosis, better insight into psychosis, and lower severity of symptoms predict 12-month remission rates.[66] Therefore, timely identification and referral to mental health services are imperative to prevent adaptive decline and to improve overall functional outcomes.

Given the significant overlap in presenting symptoms between SIPD and first-episode PPD with a co-occurring substance use, long-term observation of these youth by a mental health provider experienced in psychosis is required. A premature diagnosis of SIPD has the potential to provide false comfort to patients and families, making engagement in further treatment more difficult. This future delay in treatment could result in subsequent, more severe psychotic episodes that are more difficult to treat. First-episode psychosis programs that provide intensive case management, along with psychiatric, psychological, and peer support, have proved most effective to reduce chemical use and prevent additional psychotic episodes.[67]

The subject of cannabis use remains controversial in our society. A few states recently passed laws making the use of marijuana legal. With the ever-increasing availability of cannabis products in society, education on the risks of use is imperative. Recreational use of cannabis in those who are sensitive to the psychosis-inducing effects of the substance could result in a severe and persistent mental illness in at-risk adolescents. Cannabis use is a highly modifiable risk factor to prevent the onset of PPDs in our society. Youth have reported that the most common reason for abstaining or quitting cannabis use was their concern for psychological and physical damage.[68] It is the obligation of practitioners to educate their patients, families, and communities about the risks associated with cannabis use.

Key to the prediction of clinical outcome for youth experiencing psychotic symptoms is a trusting relationship with their primary mental health provider and the education of those family members closest to them. Both of these factors require an extended relationship with patients and their families. Engagement in treatment through building a therapeutic alliance and psychoeducation should be the top priority in treating youth presenting with psychosis and substance use.

REFERENCES

1. Lambert M, Conus P, Lubman DI, et al. The impact of substance use disorders on clinical outcome in 643 patients with first-episode psychosis. Acta Psychiatr Scand 2005;112(2):141–8.
2. Addington J, Addington D. Effect of substance misuse in early psychosis. Br J Psychiatry Suppl 1998;172(33):134–6.
3. Fraser S, Hides L, Philips L, et al. Differentiating first episode substance induced and primary psychotic disorders with concurrent substance use in young people. Schizophr Res 2012;136(1–3):110–5.
4. Arendt M, Rosenberg R, Foldager L, et al. Cannabis-induced psychosis and subsequent schizophrenia-spectrum disorders: follow-up study of 535 incident cases. Br J Psychiatry 2005;187:510–5.
5. Caton CL, Hasin DS, Shrout PE, et al. Stability of early-phase primary psychotic disorders with concurrent substance use and substance-induced psychosis. Br J Psychiatry 2007;190:105–11.
6. McGorry PD. The influence of illness duration on syndrome clarity and stability in functional psychosis: does the diagnosis emerge and stabilise with time? Aust N Z J Psychiatry 1994;28(4):607–19.

7. Schwartz JE, Fennig S, Tanenberg-Karant M, et al. Congruence of diagnoses 2 years after a first-admission diagnosis of psychosis. Arch Gen Psychiatry 2000;57(6):593–600.
8. Clark RE, Teague GB, Ricketts SK, et al. Cost-effectiveness of assertive community treatment versus standard case management for persons with co-occurring severe mental illness and substance use disorders. Health Serv Res 1998; 33(5 Pt 1):1285–308.
9. Ridgely MS, Osher FC, Goldman HH, et al. Executive summary: chronic mentally ill young adults with substance abuse problems: a review of research, treatment, and training issues. Baltimore (MD): University of Maryland School of Medicine, Mental Health Services Research Center; 1987.
10. Jablensky A, McGrath J, Herrman H, et al. Psychotic disorders in urban areas: an overview of the study on low prevalence disorders. Aust N Z J Psychiatry 2000;34(2):221–36.
11. McEvoy JP, Allen TB. Substance use (including nicotine) in schizophrenic patients. Curr Opin Psychiatry 2003;16:199–205.
12. Akvardar Y, Tumuklu M, Akdede BB, et al. Substance use among patients with schizophrenia in a university hospital. BCP 2004;14(4):191–7.
13. Drake RE, Caton CL, Xie H, et al. A prospective 2-year study of emergency department patients with early-phase primary psychosis or substance-induced psychosis. Am J Psychiatry 2011;168(7):742–8.
14. Archie S, Rush BR, Akhtar-Danesh N, et al. Substance use and abuse in first-episode psychosis: prevalence before and after early intervention. Schizophr Bull 2007;33(6):1354–63.
15. McCleery A, Addington J, Addington D. Substance misuse and cognitive functioning in early psychosis: a 2 year follow-up. Schizophr Res 2006;88(1–3): 187–91.
16. Wade D, Harrigan S, Edwards J, et al. Substance misuse in first-episode psychosis: 15-month prospective follow-up study. Br J Psychiatry 2006;189:229–34.
17. Addington J, Addington D. Impact of an early psychosis program on substance use. Psychiatr Rehabil J 2001;25(1):60–7.
18. Hides L, Dawe S, Kavanagh DJ, et al. Psychotic symptom and cannabis relapse in recent-onset psychosis. Prospective study. Br J Psychiatry 2006;189:137–43.
19. Sorbara F, Liraud F, Assens F, et al. Substance use and the course of early psychosis: a 2-year follow-up of first-admitted subjects. Eur Psychiatry 2003;18: 133–6.
20. Strakowski SM, Keck PE Jr, McElroy SL, et al. Twelve-month outcome after a first hospitalization for affective psychosis. Arch Gen Psychiatry 1998;55(1):49–55.
21. Eaton DK, Kann L, Kinchen S, et al. Youth risk behavior surveillance–United States, 2007. MMWR Surveill Summ 2008;57(4):1–131.
22. Johnston LD, O'Malley PM, Bachman JG, et al. Secondary School Students (NIH Publication No. 09-7402). Monitoring the future national survey results on drug use, 1975-2008, vol. I. Bethesda (MD): National Institute on Drug Abuse; 2009. p. 1–721.
23. Andreasson S, Allebeck P, Engstrom A, et al. Cannabis and schizophrenia. A longitudinal study of Swedish conscripts. Lancet 1987;2(8574):1483–6.
24. Arseneault L, Cannon M, Poulton R, et al. Cannabis use in adolescence and risk for adult psychosis: longitudinal prospective study. BMJ 2002;325(7374): 1212–3.
25. van Os J, Bak M, Hanssen M, et al. Cannabis use and psychosis: a longitudinal population-based study. Am J Epidemiol 2002;156(4):319–27.

26. Zammit S, Allebeck P, Andreasson S, et al. Self reported cannabis use as a risk factor for schizophrenia in Swedish conscripts of 1969: historical cohort study. BMJ 2002;325(7374):1199.

27. Compton MT, Kelley ME, Ramsay CE, et al. Association of pre-onset cannabis, alcohol, and tobacco use with age at onset of prodrome and age at onset of psychosis in first-episode patients. Am J Psychiatry 2009;166(11):1251–7.

28. Weiser M, Knobler HY, Noy S, et al. Clinical characteristics of adolescents later hospitalized for schizophrenia. Am J Med Genet 2002;114(8):949–55.

29. Stefanis NC, Delespaul P, Henquet C, et al. Early adolescent cannabis exposure and positive and negative dimensions of psychosis. Addiction 2004;99(10): 1333–41.

30. Fergusson DM, Horwood LJ, Swain-Campbell NR. Cannabis dependence and psychotic symptoms in young people. Psychol Med 2003;33(1):15–21.

31. Moore TH, Zammit S, Lingford-Hughes A, et al. Cannabis use and risk of psychotic or affective mental health outcomes: a systematic review. Lancet 2007; 370(9584):319–28.

32. Henquet C, Murray R, Linszen D, et al. The environment and schizophrenia: the role of cannabis use. Schizophr Bull 2005;31(3):608–12.

33. Semple DM, McIntosh AM, Lawrie SM. Cannabis as a risk factor for psychosis: systematic review. J Psychopharmacol 2005;19(2):187–94.

34. Thomas H. A community survey of adverse effects of cannabis use. Drug Alcohol Depend 1996;42(3):201–7.

35. Fergusson DM, Poulton R, Smith PF, et al. Cannabis and psychosis. BMJ 2006; 332(7534):172–5.

36. Henquet C, Di Forti M, Morrison P, et al. Gene-environment interplay between cannabis and psychosis. Schizophr Bull 2008;34(6):1111–21.

37. Buhler B, Hambrecht M, Loffler W, et al. Precipitation and determination of the onset and course of schizophrenia by substance abuse–a retrospective and prospective study of 232 population-based first illness episodes. Schizophr Res 2002;54(3):243–51.

38. Veen ND, Selten JP, van der Tweel I, et al. Cannabis use and age at onset of schizophrenia. Am J Psychiatry 2004;161(3):501–6.

39. Mauri MC, Volonteri LS, De Gaspari IF, et al. Substance abuse in first-episode schizophrenic patients: a retrospective study. Clin Pract Epidemiol Ment Health 2006;2:4.

40. Gonzalez-Pinto A, Vega P, Ibanez B, et al. Impact of cannabis and other drugs on age at onset of psychosis. J Clin Psychiatry 2008;69(8):1210–6.

41. Ongur D, Lin L, Cohen BM. Clinical characteristics influencing age at onset in psychotic disorders. Compr Psychiatry 2009;50(1):13–9.

42. Sugranyes G, Flamarique I, Parellada E, et al. Cannabis use and age of diagnosis of schizophrenia. Eur Psychiatry 2009;24(5):282–6.

43. Foti DJ, Kotov R, Guey LT, et al. Cannabis use and the course of schizophrenia: 10-year follow-up after first hospitalization. Am J Psychiatry 2010;167(8): 987–93.

44. Barrigon ML, Gurpegui M, Ruiz-Veguilla M, et al. Temporal relationship of first-episode non-affective psychosis with cannabis use: a clinical verification of an epidemiological hypothesis. J Psychiatr Res 2010;44(7):413–20.

45. Pelayo-Teran JM, Perez-Iglesias R, Mata I, et al. Catechol-O-methyltransferase (COMT) Val158Met variations and cannabis use in first-episode non-affective psychosis: clinical-onset implications. Psychiatry Res 2010;179(3): 291–6.

46. De Hert M, Wampers M, Jendricko T, et al. Effects of cannabis use on age at onset in schizophrenia and bipolar disorder. Schizophr Res 2011;126(1–3): 270–6.
47. Large M, Sharma S, Compton MT, et al. Cannabis use and earlier onset of psychosis: a systematic meta-analysis. Arch Gen Psychiatry 2011;68(6): 555–61.
48. Addington J, Addington D. Patterns, predictors and impact of substance use in early psychosis: a longitudinal study. Acta Psychiatr Scand 2007;115(4):304–9.
49. Barnes TR, Mutsatsa SH, Hutton SB, et al. Comorbid substance use and age at onset of schizophrenia. Br J Psychiatry 2006;188:237–42.
50. Caspi A, Moffitt TE, Cannon M, et al. Moderation of the effect of adolescent-onset cannabis use on adult psychosis by a functional polymorphism in the catechol-O-methyltransferase gene: longitudinal evidence of a gene X environment interaction. Biol Psychiatry 2005;57(10):1117–27.
51. Rais M, Cahn W, Van Haren N, et al. Excessive brain volume loss over time in cannabis-using first-episode schizophrenia patients. Am J Psychiatry 2008; 165(4):490–6.
52. Giedd JN, Blumenthal J, Jeffries NO, et al. Brain development during childhood and adolescence: a longitudinal MRI study. Nat Neurosci 1999;2(10):861–3.
53. Bartzokis G, Beckson M, Lu PH, et al. Age-related changes in frontal and temporal lobe volumes in men: a magnetic resonance imaging study. Arch Gen Psychiatry 2001;58(5):461–5.
54. Andersen SL, Teicher MH. Stress, sensitive periods and maturational events in adolescent depression. Trends Neurosci 2008;31(4):183–91.
55. Spear LP. The adolescent brain and age-related behavioral manifestations. Neurosci Biobehav Rev 2000;24(4):417–63.
56. Mato S, Del Olmo E, Pazos A. Ontogenetic development of cannabinoid receptor expression and signal transduction functionality in the human brain. Eur J Neurosci 2003;17(9):1747–54.
57. Rubino T, Zamberletti E, Parolaro D. Adolescent exposure to cannabis as a risk factor for psychiatric disorders. J Psychopharmacol 2012;26(1):177–88.
58. Bossong MG, Niesink RJ. Adolescent brain maturation, the endogenous cannabinoid system and the neurobiology of cannabis-induced schizophrenia. Prog Neurobiol 2010;92(3):370–85.
59. Kreyenbuhl J, Nossel IR, Dixon LB. Disengagement from mental health treatment among individuals with schizophrenia and strategies for facilitating connections to care: a review of the literature. Schizophr Bull 2009;35(4):696–703.
60. Conus P, Lambert M, Cotton S, et al. Rate and predictors of service disengagement in an epidemiological first-episode psychosis cohort. Schizophr Res 2010; 118(1–3):256–63.
61. Turner MA, Boden JM, Smith-Hamel C, et al. Outcomes for 236 patients from a 2-year early intervention in psychosis service. Acta Psychiatr Scand 2009; 120(2):129–37.
62. Miller R, Ream G, McCormack J, et al. A prospective study of cannabis use as a risk factor for non-adherence and treatment dropout in first-episode schizophrenia. Schizophr Res 2009;113(2–3):138–44.
63. Carr JA, Norman RM, Manchanda R. Substance misuse over the first 18 months of specialized intervention for first episode psychosis. Early Interv Psychiatry 2009;3(3):221–5.
64. Levy E, Pawliuk N, Joober R, et al. Medication-adherent first-episode psychosis patients also relapse: why? Can J Psychiatry 2012;57(2):78–84.

65. Jackson HJ, McGorry PD. The recognition and management of early psychosis: a preventive approach. 2nd edition. New York: Cambridge University Press; 2009.
66. Caton CL, Hasin DS, Shrout PE, et al. Predictors of psychosis remission in psychotic disorders that co-occur with substance use. Schizophr Bull 2006;32(4): 618–25.
67. Tucker P. Substance misuse and early psychosis. Australas Psychiatry 2009; 17(4):291–4.
68. Terry-McElrath YM, O'Malley PM, Johnston LD. Saying no to marijuana: why American youth report quitting or abstaining. J Stud Alcohol Drugs 2008; 69(6):796–805.

Diagnosis and Evaluation of Hallucinations and Other Psychotic Symptoms in Children and Adolescents

Linmarie Sikich, MD

KEYWORDS

- Hallucinations • Psychosis • Differential diagnosis
- Positive and Negative Syndrome Scale • Brief Psychiatric Rating Scale for Children
- Affective psychoses • Benign hallucinations • Early-onset schizophrenia

KEY POINTS

- Many children and adolescents do not volunteer that they hallucinate but report it when asked.
- Hallucinations during childhood are frequently multimodal in nature (eg, auditory, visual).
- Delusions are typically vague and much less common than hallucinations during childhood.
- Youth with hallucinations have increased risk for psychiatric illnesses and suicidality.
- Symptoms and functioning should be monitored given the high risk for subsequent disorders.
- Families need to know that the diagnosis is challenging and that it should be reevaluated periodically.

Disclosures: All disclosures for 2009 to 2013. Dr Sikich receives or has received research funding from NIMH, NICHD, Foundation of Hope, Autism Speaks, Case Western Reserve University (subcontract from NICHD), Research Foundation for Mental Hygiene Research (subcontract from NIMH), Pfizer, and Bristol Myers-Squibb. She is participating or has participated in clinical trials with Bristol Myers-Squibb, Otsuka Research Institute, Forest Pharmaceuticals, SynapDX, Merck, Curemark, and Seaside Pharmaceuticals. She also received medication for clinical trials from Eli Lilly, Janssen, Pfizer, and Bristol Myers-Squibb, and software for a computer intervention in schizophrenia from Posit Science. She has no stock or equity in any companies that provide services to individuals with mental health problems.
ASPIRE Program, University of North Carolina at Chapel Hill, CB 7167 UNC-CH, 2218 Nelson Highway, Suite 1, Chapel Hill, NC 27599-7167, USA
E-mail address: Lsikich@med.unc.edu

Child Adolesc Psychiatric Clin N Am 22 (2013) 655–673
http://dx.doi.org/10.1016/j.chc.2013.06.005
1056-4993/13/$ – see front matter © 2013 Elsevier Inc. All rights reserved.

OVERVIEW

It is becoming increasingly clear that many psychiatric disorders emerge during childhood and adolescence. Furthermore, early recognition and effective treatment continue to hold promise of reducing the long-term disability and suffering associated with these illnesses. Despite this, epidemiologic studies consistently find that a large proportion of children with mental illness are not diagnosed and many do not receive the treatment they need. Earlier recognition and treatment of the most severe psychiatric disorders is particularly important to limit long-term disability and promote recovery. These include schizophrenia spectrum disorder (Sz), bipolar affective disorder (BP), recurrent major depression, and posttraumatic stress disorder (PTSD). These severe and persistent mental illnesses often present with nonspecific symptoms such as poor attention and school performance, social problems, and irritability. Although hallucinations and delusions may be present, they are seldom the primary reason for referral and may not be disclosed without direct questioning. Conversely, positive psychotic symptoms are not specific to these severe disorders, particularly in children. They may occur in the context of genetic and neurologic disorders, toxic exposures, and chemical imbalances. These symptoms may also indicate milder forms of mental illness and heightened risk for suicide or serious mental illness later. Finally, the symptoms may represent normal developmental responses. This article focuses on the recognition, differential diagnosis, and follow-up of positive psychotic symptoms in youth.

CHARACTERISTICS OF HALLUCINATIONS AND DELUSIONS IN YOUTH

Hallucinations are much more common than delusions in youth. Auditory hallucinations, with frequent comments and commands, are most common. Conversing voices are less common. Visual and tactile hallucinations often accompany the auditory hallucinations, resulting in a multimodal hallucination.[1,2] Children and adolescents often name their hallucinations with reference to physical characteristics (eg, "black cape guy") or to culturally referenced phenomena (eg, monsters). This may lead to confusion with imaginary companions, which are normal developmental phenomena in latency-age children. Unlike imaginary companions, youth cannot make hallucinations go away, but they may be able to ignore them. True hallucinations are usually vivid, but not detailed, and often provoke a response from the child. True hallucinations occur when fully awake.

Delusions also occur in children and adolescents, but these tend to be vague and difficult to distinguish from reality. They are often related to hallucinations. For instance, children may feel that their hallucinations are trying to hurt them or will hurt family members. Frequent grandiose delusions include the belief that simply thinking about something will make it happen. Somatic delusions may include being pregnant. However, youth younger than 16 years old seldom develop highly specific and complex delusions such as the persecutory or religious delusions seen in adults.[3–6] Frequently observed differences between the presentations of positive psychotic symptoms are summarized in **Table 1**.

EPIDEMIOLOGY OF POSITIVE PSYCHOTIC SYMPTOMS IN THE GENERAL PEDIATRIC POPULATION

A series of epidemiologic studies have shown that children and, to a lesser extent, adolescents often acknowledge positive psychotic symptoms.[7] Among community samples of 9- to 12-year-olds, the rate of those endorsing auditory hallucinations

Table 1
Differences between pediatric and adult positive psychotic symptoms

Symptom	Pediatric Manifestation	Adult Manifestation
Delusions	Usually poorly elaborated and vague May build on real experiences (eg, being teased or disliked)	Usually specific, complex
Hallucinations	Often multimodal (auditory, visual, tactile) Often given names, which may be stereotypic (eg, "the devil")	Auditory much more common than any other modality Seldom personalized
Disorganized speech	May be hard to distinguish from developmental language disability especially given premorbid disabilities	Clear difference from previous state
Disorganized behavior	Similar to adults, but parents may exert more control and minimize effects	—
Negative symptoms	May be confused with oppositionality or depression	—
Common comorbidities	Autism spectrum symptoms Attention deficit hyperactivity disorder Oppositional defiant disorder Anxiety disorders Depression	Depression Substance use Cannabis use associated with earlier adult onset, but rare before middle-teen years ASD symptoms, which occur before age 3 y

ranged from 9% to 35% with a median rate of 17%. Among 13- to 18-year-olds, the rate ranged from 5% to 11% with a median of 7.5%. Youth generally reported on symptoms occurring within the past year. Youth who endorse positive psychotic symptoms are much more likely to have current mental health problems than those who do not. Researchers in Ireland surveyed 2245 youth, 425 of whom were interviewed by expert clinicians. The 11- to 13-year-olds reporting the lowest levels of well-being were 5.5 times more likely to report hallucinations than those in the quartile reporting the highest levels (38% vs 7%). A similar pattern, but with greater specificity for distress, was observed among 14- to 16-year-olds; 19% of those with low well-being endorsed psychotic symptoms versus 1.4% in the highest quartile. Reported hallucinations were also increased with a lifetime history of psychiatric disorders. Among the younger group, 40% with two disorders and 55% with three disorders reported hallucinations; in the older group, rates were 20% and 35%, respectively. About half of the 11- to 13-year-olds and a quarter of the middle adolescents with affective and behavioral disorders reported hallucinations, compared with only 9% of those with anxiety.[8,9] Among those endorsing psychotic symptoms, 60% to 80% met lifetime criteria for an Axis I disorder with 30% to 43% having a current disorder. Compared with youth who did not report psychotic symptoms, those who reported psychotic symptoms were more likely to have been abused (odds ratio [OR] 6), witnessed domestic violence (OR 10), been bullied (OR 10), or had suicidal ideation (SI) or behavior (OR 10).[10] Nearly all (86%) the interviewed youth with both psychotic symptoms and SI had planned or attempted suicide, reflecting a 20-fold greater rate than those with SI but no psychosis.[11]

Similar results have been found in three other studies. Approximately 20% of 12-year-old twins studied reported positive psychotic symptoms, with hallucinations being four times as common as paranoia. A large number of the youth with positive symptoms had current depressive symptoms with smaller proportions having anxiety or antisocial disorders. Those with psychotic symptoms were four times as likely to harm themselves.[12] Japanese 12- to 15-year-olds with psychotic symptoms had increased rates of SI and self-harm (relative risk [RR] 2.1), severe anxiety (RR 1.4), or assaultive behavior (RR 1.3).[13,14] More than half of Dutch adolescents reporting psychotic symptoms were anxious or depressed, easily distracted, and highly irritable compared with 25% of their peers without hallucinations.[15]

Psychotic symptoms occurring during childhood and adolescence frequently disappear.[16] After 1 year, 67% of teens with hallucinations had reduced symptoms, including half who had no symptoms.[17] Despite this, youth with positive psychotic symptoms are at increased risk for multiple psychiatric disorders compared with adults. The most robust studies involve the follow-up at ages 26 and 38 of an epidemiologic cohort of 789 youth. When 11 years old, 15% had acknowledged, "hearing voices that other people could not hear." At age 26, one-third of these youth had anxiety disorders, including PTSD, 20% had depression, and 11% had Sz.[18] Half of all those diagnosed with Sz at 26 had reported psychotic symptoms at age 11. At age 38 years, those who had initially reported hallucinations remained at increased risk for Sz, PTSD, suicide attempts, and persistent anxiety. Among those with the most severe psychotic symptoms at age 11, 50% had PTSD, substance abuse, and suicide attempts; 23% had Sz; and only one was free of a diagnosable mental illness.[19]

PSYCHOTIC SYMPTOMS AMONG YOUTH IN PSYCHIATRIC CARE

Positive psychotic symptoms occur in a sizable minority of youth in psychiatric care. In a pediatric mood and anxiety clinic, nearly 10% of 2031 children, 5- to 21-years-old, had psychotic symptoms.[20] Among those, 62% had depressive disorders, 24% had BP disorder, and 14% had Sz. Among children hospitalized for depression, up to 60% have psychotic symptoms. Clinical samples of youth with BP disorder have similarly high rates, ranging from 16% to 88%.[21–23] Among those with mood disorders, children and adolescents are much more likely to hallucinate than adults. In contrast, psychotic symptoms seem to occur with similar frequencies in children (15%) and adults (20%) with PTSD and trauma histories.[24–26] There are also multiple case reports (but no systematic studies) about positive psychotic symptoms occurring in the context of other childhood psychiatric disorders, including severe anxiety, autism spectrum disorder (ASD), obsessive-compulsive disorder (OCD), and Tourette syndrome. The reports are most specific with regard to Tourette syndrome, with psychotic symptoms reported in 2.5% to 15% of affected individuals.[27] It is unclear whether co-occurrence of psychotic and OCD or ASD symptoms reflects comorbidity or diagnostic confusion (please see article by Carlson on ASD and psychosis in this publication.)

It is unclear if youth are at any greater risk for developing psychotic symptoms in the context of intoxication from street or prescribed drugs, though they are probably less likely to experience intoxication initially. Drugs of abuse associated with psychosis include ecstasy, methamphetamine, "bath salts," cocaine, "spice," cannabis, peyote, ketamine, PCP, LSD, dextromethorphan, opiates, and barbiturates.[28,29] Steroids, anticholinergics, antihistamines, isoniazid, multiple serotonergic agents, some anesthetic agents, and stimulants also may cause psychotic symptoms.[30] Substance abuse, particularly with cannabis, may precipitate a Sz spectrum disorder in individuals who have underlying vulnerability.[31–33] Among 18,478 people hospitalized for substance-induced psychosis, 46% with cannabis and 30% with amphetamine developed Sz.[34]

PEDIATRIC PREVALENCE OF PSYCHIATRIC DISORDERS THAT MAY INCLUDE PSYCHOTIC SYMPTOMS

The developmental epidemiology of various psychiatric illnesses that may include psychotic symptoms has an important effect on the likely diagnosis affecting youth with positive symptoms. In the pediatric National Comorbidity Survey,[35] anxiety disorders were highly prevalent with median onset at 6 years and gradual resolution over time. The 12-month prevalence in adolescents was approximately 25%. Other disorders including PTSD, depression, BP, and substance abuse followed the opposite pattern with lower prevalence in children than teens. Rates of PTSD increased from 4% to 7% during adolescence. Depressive disorders had a median age of onset of 13 years with a 12-month prevalence of 8.4% in young adolescents that steadily increased to 15.4% in older adolescents. The point prevalence of significant depression in children was approximately 3% and in adolescents it was approximately 8%.[36,37] BP disorders were significantly less common, affecting only about 2% of younger adolescents and 4.3% of older adolescents. Substance abuse was present in 3.7% of younger adolescents and 22% of the older teens. Sz is extremely rare (~3 per 100,000) during the first decade of life. Sz prevalence increases approximately fourfold between 10- and 14-years-old to 13 per 100,000 and approximately threefold between 14- and 18–years-old to 20 to 55 per 10,000.[3,38–40] At least 5% of individuals with Sz become ill before age 14 years and 20% to 30% have been estimated to become ill before age 18 years.[41,42] Consequently, children are much more likely to experience hallucinations in the context of mood or anxiety disorders than Sz. Adolescents with psychosis are about equally likely to have Sz or mood disorders, with lower likelihood of having an anxiety disorder or substance abuse. **Table 2** summarizes information about frequency of psychotic symptoms and associated problems.

OTHER MEDICAL CONDITIONS THAT MAY INCLUDE POSITIVE PSYCHOTIC SYMPTOMS

Psychotic symptoms may also occur in the context of neurologic disorders, genetic and metabolic disorders, infections, and autoimmune disorders. Among key neurologic disorders to consider are migraines, seizure disorders, malignancies, encephalitis, and lupus. Hallucinations may precede or accompany migraine headaches. More chronic psychotic symptoms may be present as part of a seizure disorder, in which they can occur during, after, or between seizures. Often, in such cases, the hallucinations may be limited to a single sensory modality and may be followed by somnolence.[30,43,44] Brain tumors—especially in the pituitary or frontal, temporal, or visual association cortices—may produce hallucinations or delusions. In addition, germline, ovarian, breast, and small cell lung cancers have been associated with antibodies targeting neurotransmitter receptors that lead to psychotic encephalitis.[45,46] Lupus is associated with higher rates of psychosis in youth than in adults.[47,48] Hyperthyroidism also has been associated with new-onset psychosis. Increased head injuries have also been reported in individuals with psychosis.[49,50] Similarly, several genetic disorders have been associated with psychosis, though the strength of this association is often unclear and complicated by many of the older reports referring to childhood psychosis but actually describing ASD.[51] Relatively common genetic disorders that may have psychotic manifestations include Down syndrome (prevalence 1 per 700); acute intermittent porphyria (prevalence ~1 per 1–3000); chromosome 22q11 deletion

Table 2
Pediatric psychosis by the numbers

Population	Incidence of Acknowledging Positive Psychotic Symptoms				
	Any Youth	9–12 y	11–13 y	14–16 y	13–18 y
Meta-analysis of epidemiologic studies[7]	—	9%–35% median 17%	—	—	5%–11% median 7.5%
Irish community sample[8]	—	—	21%	7%	—
Subsets of this sample with	—	—	—	—	—
Lifetime psychiatric disorder	—	—	60%	80%	—
Current psychiatric disorder	—	—	30%	43%	—
2 lifetime psychiatric illnesses	—	—	40%	20%	—
≥3 lifetime psychiatric illnesses	—	—	55%	35%	—
Top 25% of SDQ difficulties	—	—	38%	19%	—
25% with fewest Strengths and Difficulties Questionnaire (SDQ) problems	—	—	7%	1.4%	
Dunedin community sample of 11-year-old children[18]	—	—	15%	—	—
Children hospitalized for depression[21]	60%	—	—	—	—
Outpatients with BP[22,23]	16%–88%	—	—	—	—
Hospitalized adolescents with BP[23]	88%	—	—	—	—
Youth and adults with PTSD,[24–26]	15%–20%	—	—	—	—
Youth w/Tourette syndrome,[27]	2.5%–15%	—	—	—	—

Risks for Associated Problems if Acknowledged Positive Psychotic Symptoms vs No Symptoms

Population	Suicidal Actions	SI	Anxiety	Domestic Violence Exposure	Prior Abuse	Aggression	Ongoing Psychotic Symptoms
Irish community sample[10,11]	OR 20[a]	OR 10	—	OR 10	OR 6	OR 10 (bullying)	33% at 1 y 50% at 2 y
12-year-old United Kingdom twins[12]	RR 4	—	RR 1.3	—	—	RR 1.3 (assault)	—
12- to 15-year-old Japanese youth[13,14]	RR 2.1	—	—	—	—	—	—
Dutch teens,[15]	—	—	RR >2	—	—	RR 2 (irritable)	—

Prevalence of Psychiatric Disorders

Population	Schizophrenia	Anxiety	Depression	BP	PTSD	Substance Abuse
National Comorbidity Survey: teens[35]	0.01% Y	25%	8.4% Y	2% Y	4% Y	3.7% Y
Population samples[3,38–40]	0.2%–0.6% O	>25% children	15.4% O	4.3% O	7% O	22% O
Outpatients in mood clinic reporting psychosis[20] (10% clinic population)	14%	62%	—	—	24%	—
Dunedin psychosis at age 11 assessed at age 26[18]	11%, RR 12	20% (with PTSD)	Half with psychosis at this time had reported psychosis at age 11			
Dunedin psychosis at 11 assessed at age 38[19]	23%	—	—	—	50%	Only 1 free of illness
Youth hospitalized for cannabis-induced psychosis[34]	46%	—	—	—	—	—
Youth hospitalized for amphetamine-induced psychosis[34]	30%	—	—	—	—	—

Abbreviations: O, older adolescents 16–19 years old; Y, younger adolescents 13–15 years old.
[a] If patient has both SI and psychosis compared with SI without psychosis.

syndrome (22q11DS), also called velocardiofacial syndrome (VCFS) or DiGeorge syndrome (prevalence 1 per 4000); Marfan syndrome (1 per 3500–5000); and Huntington disease (prevalence 1 per 12,500). Of these, 22q11DS may be the most important to recognize because approximately 25% of affected individuals become psychotic during adolescence, with most experiencing Sz.[52–55] Furthermore, the incidence of 22q11DS in individuals with Sz has been reported to be between 0.5% and 6%.[56–59] The two adolescents with 22q11DS shown in **Fig. 1** demonstrate some of the associated dysmorphic features.

ASSESSMENT OF POSITIVE SYMPTOMS IN YOUTH

The assessment of youth who may have psychotic symptoms should initially focus on the issues of greatest concern to them and their families. These are most often nonspecific problems such as poor academic performance, new-onset oppositionality or aggression. It is important to try to determine if these problems emerge primarily when psychotic symptoms are present or are relatively independent. Factors that increase the likelihood that psychotic symptoms may underlie such behavioral problems include atypical responses to stimulants, new onset of extreme reactions to environmental stress and family history of Sz or BP. If the psychotic symptoms do not appear associated with the presenting problem, the clinician should determine if the psychotic symptoms are isolated benign phenomena. If not, the next step is to determine if a specific somatic or psychiatric disorder appears to underlie the psychotic symptoms. However, patients and families should be aware that it is quite unusual to conclusively identify a specific disorder causing psychotic symptoms. Instead, clinicians generally provide a working diagnosis based on clinical judgment that frequently changes with time.

A full medical and psychiatric history should be obtained, including developmental issues and congenital malformations, cognitive functioning, chronic or recurrent illnesses, chronic medications, traumatic experiences, and substance use. It is essential to determine the temporal order of various psychiatric symptoms and to identify periods when symptoms occur in isolation or together. The child and family should be interviewed separately, if possible. There should also be efforts to gain information

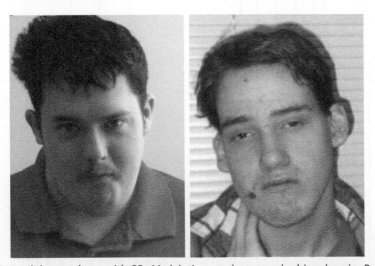

Fig. 1. Two adolescent boys with 22q11 deletion syndrome and schizophrenia. Both have low facial tone, tubular noses, and slightly low-set ears.

from the child's school. Yes-and-no questions should be avoided and examples requested whenever possible. In addition, it is often helpful to observe the child when he or she is waiting or interacting with others to assess responses to internal stimuli, affect, and social relatedness.

When speaking with families, one should ask about times when the child seemed to be persistent in telling obvious lies, which might reflect delusional beliefs, and times when the child has asked if the parent has said something or called for the child when they have not. Parents will also frequently report that the child justifies aggression based on derogatory statements made by others when there is no evidence that the other person said anything. Parents may also be able to provide information about increased social isolation such as sleeping after school and then getting up at night when others are sleeping. If there are indications that the child may be paranoid, it is often helpful to try to get collateral information from other sources, such as teachers or peers, to try to determine whether the child's perceptions are reality-based or not.

When interviewing the child, it is important to avoid jargon and to normalize potentially psychotic behaviors as much as possible. The clinician should verify that the child has understood the questions. For instance, rather than asking if the child has ever had hallucinations or heard voices, it is often much more useful to ask if he or she has ever heard something but could not figure out who was talking or noticed that others acted like they did not hear anything. Because psychotic symptoms are often heightened during periods of stress or extreme emotion, it may also be useful to ask about misperceptions occurring when the child is really angry, sad, or upset. If psychotic symptoms are elicited, ask the child to provide as full a description of the events and their precipitants as possible. It is also important to ask the child if these experiences are different from imagining or remembering and, if so, to explain how they are different. Similarly, there may be variability in the extent of the youth's insight. When less ill, the youth may recognize that the hallucination is unlikely to be real, may be caused by something in his or her brain, or is not accepted by others. Finally, it is important to determine when these perceptions have occurred and how long they have persisted. In most cases, identification of positive psychotic symptoms depends on the youth's self-report. Parents are frequently unaware the child has experienced any psychotic symptoms.

If the child seems guarded, it is often helpful to ask if she or he is being told not to respond or if she or he is afraid of something happening if she or he does respond. Thought disorder in early-onset Sz is reflected by contradictory statements, loose associations or poor cohesion, efforts to avoid answering, and/or marked latency in responses.[60] If the clinician has difficulty following the child's thought processes, it is often helpful to ask her or him to explain it in a different way. Most children can readily do this, whereas those with psychosis cannot.

In addition, the clinician should push for descriptions of the patient's affective state rather than relying on labels such as sad, depressed, mood swings, or manic. Youth with Sz tend to report feeling blah, numb, or empty. In contrast, youth with depression often provide graphic descriptions of how bad they feel. One should determine whether hallucinations and delusions are mood congruent.

USE OF RATING SCALES

Screening instruments such as the Youth Self-Report, Child Behavior Checklist, Behavior Assessment System for Children (BASC),[61] or Brief Psychiatric Report for Children (BPRS-C)[62] can be useful in identifying potentially concerning experiences that might reflect positive psychotic symptoms as well as suggesting other psychiatric or behavioral problems. Kelleher and colleagues[63] examined the usefulness of various questions from the Kiddie-Schedule for Affective Disorders and Schizophrenia (K-SADS) for detecting hallucinations and delusions among the general population. The most frequently endorsed was "Do you ever hear things that other people don't hear," whereas none of the youth in this sample endorsed feeling like "something had gotten into or changed in my body." A large proportion of the general population who were not thought to be probably or definitely experiencing psychotic symptoms also endorsed the question about feeling that people were paying special attention to them or looking at them, which raises question about the extent to which this reflects typical adolescent self-consciousness. Projective psychological testing may be useful in confirming suspected cognitive disorganization. However, failure to demonstrate psychotic disorganization during projective testing is not sufficient to reject the diagnosis.

Once the clinician has determined that psychotic symptoms are present, it is often useful to track symptoms over time by using existing rating scales. The most widely used scales in child and adolescent psychiatry are the Positive and Negative Syndrome Scale,[64] and the BPRS-C. In older adolescents, the Scale Assessing Positive Symptoms and the Scale for Assessing Negative Symptoms may also be used.[65] For youth with psychosis occurring in the context of BP affective disorder, the Young Mania Rating Scale may be more useful for tracking response to treatment.[66] Frequently, these scales show a rapid reduction in the severity of very specific positive symptoms with treatment, whereas the more general or negative symptoms queried may provide more information about persistent or emerging functional problems associated with the illness. Another scale that has not been widely used in youth but which seems potentially useful for tracking the response to treatment is the Psychotic Symptom Rating Scale, which assesses the frequency, intensity, and level of distress associated with hallucinations and delusions.[67,68]

DIFFERENTIAL DIAGNOSIS

Table 3 summarizes potential components of the organic work-up of hallucinations in children and adolescents. Many of the organic causes of positive psychotic symptoms are rare, but recognition of them is important because some have specific treatments. Furthermore, these treatments may both treat psychotic symptoms and prevent the development of progressive or permanent neurologic sequelae. In other cases, no treatments are currently available but they might be developed in the future. Key elements of the work-up include a comprehensive neurologic examination; blood tests for sodium, calcium, magnesium, leukocytosis, and inflammation; and urine toxicology. If dysmorphologies, intellectual disability, or congenital malformations are present, it is essential to obtain a genetic consult and consider microarray testing. Microarray testing may become more widely recommended as its cost is reduced.

Distinction of between psychiatric illnesses with positive psychotic features usually depends on associated features. In Sz, there is more likely to be a history of longstanding subtle issues with social relationships, attention, and behavioral issues. Pediatric BP may also have a chronic course. In such cases, the distinctions may be related to apparent cyclicity in symptoms and intensity of affective experiences other than anger or irritability. In considering whether the symptoms are occurring in the context of depression, there is considerable emphasis on the child's description of sadness or dysphoria, as well as whether the illness is more episodic. In making this distinction, it is important to recognize that individuals with Sz may have had a true depressive illness previously.[69–72] Perhaps more important is examination of the temporal

Table 3
Proposed workup for psychotic symptoms

Assessment	Indication	Priority of Assessment	Potential Alternative Diagnoses if Positive	Specific Treatment Possibly
Detailed neurologic examination	• Psychotic symptoms	Mandatory	• Structural brain lesion • Genetic disorder • Metabolic disorder • Delirium often secondary to toxic ingestion • CNS infection, consider lumbar puncture	• Possibly • Possibly enzyme replacement or stem cell transplant • Possibly, dietary change, Miglustat in Niemann-Pick disease • Supportive • Antibiotics
Neurology consult	• Possibly psychotic symptoms • Neurologic findings • Dysmorphology	Strongly suggested Mandatory if indicators (not universal practice)	• As above	• As above
Genetics consult	• Possibly psychotic symptoms • Possibly positive family history • Neurologic findings • Dysmorphology • Hepatomegaly, splenomegaly	Suggested mandatory if indicators (currently uncommon practice)	• Genetic disorder • Metabolic disorder	• Possibly enzyme replacement or stem cell transplant • Possibly, dietary change, miglustat in Niemann-Pick disease
Na^+, Ca^{++}, Mg^{++}, glucose	• Psychotic symptoms	Mandatory	• Hypernatremia • Low Na^+, Ca^{++}, Mg^{++}, hypoglycemia	• Hydration • Supplementation
Complete blood count	• Psychotic symptoms	Mandatory	• Infection	• Antibiotics
Liver function tests	• Psychotic symptoms	Mandatory	• Metabolic disorders	• Possibly further work-up

(continued on next page)

Table 3
(continued)

Assessment	Indication	Priority of Assessment	Potential Alternative Diagnoses if Positive	Specific Treatment Possibly
Urine toxicology	• Psychotic symptoms	Mandatory	• Substance-induced psychosis • Comorbidity	• Detoxification • Substance abuse treatment
TSH, free T4	• Psychotic symptoms	Mandatory	• Hyperthyroidism	• Ablative therapy
Erythrocyte sedimentation rate	• Psychotic symptoms	Strongly suggested	• Autoimmune disorder especially lupus	• Immunosuppression
Ceruloplasmin (low), 24 h urine copper (increased)	• Kayser-Fleischer rings • Hepatomegaly, elevated LFTs	• Mandatory if indicators • Suggested if only psychosis	• Wilson disease • Aceruloplasminemia	• Copper sequestration
Electroencephalogram 24–48 h if possible, sleep-deprived otherwise	• Episodic psychotic symptoms • Postepisode sedation • Automatisms • Single-modality hallucinations	• Mandatory if indicators • Optional if only psychosis	• Complex partial seizures • Interictal psychosis • Postictal psychosis	• Anticonvulsants
MRI (preferably with contrast)	• Neurologic symptoms • History of head trauma	• Mandatory if indicators • Optional if only psychosis	• Tumors • Hematoma • Vascular malformations	• Oncological treatment • Possible surgery • Unlikely
Microarray and karyotype	• Dysmorphology • Intellectual disabilities • Significant cognitive decline • Small or marfanoid stature • Congenital abnormalities	• Mandatory if indicators • Optional if only psychosis	• Genetic disorder • Metabolic disorder	• Possibly enzyme replacement or stem cell transplant • Possibly, dietary restriction, miglustat in Niemann-Pick disease

Spot urinary porphobilinogens	• Psychosis with intermittent severe abdominal pain, motor neuropathies, or red or brown urine • Episodic psychosis	• Mandatory if indicators • Optional if only psychosis	• Acute intermittent porphyria • Other porphyrias	• Carbohydrate loading • Hemin • Consider relation to menstrual cycle • Consider drug interactions
Arylsulfatase A	• Psychosis with dystonia or progressive muscle weakness	• Mandatory if indicators • Optional if only psychosis	• Metachromatic leukodystrophy	• Stem cell transplant • Possibly enzyme replacement
Urine and serum amino acids	• Psychosis with marked progressive cognitive dysfunction, frequent seizures	• Mandatory if indicators • Optional if only psychosis	• Inborn errors of metabolism including urea cycle disorders, MTHFR deficiency, cystathionine B-synthase	• Dietary manipulation • Stem cell transplant • Enzyme replacement
Urine organic acids	• Psychosis with progressive cognitive dysfunction	• Mandatory if indicators • Optional if only psychosis	• Nonketotic hyperglycinemia	• Dietary manipulation • Correct acid base imbalances
Very-long-chain fatty acids	• Psychosis with neurologic signs or seizures	• Mandatory if indicators • Optional if only psychosis	• Adrenoleukodystrophy	• Correction of adrenal insufficiency • Dietary manipulation • Gene therapy
Antinuclear antibody	• Other signs of lupus • Elevated ESR	• Strongly suggested if indicators	• Lupus	• Immunosuppression
Anti-NMDA receptor Antibody	• Psychosis in presence of cancer or elevated ESR • Sudden onset of symptoms	• Only if indicators or somatic symptoms suggesting cancer	• Anti-NMDA receptor encephalitis	• Treatment of cancer • Immunosuppression

Abbreviations: CNS, central nervous system; ESR, erythrocyte sedimentation rate; LFTs, liver function tests; MTHFR, methylenetetrahydrofolate reductase; TSH, thyrotropin.

relationship between psychotic and mood symptoms. In Sz, there should be psychotic symptoms at some time when there are not mood symptoms. In affective psychoses, the hallucinations and delusions should be limited to periods with clear mood symptoms. Typically, formal thought disorder is not part of depression and is less likely to be part of BP than Sz.

The two anxiety disorders that are most likely to be confused with Sz are PTSD and OCD. In each case, the primary question is whether only the anxiety disorder or Sz is present or whether the two conditions are comorbid. Individuals with PTSD and without comorbid Sz frequently present with very detailed hallucinations that tend to occur transiently during periods of stress. There is conflicting information about the extent to which the content of hallucinations is restricted to earlier trauma, but most current evidence suggests this is not the case.[73] Youth may also experience dissociative episodes in which they may seem delusional. Functioning between these episodes is generally fair with some preservation of academic functioning. Youth with apparent OCD symptoms in the context of a Sz diagnosis are usually distinguished by more severe and pervasive premorbid difficulties, more bizarre compulsive behaviors, less relief when they have completed a behavior, and other fears that they cannot easily explain. They may show variability in describing their obsessions as thoughts or voices. They typically will have other sorts of psychotic experiences, including visual hallucinations and thought disorder. In contrast, those with severe OCD may be more likely to have repetitive or superstitious behaviors and speak of "needing" to do things as opposed to being commanded to do things.[74–76]

There is a complex relationship between ASD and Sz that involves shared genetic vulnerabilities, premorbid developmental problems in Sz, and true comorbidity.[77–80] There should be hallucinations or delusions for Sz to be diagnosed in addition to ASD. In most cases, the premorbid features of Sz do not include repetitive behaviors. Youth with ASD tend to describe their possibly psychotic symptoms in highly perseverate ways but do not have formal thought disorder. There are also marked differences in course. Youth with ASD often show some improvement in functioning as they mature, whereas those with Sz show deterioration.

SUMMARY

Hallucinations and poorly formed delusions are relatively common in childhood and adolescence. However, they are seldom volunteered. These symptoms may reflect a wide range of medical and psychiatric disorders, signal heightened risk for future psychiatric disorders, or be transient benign phenomena. Consequently, clinicians should specifically inquire about positive psychotic symptoms using developmentally and culturally appropriate language. Failure to accurately diagnosis psychiatric and medical illnesses when present may lead to delays in effective treatment and worse prognosis.

REFERENCES

1. Remschmidt H, Theisen FM. Schizophrenia and related disorders in children and adolescents. J Neural Transm Suppl 2005;(69):121–41.
2. Masi G, Mucci M, Pari C. Children with schizophrenia: clinical picture and pharmacological treatment. CNS Drugs 2006;20(10):841–66.
3. Remschmidt HE, Schulz E, Martin M, et al. Childhood-onset schizophrenia: history of the concept and recent studies. Schizophr Bull 1994;20(4):727–45.
4. Russell AT. The clinical presentation of childhood-onset schizophrenia. Schizophr Bull 1994;20(4):631–46.

5. Spencer EK, Campbell M. Children with schizophrenia: diagnosis, phenomenology, and pharmacotherapy. Schizophr Bull 1994;20(4):713–25.
6. Werry JS, McClellan JM, Andrews LK, et al. Clinical features and outcome of child and adolescent schizophrenia. Schizophr Bull 1994;20(4):619–30.
7. Kelleher I, Connor D, Clarke MC, et al. Prevalence of psychotic symptoms in childhood and adolescence: a systematic review and meta-analysis of population-based studies. Psychol Med 2012;42(9):1857–63.
8. Kelleher I, Keeley H, Corcoran P, et al. Clinicopathological significance of psychotic experiences in non-psychotic young people: evidence from four population-based studies. Br J Psychiatry 2012;201(1):26–32.
9. Kelleher I, Murtagh A, Molloy C, et al. Identification and characterization of prodromal risk syndromes in young adolescents in the community: a population-based clinical interview study. Schizophr Bull 2012;38(2):239–46.
10. Kelleher I, Harley M, Lynch F, et al. Associations between childhood trauma, bullying and psychotic symptoms among a school-based adolescent sample. Br J Psychiatry 2008;193(5):378–82.
11. Kelleher I, Lynch F, Harley M, et al. Psychotic symptoms in adolescence index risk for suicidal behavior: findings from 2 population-based case-control clinical interview studies. Arch Gen Psychiatry 2012;69(12):1277–83.
12. Polanczyk G, Moffitt TE, Arseneault L, et al. Etiological and clinical features of childhood psychotic symptoms: results from a birth cohort. Arch Gen Psychiatry 2010;67(4):328–38.
13. Nishida A, Tanii H, Nishimura Y, et al. Associations between psychotic-like experiences and mental health status and other psychopathologies among Japanese early teens. Schizophr Res 2008;99(1–3):125–33.
14. Nishida A, Sasaki T, Nishimura Y, et al. Psychotic-like experiences are associated with suicidal feelings and deliberate self-harm behaviors in adolescents aged 12-15 years. Acta Psychiatr Scand 2010;121(4):301–7.
15. Lataster T, van Os J, Drukker M, et al. Childhood victimisation and developmental expression of non-clinical delusional ideation and hallucinatory experiences: victimisation and non-clinical psychotic experiences. Soc Psychiatry Psychiatr Epidemiol 2006;41(6):423–8.
16. Rubio JM, Sanjuan J, Florez-Salamanca L, et al. Examining the course of hallucinatory experiences in children and adolescents: a systematic review. Schizophr Res 2012;138(2–3):248–54.
17. Simon AE, Cattapan-Ludewig K, Gruber K, et al. Subclinical hallucinations in adolescent outpatients: an outcome study. Schizophr Res 2009;108(1–3): 265–71.
18. Poulton R, Caspi A, Moffitt TE, et al. Children's self-reported psychotic symptoms and adult schizophreniform disorder: a 15-year longitudinal study. Arch Gen Psychiatry 2000;57(11):1053–8.
19. Fisher HL, Caspi A, Poulton R, et al. Specificity of childhood psychotic symptoms for predicting schizophrenia by 38 years of age: a birth cohort study. Psychol Med 2013;10:1–10.
20. Ulloa RE, Birmaher B, Axelson D, et al. Psychosis in a pediatric mood and anxiety disorders clinic: phenomenology and correlates. J Am Acad Child Adolesc Psychiatry 2000;39(3):337–45.
21. Kowatch RA, Youngstrom EA, Danielyan A, et al. Review and meta-analysis of the phenomenology and clinical characteristics of mania in children and adolescents. Bipolar Disord 2005;7(6):483–96.

22. Tillman R, Geller B, Klages T, et al. Psychotic phenomena in 257 young children and adolescents with bipolar I disorder: delusions and hallucinations (benign and pathological). Bipolar Disord 2008;10(1):45–55.

23. McGlashan TH. Adolescent versus adult onset of mania. Am J Psychiatry 1988; 145(2):221–3.

24. Freeman D, Fowler D. Routes to psychotic symptoms: trauma, anxiety and psychosis-like experiences. Psychiatry Res 2009;169(2):107–12.

25. Scott JG, Nurcombe B, Sheridan J, et al. Hallucinations in adolescents with post-traumatic stress disorder and psychotic disorder. Australas Psychiatry 2007;15(1):44–8.

26. Hlastala SA, McClellan J. Phenomenology and diagnostic stability of youths with atypical psychotic symptoms. J Child Adolesc Psychopharmacol 2005;15(3): 497–509.

27. Kerbeshian J, Peng CZ, Burd L. Tourette syndrome and comorbid early-onset schizophrenia. J Psychosom Res 2009;67(6):515–23.

28. Fraser S, Hides L, Philips L, et al. Differentiating first episode substance induced and primary psychotic disorders with concurrent substance use in young people. Schizophr Res 2012;136(1–3):110–5.

29. Fiorentini A, Volonteri LS, Dragogna F, et al. Substance-induced psychoses: a critical review of the literature. Curr Drug Abuse Rev 2011;4(4):228–40.

30. Sosland MD, Edelsohn GA. Hallucinations in children and adolescents. Curr Psychiatry Rep 2005;7(3):180–8.

31. Griffith-Lendering MF, Wigman JT, Prince van Leeuwen A, et al. Cannabis use and vulnerability for psychosis in early adolescence-a TRAILS study. Addiction 2013;108(4):733–40.

32. Compton MT, Kelley ME, Ramsay CE, et al. Association of pre-onset cannabis, alcohol, and tobacco use with age at onset of prodrome and age at onset of psychosis in first-episode patients. Am J Psychiatry 2009;166(11):1251–7.

33. Minozzi S, Davoli M, Bargagli AM, et al. An overview of systematic reviews on cannabis and psychosis: discussing apparently conflicting results. Drug Alcohol Rev 2010;29(3):304–17.

34. Niemi-Pynttari JA, Sund R, Putkonen H, et al. Substance-induced psychoses converting into schizophrenia: a register-based study of 18,478 finnish inpatient cases. J Clin Psychiatry 2013;74(1):e94–9.

35. Merikangas KR, He JP, Brody D, et al. Prevalence and treatment of mental disorders among US children in the 2001-2004 NHANES. Pediatrics 2010;125(1): 75–81.

36. Kessler RC, Avenevoli S, Ries Merikangas K. Mood disorders in children and adolescents: an epidemiologic perspective. Biol Psychiatry 2001;49(12): 1002–14.

37. Lewinsohn PM, Clarke GN, Seeley JR, et al. Major depression in community adolescents: age at onset, episode duration, and time to recurrence. J Am Acad Child Adolesc Psychiatry 1994;33(6):809–18.

38. Hafner H, Nowotny B. Epidemiology of early-onset schizophrenia. Eur Arch Psychiatry Clin Neurosci 1995;245(2):80–92.

39. Maziade M, Gingras N, Rodrigue C, et al. Long-term stability of diagnosis and symptom dimensions in a systematic sample of patients with onset of schizophrenia in childhood and early adolescence. I: nosology, sex and age of onset. Br J Psychiatry 1996;169(3):361–70.

40. Thomsen PH. Schizophrenia with childhood and adolescent onset–a nationwide register-based study. Acta Psychiatr Scand 1996;94(3):187–93.

41. Schimmelmann BG, Conus P, Cotton S, et al. Pre-treatment, baseline, and outcome differences between early-onset and adult-onset psychosis in an epidemiological cohort of 636 first-episode patients. Schizophr Res 2007; 95(1–3):1–8.

42. Luoma S, Hakko H, Ollinen T, et al. Association between age at onset and clinical features of schizophrenia: the Northern Finland 1966 birth cohort study. Eur Psychiatry 2008;23(5):331–5.

43. Caplan R, Shields WD, Mori L, et al. Middle childhood onset of interictal psychosis. J Am Acad Child Adolesc Psychiatry 1991;30(6):893–6.

44. Sakakibara E, Nishida T, Sugishita K, et al. Acute psychosis during the postictal period in a patient with idiopathic generalized epilepsy: postictal psychosis or aggravation of schizophrenia? A case report and review of the literature. Epilepsy Behav 2012;24(3):373–6.

45. Mann A, Machado NM, Liu N, et al. A multidisciplinary approach to the treatment of anti-NMDA-receptor antibody encephalitis: a case and review of the literature. J Neuropsychiatry Clin Neurosci 2012;24(2):247–54.

46. Ginory A, Horst I, Patnaik M, et al. New onset psychosis and limbic encephalitis. J Neuropsychiatry Clin Neurosci 2012;24(2):E25.

47. Yu HH, Lee JH, Wang LC, et al. Neuropsychiatric manifestations in pediatric systemic lupus erythematosus: a 20-year study. Lupus 2006;15(10):651–7.

48. Sibbitt WL Jr, Brandt JR, Johnson CR, et al. The incidence and prevalence of neuropsychiatric syndromes in pediatric onset systemic lupus erythematosus. J Rheumatol 2002;29(7):1536–42.

49. David AS, Prince M. Psychosis following head injury: a critical review. J Neurol Neurosurg Psychiatr 2005;76(Suppl 1):i53–60.

50. Harrison G, Whitley E, Rasmussen F, et al. Risk of schizophrenia and other non-affective psychosis among individuals exposed to head injury: case control study. Schizophr Res 2006;88(1–3):119–26.

51. Lauterbach MD, Stanislawski-Zygaj AL, Benjamin S. The differential diagnosis of childhood- and young adult-onset disorders that include psychosis. J Neuropsychiatry Clin Neurosci 2008;20(4):409–18.

52. Jolin EM, Weller RA, Weller EB. Psychosis in children with velocardiofacial syndrome (22q11.2 deletion syndrome). Curr Psychiatry Rep 2009;11(2): 99–105.

53. Stoddard J, Niendam T, Hendren R, et al. Attenuated positive symptoms of psychosis in adolescents with chromosome 22q11.2 deletion syndrome. Schizophr Res 2010;118(1–3):118–21.

54. Murphy KC, Jones LA, Owen MJ. High rates of schizophrenia in adults with velocardio-facial syndrome. Arch Gen Psychiatry 1999;56(10):940–5.

55. Bassett AS, Chow EW, AbdelMalik P, et al. The schizophrenia phenotype in 22q11 deletion syndrome. Am J Psychiatry 2003;160(9):1580–6.

56. Arinami T, Ohtsuki T, Takase K, et al. Screening for 22q11 deletions in a schizophrenia population. Schizophr Res 2001;52(3):167–70.

57. Hoogendoorn ML, Vorstman JA, Jalali GR, et al. Prevalence of 22q11.2 deletions in 311 Dutch patients with schizophrenia. Schizophr Res 2008;98(1–3): 84–8.

58. Roos JL, Pretorius HW, Karayiorgou M. Clinical characteristics of an Afrikaner founder population recruited for a schizophrenia genetic study. Ann N Y Acad Sci 2009;1151:85–101.

59. Sporn A, Addington A, Reiss AL, et al. 22q11 deletion syndrome in childhood onset schizophrenia: an update. Mol Psychiatry 2004;9(3):225–6.

60. Caplan R, Guthrie D, Tang B, et al. Thought disorder in childhood schizophrenia: replication and update of concept. J Am Acad Child Adolesc Psychiatry 2000; 39(6):771–8.

61. Kamphaus RW, Petoskey MD, Cody AH, et al. A typology of parent rated child behavior for a national U.S. sample. J Child Psychol Psychiatry 1999;40(4): 607–16.

62. Hughes CW, Rintelmann J, Emslie GJ, et al. A revised anchored version of the BPRS-C for childhood psychiatric disorders. J Child Adolesc Psychopharmacol 2001;11(1):77–93.

63. Kelleher I, Harley M, Murtagh A, et al. Are screening instruments valid for psychotic-like experiences? A validation study of screening questions for psychotic-like experiences using in-depth clinical interview. Schizophr Bull 2011;37(2):362–9.

64. Kay SR, Fiszbein A, Opler LA. The Positive and Negative Syndrome Scale (PANSS) for schizophrenia. Schizophr Bull 1987;13:262–76.

65. Andreasen NC. Methods for assessing positive and negative symptoms. Mod Probl Pharmacopsychiatry 1990;24:73–88.

66. Young RC, Biggs JT, Ziegler VE, et al. A rating scale for mania: reliability, validity and sensitivity. Br J Psychiatry 1978;133:429–35.

67. Haddock G, McCarron J, Tarrier N, et al. Scales to measure dimensions of hallucinations and delusions: the psychotic symptom rating scales (PSYRATS). Psychol Med 1999;29(4):879–89.

68. Steel C, Garety PA, Freeman D, et al. The multidimensional measurement of the positive symptoms of psychosis. Int J Methods Psychiatr Res 2007;16(2):88–96.

69. Naz B, Craig TJ, Bromet EJ, et al. Remission and relapse after the first hospital admission in psychotic depression: a 4-year naturalistic follow-up. Psychol Med 2007;37(8):1173–81.

70. Ruggero CJ, Kotov R, Carlson GA, et al. Diagnostic consistency of major depression with psychosis across 10 years. J Clin Psychiatry 2011;72(9): 1207–13.

71. Varghese D, Scott J, Welham J, et al. Psychotic-like experiences in major depression and anxiety disorders: a population-based survey in young adults. Schizophr Bull 2011;37(2):389–93.

72. Bromet EJ, Kotov R, Fochtmann LJ, et al. Diagnostic shifts during the decade following first admission for psychosis. Am J Psychiatry 2011;168(11):1186–94.

73. Jessop M, Scott J, Nurcombe B. Hallucinations in adolescent inpatients with post-traumatic stress disorder and schizophrenia: similarities and differences. Australas Psychiatry 2008;16(4):268–72.

74. Faragian S, Fuchs C, Pashinian A, et al. Age-of-onset of schizophrenic and obsessive-compulsive symptoms in patients with schizo-obsessive disorder. Psychiatry Res 2012;197(1–2):19–22.

75. Cunill R, Castells X, Simeon D. Relationships between obsessive-compulsive symptomatology and severity of psychosis in schizophrenia: a systematic review and meta-analysis. J Clin Psychiatry 2009;70(1):70–82.

76. Poyurovsky M, Faragian S, Shabeta A, et al. Comparison of clinical characteristics, co-morbidity and pharmacotherapy in adolescent schizophrenia patients with and without obsessive-compulsive disorder. Psychiatry Res 2008;159(1–2): 133–9.

77. Yan WL, Guan XY, Green ED, et al. Childhood-onset schizophrenia/autistic disorder and t(1;7) reciprocal translocation: identification of a BAC contig spanning the translocation breakpoint at 7q21. Am J Med Genet 2000;96(6):749–53.

78. Rapoport J, Chavez A, Greenstein D, et al. Autism spectrum disorders and childhood-onset schizophrenia: clinical and biological contributions to a relation revisited. J Am Acad Child Adolesc Psychiatry 2009;48(1):10–8.
79. Reaven JA, Hepburn SL, Ross RG. Use of the ADOS and ADI-R in children with psychosis: importance of clinical judgment. Clin Child Psychol Psychiatry 2008; 13(1):81–94.
80. Sprong M, Becker HE, Schothorst PF, et al. Pathways to psychosis: a comparison of the pervasive developmental disorder subtype Multiple Complex Developmental Disorder and the "At Risk Mental State". Schizophr Res 2008;99(1–3): 38–47.

Genetics of Childhood-onset Schizophrenia

Robert F. Asarnow, PhD[a,b,*], Jennifer K. Forsyth, MA[b]

KEYWORDS

- Childhood-onset schizophrenia • Genetics • Common alleles • GWAS
- Copy number variants • Rare alleles • Autism

KEY POINTS

- Childhood-onset schizophrenia (COS) shares considerable genetic overlap with adult-onset schizophrenia (AOS).
- Causal genes for COS seem to involve both common and rare genetic variants.
- COS is associated with greater familial aggregation of schizophrenia spectrum disorders and a higher rate of rare allelic variants than AOS.
- COS shares genetic overlap with autism.
- The current usefulness of genetic screening for diagnosis and individualized treatment is limited; however, identifying common neural pathways on which multiple genetic variants act offers great promise toward developing novel pharmacologic interventions.

OVERVIEW

Childhood-onset schizophrenia (COS) is an early-onset variant of the more common adult-onset schizophrenia (AOS). Schizophrenia with onset before age 12 years is infrequent. The prevalence rate of COS is fewer than 1 in 10,000.[1] In contrast, the lifetime prevalence of AOS is 4.0 in 1000.[2] Before the Diagnostic and Statistical Manual of Mental Disorders, Third Edition (DSM-III), there were no uniform diagnostic criteria for COS. Thus, early studies of COS included children who today would receive DSM-IV[3] diagnoses of autistic disorder, pervasive developmental disorders (PDDs),

Funding Sources: Della Martin Foundation, NIMH grant MH 72697 (R.F. Asarnow); Della Martin Foundation (J.K. Forsyth).
Conflicts of Interest: None.
[a] Department of Psychiatry and Biobehavioral Sciences, University of California at Los Angeles, Los Angeles, CA 90024, USA; [b] Department of Psychology, University of California at Los Angeles, Los Angeles, CA 90024, USA
* Corresponding author. Department of Psychiatry and Biobehavioral Sciences, University of California at Los Angeles, Los Angeles, CA 90024.
E-mail address: rasarnow@mednet.ucla.edu

Child Adolesc Psychiatric Clin N Am 22 (2013) 675–687
http://dx.doi.org/10.1016/j.chc.2013.06.004
1056-4993/13/$ – see front matter © 2013 Elsevier Inc. All rights reserved.

childpsych.theclinics.com

schizophrenia, or disintegrative psychosis. In addition, there were significant variations among clinicians in how childhood schizophrenia was diagnosed.[4]

Epidemiologic and family studies indicate that genetic variations play a major role in the cause of AOS. Because of the low prevalence of COS, less is known about the role of genetic variations in COS. This article summarizes what is known about the role of genetic variations as risk factors for COS and compares results of genetic studies of COS with those of AOS. Genetic studies of COS parallel genetic studies of the more common AOS. Many genetic studies of COS were designed to determine whether the same genetic risk factors present in AOS occur in COS. The question underlying many of these studies was whether COS was a variant of AOS. To highlight the historical evolution of genetic studies of COS, this article reviews 3 classes of genetic studies: familial aggregation studies, common allele studies, and rare allele studies, in the order in which they historically occurred. The siblings of probands with COS typically have not entered the classic age of risk for schizophrenia. As a result, this review of familial aggregation of schizophrenia-related diagnoses and neurobiological abnormalities in relatives of AOS and COS probands focuses on studies of risk in parents of probands separately from risk in siblings.

FAMILIAL AGGREGATION STUDIES

The first genetic studies of AOS and COS examined family members of patients with AOS or COS to test the hypothesis that schizophrenia, schizophrenia spectrum disorders, and neurobiological abnormalities related to schizophrenia showed familial transmission.

Familial Aggregation of Schizophrenia

Every modern study that has used narrow, operationalized criteria for schizophrenia and collected data through both personal interview and interviews of family members has found that schizophrenia strongly aggregates in families of patients with AOS relative to families of community controls. Adoption and twin studies suggest that genetic factors greatly increase the risk of schizophrenia.[5] Modern family studies showed a 3-fold increase in the relative risk (RR; ie, risk in relatives of AOS probands vs risk in relatives of community controls) for schizophrenia in parents of schizophrenia probands.[5] The morbid risk for parents of AOS probands is 6% compared with 9% for siblings.[6] Thus, there are significant differences in the risk for schizophrenia in the parents and siblings of probands with AOS.

Two early studies[7,8] that used different diagnostic criteria for COS than were used by modern studies found that rates of schizophrenia in families of COS probands were comparable with rates in AOS probands. One study[7] did not use operationalized criteria for schizophrenia but simply stated that the children had psychotic symptoms. Although the other study[8] predated DSM-III it required that, to be diagnosed with COS, children had hallucinations, delusions, or formal thought disorder, but the criteria for these symptoms were not operationalized. An early twin study[7] found a concordance for COS diagnosis for monozygotic twins of 88.2% compared with a concordance of 22.3% in dizygotic twins, resulting in an estimate of heritability of 84.5%. Two modern studies used DSM-III Revised (DSM-III-R) and collected data through both personal interview and interviews of family members. The UCLA study[9] found an RR of 17 for schizophrenia in parents of COS probands. The National Institutes of Mental Health (NIMH) Child Psychiatry Branch[10] study of 95 patients with COS found only 1 case of schizophrenia in parents of COS probands and none in parents of community control probands.

Familial Aggregation of Schizophrenia Spectrum Disorders

Modern family studies find that, in addition to schizophrenia, several other psychiatric disorders tend to aggregate in families of AOS probands. These disorders are termed schizophrenia spectrum disorders. The narrow schizophrenia spectrum includes schizoaffective disorder (depressed type), schizotypal personality disorder, schizophreniform and atypical psychosis, and paranoid personality disorder. The only two studies that determined the RR of schizophrenia spectrum disorders separately for parents (ie, not combined with siblings) of AOS probands found RRs of schizotypal personality and/or paranoid personality disorders of 6.6[11] and 3.0[12] in parents of AOS probands.

In the two modern family studies of COS probands, the RR for schizotypal personality and/or paranoid personality disorders in parents was 10.5[9] and 15.2.[10] In addition, there was an RR of 5.6 for avoidant personality disorder.[9] When schizophrenia was included as a schizophrenia spectrum disorder, the RR for schizophrenia spectrum disorders was 16.9[9] and 15.9[10] in parents of COS probands. The RR for just schizophrenia, schizotypal, or paranoid personality disorders was 15.1 in parents of COS probands.[9] Compared with the RR of 5.8 for schizophrenia, schizotypal, or paranoid personality disorder in a large family study of AOS probands that used similar diagnostic approaches to the UCLA study,[11] the RR risk of schizophrenia and schizophrenia spectrum disorders seems to be greater in parents of COS probands than in parents of AOS probands. The increased rate of schizophrenia spectrum disorders of COS probands is consistent with familial transmission. The greater concordance for schizophrenia in monozygotic than dizygotic twins in the Kallman and Roth[7] twin study suggests that schizophrenia is highly heritable in COS.

Familial Aggregation of Neurobiological Abnormalities

Several neurobiological abnormalities present in patients with AOS are also present in a substantial number of their nonpsychotic first-degree relatives. These abnormalities are sometimes referred to as endophenotypes. Endophenotypes are features that lie intermediate to the phenotype and genotype of schizophrenia[13] and are therefore hypothesized to be closer to the effects of schizophrenia genes than are DSM-IV[3] symptoms of schizophrenia. Given the complexity of the genetic architecture and the heterogeneity of schizophrenia, some have argued that identifying endophenotypes may help in elucidating the causal pathways between putative risk genes and their expression as a clinically identifiable phenotype.[14]

Abnormalities found in the nonpsychotic first-degree relatives of patients with AOS include impairments in neurocognitive functioning, abnormalities in smooth-pursuit eye movements, brain structure, brain electrical activity, and autonomic activity. Many of the abnormalities found in nonpsychotic relative of AOS probands are also found in the nonpsychotic relatives of COS probands. For example, a combination of scores on 3 tests that detect neurocognitive deficits in nonpsychotic relatives of AOS probands identified 20% of mothers and fathers of COS probands compared with 0% of the mothers or fathers of community control probands. There was some diagnostic specificity of the neurocognitive impairments: 12% of mothers of COS probands were identified compared with 0% of attention-deficit/hyperactivity disorder (ADHD) mothers. A cutoff that identified 2% of the fathers of ADHD probands similarly classified 17% of the fathers of COS probands.[15] Nonpsychotic first-degree relatives of patients with COS showed impairments on a measure of attention/executive function[16] and in smooth-pursuit eye tracking,[17] and nonpsychotic siblings of COS probands showed deficits on a procedural skill learning task supported by a cortical-striatal network.[18] A longitudinal study[19] found that before adolescence the nonpsychotic siblings of patients with COS show reduced cortical gray matter in the superior temporal prefrontal areas, but that this reduction normalizes during adolescence. In general, the first-degree relatives of patients with COS show subtle impairments on some of the tasks identified as potential endophenotypes in studies of relatives of patients with AOS.

The presence of these neurobiological abnormalities in nonpsychotic relatives of patients with COS indicates that they do not merely reflect the effects of psychosis. Moreover, a family study of first-degree and second-degree relatives of community control probands with and without family histories of schizophrenia[15] found that impairments in neurocognitive functioning and schizophrenia spectrum disorders were independent expressions of familial liability to schizophrenia. Given that schizophrenia is a complex, polygenic disorder, the genes associated with neurobiological endophenotypes may not be the same set of genes that are associated with psychotic symptoms.

Paralleling the heterogeneity of findings in studies of patients with COS and AOS, many first-degree relatives of patients with schizophrenia do not have neurobiological abnormalities. In addition, there is considerable heterogeneity among relatives who do show neurobiological abnormalities in what abnormalities they have. Not all relatives show the same abnormalities. The neurobiological abnormalities identified in nonpsychotic relatives of patients with COS seem to tap diverse neural networks. It remains to be seen whether there is a common pathway for the neural networks underlying these neurobiological abnormalities. An alternative is that the heterogeneity of neurobiological abnormalities may indicate that impairments in specific neural networks are associated with different sets of susceptibility genes. If this is the case, endophenotypes might identify biologically meaningful subtypes of schizophrenia linked to specific genotypes, thereby providing a clearer link between genetic and phenotypic variation.[20]

STUDIES OF COMMON ALLELES

Studies of complex diseases, including AOS, have been guided until recently by the common disease/common variant hypothesis. This hypothesis proposes that common polymorphisms, classically defined as genetic variants present in more than 1% of the population, might contribute to susceptibility to common diseases.[21] The common disease/common variant hypothesis was stimulated by findings from population genetics that humans have limited genetic variation: most genetic variation in an individual is shared with other members of the species. Studies of some common genetic variants for diseases such as age-related macular degeneration, type 2 diabetes, and Crohn disease have identified numerous common variants associated with increased risk for these complex, polygenic diseases.[21] However, in most complex polygenic disorders, each variation has a small effect on the disease phenotype. It is thought that one of the reasons these polygenic diseases are not rapidly removed through selection is that so many genes influence the phenotype.

Because of the low incidence of COS there are few molecular genetic studies of COS. Of the existing studies, most used a candidate gene approach to examine whether common genetic polymorphisms are associated with COS. The candidate gene approach used a limited number of single-nucleotide polymorphisms (SNPs) to tag common variations in genes selected on an a priori basis. Candidate genes selected for investigation in these studies were chosen largely based on positive associations in AOS samples. A summary of the positive gene associations with COS is shown in **Table 1**.

Table 1
Genes associated with childhood-onset and early-onset schizophrenia in candidate gene studies

Investigators and Year	Study Design	Sample	Significant Associations	Smallest P
Addington et al,[22] 2004	Family-based transmission disequilibrium for 8 G72/G30 locus and 2-marker haplotypes and DAO SNPs	53 COS proband trios, 11 COS proband dyads, 16 psychosis NOS proband trios, 8 psychosis NOS dyads (mixed ethnicity)	3 G72/G30 locus SNPs associated with COS; two 2-marker G72/G30 SNP haplotypes associated with COS; no DAO SNPs associated with COS	.015
Addington et al,[23] 2005	Family-based transmission disequilibrium for 14 GAD1, all haplotypes with 2, 3, and 4 SNPs, and 3 GAD2 SNPs	55 COS + psychosis NOS trios, 11 COS + psychosis NOS dyads (mixed ethnicity)	3 GAD1 SNPs associated with COS; one 4 SNP haplotype associated with COS	.005
Gornick et al,[24] 2005	Family-based transmission disequilibrium for 14 dysbindin SNPs	73 COS + psychosis NOS proband trios, 19 COS + psychosis NOS proband dyads (mixed ethnicity)	1 dysbindin SNP associated with COS; two 2-marker haplotypes containing P3521 associated with COS	.008
Addington et al,[25] 2007	Family-based transmission disequilibrium for 56 NRG1 SNPs and 2 microsatellites	59 COS + psychosis NOS proband trios, 11 COS + psychosis NOS proband dyads (mixed ethnicity)	Several NRG1 SNPs associated with COS; several 2, 3, and 4 SNP haplotypes associated with COS	.0004
Sekizawa et al,[26] 2004	Childhood-onset case vs control design for tryptophan hydroxylase gene polymorphism	51 COS (onset before 16 y) vs 148 healthy controls (Japanese)	AA genotype associated with COS (OR = 1.97)	.0058
Pakhomova et al,[27] 2011	Early-onset case vs control design for BDNF Val/Met polymorphism, 5-HTTLPR, type 2A serotonin receptor, T 102c, D2 dopamine receptor (Taq1A)	65 EOS (onset before 15 y) vs 111 healthy controls (Russian)	ValVal BDNF polymorphism associated with EOS	.03

Abbreviation: OR, odds ratio.

The NIMH Child Psychiatry Branch COS study is the largest and most thoroughly characterized sample of individuals with COS to date. Initiated in 1990, the investigators genotyped COS probands and their parents to determine whether specific genetic polymorphisms were associated with proband status using family-based transmission tests. Results indicated that COS was significantly associated with common polymorphisms in G72/G30,[22] GAD1,[23] dysbindin,[24] and NRG1.[25] Polymorphisms in these genes were also associated with neurobiological and clinical features in COS probands. Individuals with COS with the NRG1 risk alleles showed larger gray and white matter volume in childhood and a steeper rate of volume decline into adolescence relative to individuals with COS without these risk alleles.[25] GAD1 polymorphisms were similarly associated with increased rate of frontal gray matter volume loss.[23] G72/G30 risk alleles were associated with later age of onset and better premorbid functioning in these individuals.[22] In addition, the dysbindin allele was also associated with later age of onset.[24] Other candidate gene studies of individuals with COS and early-onset schizophrenia (EOS) using independent samples have compared the frequencies of gene polymorphisms in COS/EOS cases versus healthy controls. Results from these studies indicated that COS was associated with a polymorphism in the tryptophan hydroxylase gene in a Japanese sample[26] and with the ValVal polymorphism of the BDNF gene in a Russian sample.[27]

Genome-wide Association Studies of AOS

In contrast with candidate gene studies, which examine a limited number of SNPs, genome-wide association studies (GWASs) use a broader array of SNPs to systematically examine the genome independently of any prior hypotheses about susceptibility genes. GWAS approaches are particularly important in studies of schizophrenia because the limited knowledge about the pathobiology of this disorder severely constrains the ability to choose high-quality candidate genes. However, because of the large number of statistical comparisons that are made, strict thresholds of statistical significance are required that place a premium on large sample sizes.[28] Taken collectively, the NIMH COS and UCLA studies have collected data from fewer than 200 patients with COS. Given that an AOS study with a sample size of 16,161 participants did not yield a genome-wide significant result,[28] the COS samples cannot yet support a GWAS study.

Given the similarity of results of familial aggregation and candidate gene studies of COS and AOS probands, it is reasonable to expect that the results of GWAS studies of patients with AOS might extend to patients with COS. Recent reviews and meta-analysis of GWAS studies of AOS probands[28,29] have concluded that:

1. There is a genome-wide significant association between AOS and the major histocompatibility locus on chromosome 6p with an odds ratio of 1.14 to 1.16, as well as with TCF4, a neuronal transcription factor implicated in neurogenesis.
2. The data support a polygenic model of AOS, involving hundreds of genes with small individual effects; polygenic variants collectively account for approximately 30% of the total variation in genetic liability to schizophrenia, and much of the genetic variation in schizophrenia is not accounted for by variations in common alleles.
3. GWAS results have frequently not supported prior reports of associations with classic candidate genes.
4. There is genetic overlap of schizophrenia with autism and bipolar disorder.

STUDIES OF RARE ALLELES

An alternative to the common disease/common allele model is the common disease/rare variant model.[30] Rare alleles are classically defined as genetic variants with a minor allele that occurs in less than 1% of the population.[30] As applied to schizophrenia this model, as discussed by Walsh and colleagues,[31] hypothesizes "that some mutations predisposing to schizophrenia are highly penetrant, individually rare, and of recent origin, even specific to single cases and families." A major focus of studies of rare variants in schizophrenia has been copy number variations (CNVs). The development of microarray-based methods for conducting genome-wide scans for structural variants allowed higher resolution exploration of the structure of chromosomes that led to the discovery that variation in the number of copies of large stretches of DNA (ie, fewer or more than the expected 2 copies) is present in the normal population and also contributes to genetic risk for complex illnesses. CNVs are stretches of genomic deletions and duplications ranging from 1 kb to several Mb, and thus are likely to have larger phenotypic effects than SNPs. Studies of CNVs have begun to change the understanding of the genetic architecture underlying psychiatric illnesses. In addition to the role of common genetic variants in the genetic architecture of AOS and COS, increasing research now points to a key role for variation in chromosomal structure as well.[32]

The first major study[31] of rare structural variants (ie, microduplications and microdeletions) in schizophrenia compared the overall frequency of CNVs in patients with AOS, COS, and ancestry-matched controls. Fifteen percent of patients with schizophrenia with onset after 18 years of age had novel structural variants compared with 5% of controls. Patients with earlier ages of onset had increased frequencies of novel structural variants. Twenty percent of patients with schizophrenia with onset before 18 years of age and 28% of patients with COS carried one or more rare structural variants. Almost every rare structural variant identified in patients was unique. Some deletions and duplications were multiple megabases in size; other variants altered only 1 or a few genes. The mutations found in patients with schizophrenia disproportionately affected genes involved in signaling networks that control brain development, especially those involving neuregulin and glutamate pathways.[31]

The NIMH COS study found that, of 96 patients with COS, 10% showed large chromosomal abnormalities, including 4 individuals with the 3-Mb 22q11.21 deletion, 3 individuals with sex chromosome abnormalities, and 2 individuals with 500-kb duplications at 16p11.2; all at rates significantly higher than those seen in the general population or in AOS.[33] Two novel duplications disrupting the MYT1L gene on chromosome 2p25.3, one 2.5-Mb deletion on chromosome 2q31.2-31.3, 1 novel 115-kb deletion on NRXN1, and one 120-kb duplication overlapping exons in the SRGAP3 gene on chromosome 3p25.3 were also found in additional patients with COS.[33] Individual case reports have identified additional rare and de novo mutations in other individuals with COS, including a novel frameshift mutation in UPF3B,[34] a de novo missense mutation in the gene encoding SHANK3[35] and a 1.58-Mb de novo 3q29 deletion encompassing numerous genes.[36]

As noted earlier, the concordance rates for schizophrenia are greater than expected in monozygotic than dizygotic twins.[7] Deleterious de novo mutations, which enter the gene pool for only a brief time because they reduce fecundity, are therefore rarely transmitted and may be the simplest way to account for large discrepancies between monozygotic and dizygotic concordance rates.[37] A similar monozygotic/dizygotic pattern is observed in twin studies of autism and AOS, disorders for which de novo variation has already been shown to be a significant contributor.[38] In line with this, most COS cases in the NIMH and UCLA cohorts are apparently sporadic even after detailed diagnostic evaluations of family members were conducted.

Furthermore, there is a strong monotonic increase in the risk for AOS with increasing paternal age. One explanation of this finding is that older fathers have a higher rate of de novo mutations. Malaspina and colleagues[39] state that sporadic cases of AOS had significantly older fathers than cases with a family history of schizophrenia "supports the hypothesis that de novo mutations contribute to the risk of sporadic schizophrenia." The effect of paternal age on risk for COS has not been rigorously examined.

GENE-ENVIRONMENT INTERACTION

A widely accepted working model of schizophrenia hypothesizes that abnormalities during embryonic brain development are caused by genetic variations. Tsuang[6] states that "Environmental insults such as fetal hypoxia during delivery and infection in the second trimester of pregnancy interact with the genotype to produce the neuropathology and cognitive deficits." In AOS, a history of obstetric complications is associated with having an earlier age of onset of schizophrenia than in patients without a history of obstetric complications.[40]

The NIMH COS study did not find an increased rate of obstetric complications in COS probands.[41] In contrast, a Japanese study[42] found increased rates of obstetric complications, particularly for boys, in patients with COS compared with children with other psychiatric disorders. Histories of obstetric complications are found in children with several neuropsychiatric conditions besides COS. Neither study examined whether obstetric complications interacted with family history of schizophrenia.

PLEIOTROPY: OVERLAP WITH AUTISM

Variation in a gene can result in multiple phenotypes. This variation is referred to as pleiotropy. For example, in humans, colon/lung cancer and familial Parkinson disease are both associated with variations in the PARK2 gene.[43] Based on phenomenological and follow-up data in DSM-IV, autism and schizophrenia are separate and distinct disorders. However, molecular genetic studies suggest considerable overlap between these disorders. Forty-five genes have been evaluated for positive associations with both autism and AOS or COS. Although failures to replicate have been common, at least 20 of these genes were positively associated with both autism and schizophrenia, 2 genes were positive for autism and not schizophrenia, 11 genes were positive for schizophrenia and not autism, and 12 genes were negatively associated with both disorders.[44] Moreover, there are increased rates of rare CNVs that sometimes overlap in children with autism and children with schizophrenia.[36,45] Thus, increasing evidence suggests some overlap in genetic risk for COS and autism.

SUMMARY

Schizophrenia (AOS and COS) is a highly heritable disorder with a heterogeneous genomic architecture. Like autism, there are at least 2 distinct genetic mechanisms for acquiring schizophrenia, one through de novo mutations resulting in rare alleles in simplex families, and one through inheritance of common alleles of small effect in multiplex families. Most of the mutations associated with schizophrenia are currently thought to be rare alleles.[46]

The adult-onset and childhood-onset forms of schizophrenia seem to overlap genetically. The differences between AOS and COS seem to be quantitative. There is a greater aggregation of schizophrenia and schizophrenia spectrum disorders in first-degree relatives of patients with COS compared with first-degree relatives of patients with AOS. In addition, the occurrence of rare alleles, mostly de novo, seems to be higher in patients with COS compared with patients with AOS. Other than these quantitative differences, genetic studies have offered little insight thus far into why, in rare cases, the first onset of schizophrenia occurs before adolescence, which is perhaps the most interesting question to be addressed in future genetic studies of COS.

The recent findings on common and rare alleles shed light on a question that has long puzzled geneticists. How has schizophrenia persisted in the gene pool given the adverse effect of this disorder on fertility? Negative selection predicts the removal of most risk alleles with major deleterious effects. In schizophrenia (and other neuropsychiatric disorders such as autism), common risk alleles have small effects and alleles with large penetrance (eg, CNVs) are rare. Multiple common alleles are required to develop schizophrenia. The increase in risk conferred by any one common allele is small. Duan and colleagues[29] state that, "Rare risk alleles are either of recent origin if highly penetrant, or older mutations with smaller effect which have not yet been eliminated by selection."

Both the common disease/common variant and rare allele models face challenges in explicating the genetic mechanisms for the transmission of schizophrenia. The common disease/common variant model accounts for a small percentage of cases, and any 1 allelic variation, with rare exceptions, confers only a small amount of risk for schizophrenia. In contrast, alleles with large penetrance (eg, CNVs) are rare, and negative selection predicts the removal of most risk alleles with major deleterious effects from the population gene pool, which suggests that the genomes of individuals with these conditions are unusually fragile.[30] However, Schork and colleagues[30] state that, "the unique phenotypes of autism, schizophrenia and bipolar disorder seem too specific for a gross molecular lesion such as global genomic instability."

The common disease/common variant and rare allele models of schizophrenia also have the challenge of explaining how either many different common alleles of small effect, or many different rare (in many cases unique) mutations can eventuate in the same clinical phenotype: schizophrenic symptoms. The corresponding challenge for both models is to account for how many of the common allelic variants and the propensity for rare variants found in schizophrenia are also frequently present in autism and bipolar disorder.

What both sets of challenges indicate is that, in schizophrenia, the pathways from genotype to phenotype are complex. Mapping the pathways from allelic variation to the symptoms of schizophrenia requires a deeper understanding of both the schizophrenia phenotype and the genetic mechanisms that increase risk for this disorder than is implied in earlier, simpler models of the genetic transmission of schizophrenia. This process has been further complicated by research suggesting that gene expression can be regulated by genes in noncoding regions of the genome and has led to interest in sequencing the noncoding regions to identify epistatic interactions with putative susceptibility genes. Thus, it is increasingly evident that a systems biology approach that, as Duan and colleagues[29] put it, "integrates genomic, transcriptomic, and proteomic data, metabolomics, gene networks, epigenetics and environmental factors" must be integrated with data on neural networks in order to elucidate the pathways from allelic variations to specific schizophrenia phenotypes. The findings briefly summarized earlier on genetic mechanisms and phenotypes in schizophrenia put in focus the necessity of this approach for both COS and AOS.

RELEVANCE OF GENETICS TO CLINICIANS/IMPLICATIONS FOR CLINICAL PRACTICE

In several areas of medicine, genetic information is beginning to be used to refine diagnoses and individualize treatment. For example, BRCA mutation in either of the BRCA1 or BRCA2 genes can result in a hereditary breast-ovarian cancer syndrome that accounts for 5% to 10% of breast cancer cases in women. Approximately 50% to 65% of women born with a deleterious mutation in BRCA1 and 40% to 57% of women with a deleterious mutation in BRCA2 develop breast cancer by age 70 years. In addition, there are implications for prognosis and treatment of having a BRAC1 versus BRAC2 mutation. For example, Imyanitov and colleagues[47] state that "multiple lines of evidence indicate that women with BRCA1-related BC may derive less benefit from taxane-based treatment than other categories of BC patients." In contrast with BRAC1 and BRAC2 mutations in breast and ovarian cancer, the allelic mutations associated with increased risk for schizophrenia detected so far offer little immediate prospect for helping to refine diagnosis or guide treatment. Each mutation in common alleles has a very small effect on risk for schizophrenia and it seems that some combination of multiple common alleles is required to substantially increase schizophrenia risk. In contrast, rare alleles may have larger effects on risk but they are idiosyncratic and therefore not useful in screening populations for schizophrenia risk. In line with this complexity and heterogeneity of genetic risk for schizophrenia, individualized treatment based on knowledge of individual genotypes seems an unrealistic goal for the foreseeable future.

In contrast, elucidating the neurobiological pathways from genes to specific schizophrenia phenotypes offers an important opportunity to identify new therapeutic targets for drug development, which is of vital interest because of the current limited understanding of the pathobiology of schizophrenia. The limited understanding of the pathobiology of schizophrenia stems from the absence of good animal or molecular models of schizophrenia. Identifying the common pathways through which multiple genes adversely affect complex neural systems offers great promise in beginning to identify new therapeutic targets for this debilitating condition.

Summary

Implications for clinical practice

- COS is a rare variant of AOS
- COS shares genetic overlap with autism
- Causal genes for COS include both common variants of small effect and rare variants with larger effect
- The current usefulness of genetic screening for COS diagnosis and individualized treatment is limited
- Identifying common neural pathways on which multiple genetic variants act offers promise toward developing novel pharmacologic interventions

REFERENCES

1. Burd L, Kerbeshian J. A North Dakota prevalence study of schizophrenia presenting in childhood. J Am Acad Child Adolesc Psychiatry 1987;26:347–50.
2. McGrath J, Saha S, Chant D, et al. Schizophrenia: a concise overview of incidence, prevalence, and mortality. Epidemiol Rev 2008;30:67–76.
3. American Psychiatric Association. Diagnostic and statistical manual of mental disorders. 4th edition. Washington, DC: Author; 1994.
4. Asarnow RF. Childhood schizophrenia. In: Beauchaine TP, Hinshaw SP, editors. Child and adolescent psychopathology;. p. 685–713.
5. Kendler KS, Diehl SR. The genetics of schizophrenia: a current, genetic-epidemiologic perspective. Schizophr Bull 1993;19:261–85.

6. Tsuang M. Schizophrenia: genes and environment. Biol Psychiatry 2000;47: 210–20.
7. Kallmann FJ, Roth B. Genetic aspects of pre-adolescent schizophrenia. Am J Psychiatry 1956;112:599–606.
8. Kolvin I, Ounsted C, Richardson L, et al. Studies in the childhood psychoses, III: the family and social background in childhood psychoses. Br J Psychiatry 1971; 118:396–402.
9. Asarnow RF, Nuechterlein KH, Fogelson D, et al. Schizophrenia and schizophrenia-spectrum personality disorders in the first-degree relatives of children with schizophrenia: the UCLA family study. Arch Gen Psychiatry 2001;58: 581–8.
10. Nicholson R, Brookner FB, Lenane M, et al. Parental schizophrenia spectrum disorders in childhood-onset and adult-onset schizophrenia. Am J Psychiatry 2003;160:490–5.
11. Kendler KS, McGuire M, Gruenberg AM, et al. The Roscommon family study: I. Methods, diagnosis of probands, and risk of schizophrenia in relatives. Arch Gen Psychiatry 1993;50:527–40.
12. Baron M, Gruen R, Asnis L, et al. Familial transmission of schizotypal and borderline personality disorders. Am J Psychiatry 1985;142:927–34.
13. Gottesman II, Shields J. Genetic theorizing and schizophrenia. Br J Psychiatry 1973;122:15–30.
14. Nenadic I, Gaser C, Sauer H. Heterogeneity of brain structural variation and the structural imaging endophenotypes in schizophrenia. Neuropsychobiology 2012; 66:44–9.
15. Asarnow RF, Nuechterlein KH, Subotnik KL, et al. Neurocognitive impairments in nonpsychotic parents of children with schizophrenia and attention-deficit/ hyperactivity disorder: the University of California, Los Angeles family study. Arch Gen Psychiatry 2002;59:1053–60.
16. Gochman PA, Greenstein D, Sporn A, et al. Childhood onset schizophrenia: familial neurocognitive measures. Schizophr Res 2004;71:43–7.
17. Sporn A, Greenstein D, Gogtay N, et al. Childhood-onset schizophrenia: smooth pursuit eye-tracking dysfunction in family members. Schizophr Res 2005;73: 243–52.
18. Wagshal D, Knowlton BJ, Cohen JR, et al. Deficits in probabilistic classification learning and liability for schizophrenia. Psychiatry Res 2012;200: 167–72.
19. Mattai AA, Weisinger B, Greenstein D, et al. Normalization of cortical gray matter deficits in nonpsychotic siblings of patients with childhood-onset schizophrenia. J Am Acad Child Adolesc Psychiatry 2011;50:697–704.
20. Greenwood TA, Lazzeroni LC, Murray SS, et al. Analysis of 94 candidate genes and 12 endophenotypes for schizophrenia from the Consortium on the Genetics of Schizophrenia. Am J Psychiatry 2011;168:930–46.
21. Altshuler D, Daly MJ, Lander ES. Genetic mapping in human disease. Science 2008;322:881–8.
22. Addington AM, Gornick M, Sporn AL, et al. Polymorphisms in the 13q33.2 gene G72/G30 are associated with childhood-onset schizophrenia and psychosis not otherwise specified. Biol Psychiatry 2004;55:976–80.
23. Addington AM, Gornick M, Duckworth J, et al. GAD1 (2q31.1), which encodes glutamic acid decarboxylase (GAD-sub-6-sub-7), is associated with childhood-onset schizophrenia and cortical gray matter volume loss. Mol Psychiatry 2005; 10:581–8.

24. Gornick MC, Addington AM, Sporn A, et al. Dysbindin (DTNBP1, 6p22.3) is associated with childhood-onset psychosis and endophenotypes measured by the Premorbid Adjustment Scale (PAS). J Autism Dev Disord 2005;35:831–8.
25. Addington AM, Gornick MC, Shaw P, et al. Neuregulin 1 (8p12) and childhood-onset schizophrenia: susceptibility haplotypes for diagnosis and brain developmental trajectories. Mol Psychiatry 2007;2:195–205.
26. Sekizawa T, Iwata Y, Nakamura K, et al. Childhood-onset schizophrenia and tryptophan hydroxylase gene polymorphism. Am J Med Genet B Neuropsychiatr Genet 2004;128B:24–6.
27. Pakhomova SA, Korovaitseva GI, Monchakovskaya MY, et al. Molecular genetic studies of early-onset schizophrenia. Neurosci Behav Physiol 2011;41:532–5.
28. Gejman PV, Sanders AR, Kendler KS. Genetics of schizophrenia: new findings and challenges. Annu Rev Genomics Hum Genet 2011;12:121–44.
29. Duan J, Sanders AR, Gejman PV. Genome-wide approaches to schizophrenia. Brain Res Bull 2010;83:93–102.
30. Schork NJ, Murray SS, Frazer KA, et al. Common vs. rare allele hypotheses for complex diseases. Curr Opin Genet Dev 2009;19:212–9.
31. Walsh T, McClellan JM, McCarthy SE, et al. Rare structural variants disrupt multiple genes in neurodevelopmental pathways in schizophrenia. Science 2008; 320:539–43.
32. Hoffman EJ, State MW. Progress in cytogenetics: implications for child psychopathology. J Am Acad Child Adolesc Psychiatry 2010;49:736–51.
33. Addington AM, Rapoport JL. The genetics of childhood-onset schizophrenia: when madness strikes the prepubescent. Curr Psychiatry Rep 2009;11: 156–61.
34. Addington AM, Gauthier J, Piton A, et al. A novel frameshift mutation in UPF3B identified in brothers affected with childhood onset schizophrenia and autism spectrum disorders. Mol Psychiatry 2011;16:238–9.
35. Gauthier J, Champagne N, Lafreniere RG, et al. De novo mutations in the gene encoding the synaptic scaffolding protein SHANK3 in patients ascertained for schizophrenia. Proc Natl Acad Sci U S A 2010;107:7863–8.
36. Sagar A, Bishop JR, Tessman C, et al. Co-occurrence of autism, childhood psychosis, and intellectual disability associated with a de novo 3q29 microdeletion. Am J Med Genet A 2013;161:845–9.
37. Zhao X, Leotta A, Kustanovich V, et al. A unified genetic theory for sporadic and inherited autism. Proc Natl Acad Sci U S A 2007;104:12831–6.
38. El-Fishawy P, State M. The genetics of autism: key issues, recent findings and clinical implications. Psychiatr Clin North Am 2010;33:83–105.
39. Malaspina D, Corcoran C, Fahim C, et al. Paternal age and sporadic schizophrenia: evidence for de novo mutations. Am J Med Genet 2002;114:299–303.
40. Geddes JR, Lawrie S. Obstetric complications and schizophrenia: a meta-analysis. Br J Psychiatry 1995;167:786–93.
41. Rapoport JL, Addington AM, Frangou S. The neurodevelopmental model of schizophrenia: update 2005. Mol Psychiatry 2005;10:439–49.
42. Matsumoto H, Takei N, Saito H, et al. Childhood-onset schizophrenia and obstetric complications: a case-control study. Schizophr Res 1999;38:93–9.
43. Veeriah S, Taylor BS, Meng S, et al. Somatic mutations of the Parkinson's disease-associated gene PARK2 in glioblastoma and other human malignancies. Nat Genet 2010;42:77–82.
44. Crespi B, Stead P, Elliott M. Comparative genomics of autism and schizophrenia. Proc Natl Acad Sci U S A 2010;107:1736–41.

45. Rapoport J, Chavez A, Greenstein D, et al. Autism spectrum disorders and childhood-onset schizophrenia: clinical and biological contributions to a relation revisited. J Am Acad Child Adolesc Psychiatry 2009;48:10–8.
46. Akil H, Brenner S, Kandel E, et al. The future of psychiatric research: genomes and neural circuits. Science 2010;327:1580–1.
47. Imyanitov EN, Moiseyenko VM. Drug therapy for hereditary cancers. Hered Cancer Clin Pract 2011;9:5.

Gray Matter Alterations in Schizophrenia High-Risk Youth and Early-Onset Schizophrenia

A Review of Structural MRI Findings

Benjamin K. Brent, MD, MS[a,b,c,d,*],
Heidi W. Thermenos, PhD[a,b,c,d,e], Matcheri S. Keshavan, MD[a,b,c],
Larry J. Seidman, PhD[a,b,c,d]

KEYWORDS

- Schizophrenia • Structural MRI • Genetic high-risk • Prodrome
- Early-onset schizophrenia • Childhood-onset schizophrenia

KEY POINTS

- Structural magnetic resonance imaging (MRI) evidence indicates that the adolescent/young adult development of individuals at genetic and clinical high risk for schizophrenia, as well as of persons with early-onset schizophrenia, is associated with smaller brain volumes, particularly in frontotemporal cortical areas.
- There is evidence implicating the disruption of both early (ie, perinatal) and late (ie, adolescent) normal neurodevelopmental processes, which lends support to the 2-hit neurodevelopmental model of schizophrenia.
- Future longitudinal studies that control for diagnostic variability, age and gender effects, and that examine the evolution of structural brain changes in at-risk youth/young adults in the context of evolving changes of white matter, brain function, and neurocognition will contribute to improving the clinical applicability of structural MRI findings during the premorbid and prodromal periods to early intervention strategies for illness prevention.

Grant Support: This project was supported in part by a KL2 Medical Research Investigator Training (MeRIT) award from Harvard Catalyst and The Harvard Clinical and Translational Science Center, NIH KL2 RR 025757 (B.K. Brent), NIMH MH081928, MH065571, and MH092840, and the Commonwealth Research Center of the Massachusetts Department of Mental Health, SCDMH82101008006 (L.J. Seidman), and by NIMH RO1 64023, 78113 and, KO2 01180 (M.S. Keshavan).
Disclosures: The authors report no financial disclosures or conflicts of interest.
[a] Harvard Medical School, Boston, MA 02115, USA; [b] Division of Public Psychiatry, Massachusetts Mental Health Center, 75 Fenwood Road, Boston, MA 02115, USA; [c] Department of Psychiatry, Beth Israel Deaconess Medical Center, 330 Brookline Avenue, Boston, MA 02215, USA; [d] Department of Psychiatry, Massachusetts General Hospital, Boston, MA 02114, USA; [e] Athinoula A. Martinos Imaging Center, Building 149, 2nd Floor, Room 2602E, 13th Street, Charlestown, MA 02129, USA
* Corresponding author. Department of Psychiatry, Beth Israel Deaconess Medical Center, 330 Brookline Avenue, Boston, MA 02215.
E-mail address: bbrent@bidmc.harvard.edu

INTRODUCTION

Neuroimaging studies over the last 4 decades have provided overwhelming evidence that schizophrenia is a disorder involving widespread abnormalities of brain structure.[1] It is believed that the neurobiological processes underlying these structural abnormalities are central to the pathophysiology of schizophrenia.[2] However, the specific mechanisms involved in producing the structural deficits of schizophrenia remain incompletely understood. Although no focal brain abnormality has been identified unequivocally, structural abnormalities, including enlargement of the lateral and third ventricles, and reduced lateral temporal cortical, medial temporal, and prefrontal lobe volumes, are consistently reported in persons with schizophrenia.[1] Further, alterations of brain structure are linked with key psychotic symptoms (eg, auditory hallucinations,[3] delusions[4]), neurocognitive deficits,[5] and social dysfunction[6] in schizophrenia.

Neurodevelopmental models hypothesize that pathologic processes occurring during early (ie, perinatally) or late (ie, adolescent/young adult) brain development (eg, aberrant migration of neuronal precursor cells during gestation or excessive dendritic pruning during adolescence) may be key to the emergence of the brain structural alterations occurring in schizophrenia.[7,8] Growing evidence from studies of typically developing children shows that brain maturational processes continue well into adolescence.[9] Neuroimaging studies, for example, reveal changes in the rates of gray matter (GM) to white matter (WM) during the second decade of life, with increases in WM (largely comprising myelinated axon bundles) accompanied by reductions in GM (an index of cellular and unmyelinated fiber density).[10,11] It is believed that, at least in part, these findings indicate changes in cellular-level processes, such as myelinization by oligodendrocytes (increased WM) and neuronal apoptosis, resulting in dendritic pruning (GM reduction), which together contribute to improved regional communication and more efficient neuronal coding over the course of adolescence.[12] In addition, several studies suggest a characteristic temporal pattern of GM reduction, with structural decrements proceeding from posterior cortical areas (eg, parietal cortex) during childhood to anterior brain regions (eg, prefrontal cortex [PFC]) during late adolescence and early adulthood.[13,14] It has been hypothesized that this lag in PFC GM maturation may result in an imbalance during adolescence between earlier developing mesolimbic structures mediating responses to pleasurable stimuli (ie, the reward circuitry of the brain) and less fully developed prefrontal brain areas involved in response inhibition and cognitive control.[12] Thus, the trajectories of structural brain changes in normal development are increasingly believed to provide a neurobiological basis for the increase in impulsivity and risk-taking behavior that contributes to making adolescence a period of heightened risk for the emergence of a broad range of psychopathology, including schizophrenia.[15]

Several lines of evidence provide substantial support for the neurodevelopmental hypothesis that alterations of normal brain maturational processes are implicated in the characteristic structural abnormalities of schizophrenia. This evidence, reviewed extensively elsewhere,[2,16,17] includes:

1. Neuropathologic findings in schizophrenia consistent with microneuroanatomical alterations (eg, abnormal laminal organization and orientation of neurons) associated with gestational development in the prefrontal, cingulate, and lateral temporal cortices, as well as the hippocampus.[18–20]
2. Structural magnetic resonance imaging (MRI) observations of abnormal prefrontal or temporal cortical surface morphology in adult-onset[21] and early-onset schizophrenia (EOS),[22] as well as in adolescents at genetic high risk (GHR) for

schizophrenia,[23] that are believed to reflect perturbations of gyrification during early development.

3. Reduced cortical neuropil and somal size found in postmortem studies of schizophrenia,[24,25] suggestive of dysregulated apoptosis or synaptic pruning in adolescence.

4. Immunohistochemical and genetic linkage and association studies[26] implicating gene mutations in persons with schizophrenia that are believed to disrupt normal cortical developmental processes (eg, early synaptogenesis [eg, RELN[27]] and changes in dendritic spines during adolescence [eg, DISC 1[28]]).

5. Animal models showing that early alterations of GM development produce later abnormalities of adolescent cortical function, which are analogous to those observed in schizophrenia.[29]

Despite the accumulating evidence for brain dysmaturation during childhood and adolescent development in schizophrenia, many questions regarding the pathophysiology of the structural brain abnormalities of schizophrenia remain unanswered. For example, it is not clear when GM loss first begins during development[1] (eg, whether less GM in schizophrenia is the product of primarily early [intrauterine/perinatal], or late [periadolescent/early adult] dysmaturational processes, or some combination of the 2). Further, how environmental, or epigenetic risk or protective factors might influence the course of neurodevelopment, or how alterations of brain structure are specifically linked to the emergence of psychotic symptoms has yet to be determined. In addition, it is acknowledged that although there has been significant growth in neuroscientific understanding of normal brain development, few studies have focused directly on youth (age <18 years) who develop schizophrenia (ie, EOS),[30] or adolescents or young adults (age <30 years) at risk for the illness (whether by virtue of family relatedness to a person with schizophrenia (GHR), or as a result of symptoms or functional decline believed to indicate clinical high risk (CHR) for full-blown psychosis). Characterizing the structural brain changes observed in studies of youth/young adults as GHR or CHR for schizophrenia, as well as in EOS, may be critical to refining current understanding of the timing and pathophysiology of these alterations. It may also help us to identify individuals who could benefit from early treatment interventions. Toward this end, this article provides a selective review of structural MRI findings in pediatric at-risk populations and EOS. The goal is to identify the common findings and gaps in current knowledge regarding structural brain changes associated with the trajectory of schizophrenia risk in youth and young adult development to provide future directions for research.

STRUCTURAL MRI FINDINGS IN GHR FOR SCHIZOPHRENIA INDIVIDUALS

Based on the evidence regarding the strong heritability of schizophrenia, approximately 60% to 80% of the liability to schizophrenia is caused by genes[31] – GHR structural MRI research has focused on the identification of neural abnormalities during the adolescent and young adult development of nonpsychotic, first-degree relatives of persons with schizophrenia. This work is motivated by the drive to understand brain development before psychosis and to observe it largely without medication and illness state–related confounds that commonly complicate schizophrenia research. According to the GHR model,[32] it is hypothesized that schizophrenia results from the cumulative vulnerability of multiple genetic and environmental factors, each associated with small effects. Before the onset of psychosis, subclinical neuroanatomical, or other abnormalities (eg, reduced hippocampal GM volume, or neurocognitive deficits) are believed to be reliably detectable and expressed in nonpsychotic, first-degree relatives of patients, who on average share 50% of genes with their affected family member.[33] A particular strength of the GHR approach is that it allows for the identification of neural markers of schizophrenia risk preceding psychosislike symptoms. Findings from GHR research, therefore, could contribute to greater understanding of pathophysiologic processes associated with early development, as well as to the identification of vulnerability markers that may be particularly useful for early detection strategies for psychosis prevention.[7,34] In addition, longitudinal GHR research in children and adolescents may be able to distinguish temporally distal neuroanatomical abnormalities associated with schizophrenia risk from those more closely linked to the timing of psychosis onset.[7]

Recently, our group has performed a comprehensive review[35] of all GHR MRI studies involving individuals 30 years of age or younger, bringing together the results from 14 independent research groups, 12 of which have contributed structural MRI data (**Table 1**). Studies included in this review used a variety of MRI morphometric techniques (eg, voxel-based morphometry and manual parcellation), as well as differing MRI software packages (eg, Statistical Parametric Mapping [SPM (Wellcome Department of Imaging Neuroscience, University College London, UK)], FreeSurfer [Athinoula A. Martinos Center for Biomedical Imaging, Charlestown, MA]) and methods to correct for multiple comparisons (eg, whole brain vs region-of-interest (ROI)). The main findings are summarized in the following sections.

Cross-Sectional Findings

In cross-sectional analyses, GHR youth have most consistently shown evidence for smaller PFC GM, including reduced cortical thickness,[36–38] volume (inferior frontal gyrus,[39–42] frontal pole,[43] medial PFC[43]), or gyral surface area[44] compared with controls. Other brain areas where GHR has reliably shown less GM compared with controls include: temporal cortex (decreased bilateral superior temporal gyrus [STG] volume[45,46] and surface area,[47] bilateral temporal lobe cortical thinning[36,37]), parietal cortex (decreased GM volume[37,42,48] and reduced cortical thickness[38,49]), and medial temporal/limbic regions (hippocampus,[50–55] parahippocampus,[36,56] anterior cingulate cortex[36,57]). More variable findings have been reported with respect to smaller GM in GHR versus controls in occipital cortex, cerebellum, amygdala, thalamus, and basal ganglia.[35] Significant associations between higher levels of attenuated psychotic symptoms and smaller GM in PFC,[57–59] temporal cortex,[60–62] parietal cortex,[59] amygdala,[59,61,62] and cerebellum[61,62] in GHR youth or young adults have been reported. Regarding age-related neural alterations, significantly less GM has been observed in GHR samples with children as young as 7 years.[48] However, there are insufficient data regarding neural alterations at specific ages, or developmental periods (eg, middle childhood vs adolescence), to draw firm conclusions about the onset of GM loss in GHR youth.[35] Only 1 research group has found greater GM in GHR youth compared with controls.[40] This finding included increased cortical thickness of PFC (inferior orbital, middle frontal gyri), temporal cortex (right STG), and parietal cortex (angular gyrus, inferior parietal cortex).[40] Thus, there is substantial evidence, most consistently involving PFC and hippocampus, of less GM volume in high-risk (HR) individuals than controls.

Longitudinal Findings

Two research groups (Pittsburgh High Risk (PHR) and Edinburgh (EHR)) have performed longitudinal studies of GHR first-degree adolescent or young adult relatives of patients with adult-onset schizophrenia. Consistent with the cross-sectional findings, both groups showed progressive reductions of PFC volume over time (1 year follow-up [PHR], and 10 year follow-up [EHR]) in GHR compared with controls.[49,58,63]

Further, progressive decline in PFC GM has been linked with greater symptom levels in GHR individuals, including those who developed schizophrenia.[59,63] Similar associations between increasing levels of symptoms and significant deceases in temporal cortical GM volume over time have also been reported.[59,63] An association between greater symptom severity and progressive decline in parietal cortex volume was reported in 1 study.[59]

A third research group has performed a longitudinal GHR study focused on the development of brain structure in the very healthy siblings of individuals with childhood-onset schizophrenia (COS) (ie, schizophrenia occurring in affected individuals <age 13 years). As with GHR studies involving first-degree relatives of people with adult-onset schizophrenia, COS relatives initially show significant GM reductions of PFC, temporal, and parietal cortex.[37,38] However, over time, these structural alterations were found to normalize, with no significant GM cortical decrements detected among COS relatives compared with controls by the end of adolescence (ages 17–20 years).[38] None of the nonaffected COS siblings developed psychosis during the follow-up period and, thus, may have comprised particularly resilient individuals. By contrast, findings from studies involving families with strong evidence of genetic loading (ie, EHR, in which relatives had at least 2 affected family members[63]), or in the offspring of persons with schizophrenia (ie, PHR[49]), there is mounting evidence for accelerated reduction in PFM GM in GHR individuals, particularly those who become symptomatic or go on to develop schizophrenia (~10%).

STRUCTURAL MRI FINDINGS IN CHR INDIVIDUALS

CHR studies have provided an alternative approach to the investigation of alterations of neural structure associated with schizophrenia risk in adolescents and young adults based on the presence of clinical risk syndromes that indicate the need for care[64] (ie, low-level, attenuated positive symptoms; brief intermittent psychotic symptoms; or genetic risk accompanied by functional decline).[64] Because approximately 20% of persons meeting prodromal criteria convert to psychosis within 1 year of initial assessment, and 35% over about 3 years,[65] CHR studies provide a method for examining brain structural alterations proximal to the emergence of frank psychosis, which could elucidate pathophysiologic processes most closely associated with illness onset.[7] Structural MRI findings in CHR studies have been the subject of several recent systematic and critical reviews.[66,67] As with the GHR literature, structural MRI studies of CHR individuals have used a wide range of imaging methods, and MRI morphometric analytical techniques. Here, the structural MRI findings in CHR youth from 11 independent research groups and 1 multicenter study are summarized, as well as from 2 meta-analyses (**Table 2**).

Cross-Sectional Findings

Overall, studies of CHR individuals show brain structural alterations that are neuroanatomically similar to, but less severe than, those commonly reported in established schizophrenia.[68] For example, compared with controls, CHR groups have shown both smaller GM volume and cortical thinning in PFC,[69–76] lateral temporal cortex[69,72,73,75–80] (particularly STG), and, to a lesser extent, parietal cortex.[72,81] Further, in the largest structural MRI study of CHR to date,[82] which involved data collected from 5 clinical sites, CHR individuals showed significantly less GM in the PFC bilaterally compared with controls. Less PFC GM has also been associated with impaired executive function[74] and greater severity of symptoms[71] in CHR, whereas smaller STG GM has been linked with deficits involving semantic fluency.[77]

Table 1
Structural MRI findings from studies of GHR for schizophrenia individuals younger than 30 years

Group	Reference	Study Type	Results
Pittsburgh	Keshavan et al,[53] 1997	Cross-sectional	Smaller L amygdala and enlarged third ventricle
	Keshavan et al,[52] 2002	Cross-sectional	Smaller bilateral amygdala-hippocampal complex and intracranial volume
	Rajarethinam et al,[46] 2004	Cross-sectional	Smaller STG bilaterally
	Jou et al,[23] 2005	Cross-sectional	Altered gyrification of L anterior cortical surface
	Diwadkar et al,[57] 2006	Cross-sectional	GHR showed smaller PFC GM
			GHR with symptoms showed smaller PFC, thalamus, and cuneus GM vs GHR without symptoms
	Bhojraj et al,[42] 2009	Cross-sectional	Smaller L PT, R Heschl gyrus, L supramarginal and R angular gyri
			Reversed PT asymmetry, exaggerated Heschl gyrus asymmetry, attenuated supramarginal/angular gyri
	Prasad et al,[49] 2010	Longitudinal	Reduced gyral surface area in frontoparietal lobes
			Increased gyral cortical thinning
			Shrinkage of total surface area (bilateral frontal/occipital cortices) at 1-y follow-up
	Bhojraj et al,[45] 2010	Cross-sectional	Smaller bilateral lateral temporal, R inferior parietal, and L posterior cingulate cortices
			Smaller bilateral precuneus and R DLPFC
	Bhojraj et al,[59] 2011	Longitudinal	Reduced bilateral lateral orbitofrontal, L rostral anterior cingulate, L medial PFC, R inferior frontal gyrus, and L frontal pole over time in GHR
			Smaller volumes predicted greater severity of symptoms at baseline and at follow-up
			Smaller baseline volumes and longitudinal decrease in volumes predicted greater severity of prodromal symptoms over time
	Bhojraj et al,[47] 2011	Longitudinal	L surface area in auditory association cortex and laterality index showed decline over time in GHR
Edinburgh	Lawrie et al,[54] 1999	Cross-sectional	Smaller L amygdala-hippocampal complex volume and bilateral thalamus in GHR
	Harris et al,[58] 2004	Cross-sectional	Increased R PFC gyrification index in GHR who developed schizophrenia
	Job et al,[62] 2005	Longitudinal	GHR with symptoms showed reduction in L superior lateral hippocampal surface, L fusiform gyrus, L uncus, L inferior temporal gyrus, and L STG
	Job et al,[61] 2006	Longitudinal	Changes over time in inferior temporal gyrus were significantly predictive of developing schizophrenia in GHR
	Lymer et al,[60] 2006	Cross-sectional	L STG GM density associated with schizotypal symptoms in GHR
	McIntosh et al,[63] 2011	Longitudinal	Smaller bilateral PFC volume in GHR vs controls at baseline
			GHR who transition to psychosis show significant reduction in bilateral PFC volume
			GHR as a whole show significant reductions in whole-brain volume, L and R temporal lobes, and L frontal lobe volume

NIMH	Gogtay et al,[48] 2003	Cross-sectional	Smaller total cerebral, frontal and parietal lobe GM volume in GHR
	Gogtay et al,[37] 2007	Cross-sectional	Smaller GM in L PFC and bilateral temporal cortices in GHR
	Mattai et al,[38] 2011	Longitudinal	Smaller baseline GM in bilateral PFC, L temporal cortex, and parietal cortex that normalized by age 17 y
NYU	Li et al,[40] 2012	Cross-sectional	Thinning of inferior frontal gyrus GM volume in GHR; Increased cortical thickness in PFC, temporal and parietal cortices in GHR
Iowa	Ho & Magnotta,[51] 2010	Cross-sectional	Smaller bilateral hippocampal volume in GHR
WU	Harms et al,[39] 2010	Cross-sectional	Smaller inferior frontal gyrus GM in GHR
	Karnik-Henry et al,[56] 2012	Cross-sectional	Thinner parahippocampal volume in GHR
Harvard AHRS	Rosso et al,[43] 2010	Cross-sectional	Smaller bilateral vmPFC and frontal pole GM volume in GHR; vmPFC volume negatively correlated with schizotypal symptoms in GHR
UNC	Dougherty et al,[50] 2012	Cross-sectional	Greater positive association between age and hippocampal and basal gangliar volumes in GHR
Turkey	Sismanlar et al,[55] 2010	Cross-sectional	Smaller bilateral hippocampal volume in GHR
Korea	Byun et al,[36] 2012	Cross-sectional	Cortical thinning in R anterior cingulate, L paracingulate, PCC, bilateral frontal pole, vmPFC, and occipital cortex
Harvard LHRS	Francis et al,[41] 2012	Cross-sectional	Smaller L pars triangularis and R pars orbitalis volumes in GHR with reversal of L>R pars orbitalis lateralization

For a comprehensive listing of all structural MRI findings in GHR individuals, see Ref.[35]

Abbreviations: AHRS, Adolescent High-Risk Study; DLPFC, dorsolateral prefrontal cortex; L, left; LHRS, Language High-Risk Study; NYU, New York University; PCC, posterior cingulate cortex; PT, pars triangularis; R, right; STG, superior temporal gyrus; UNC, University of North Carolina; vmPFC, ventromedial prefrontal cortex; WU, Washington University.

Table 2
Structural MRI findings from studies of CHR for schizophrenia individuals

Group	Reference	Study Type	Results
Melbourne	Phillips et al,[84] 2002	Cross-sectional	Smaller hippocampal volume bilaterally in CHR Larger L hippocampal volume in CHR-t vs CHR-n, but no differences compared with controls
	Pantelis et al,[76] 2003	Longitudinal	Smaller GM in R medial temporal, lateral temporal, and inferior frontal and bilateral cingulate cortices at baseline CHR-t showed reduced GM in L parahippocampal, fusiform, orbitofrontal, and cerebellar cortices and cingulate gyri over time CHR-n showed reduced cerebellar GM
	Yucel et al,[90] 2003	Cross-sectional	Interrupted L anterior cingulate sulcus in CHR vs controls, but no differences between CHR-t and CHR-n
	Garner et al,[105] 2005	Cross-sectional	Larger baseline pituitary volume in CHR-t vs CHR-n
	Wood et al,[87] 2005	Cross-sectional	Smaller hippocampal volume and less L anterior cingulate folding in CHR with GHR vs CHR without GHR
	Velakoulis et al,[100] 2006	Cross-sectional	Normal baseline hippocampal and amygdala volume in CHR Smaller whole-brain volumes in CHR vs controls
	Fornito et al,[89] 2008	Longitudinal	Bilateral thinning of anterior cingulate in CHR-t also associated with negative symptoms Baseline anterior cingulate differences in CHR-t vs CHR-n predicted time to psychosis onset
	Takahashi et al,[99] 2008	Cross-sectional	No increased prevalence of cavum septi pellucidi enlargement in CHR
	Walterfang et al,[108] 2008	Cross-sectional	Smaller anterior corpus callosum in CHR-t vs CHR-n
	Sun et al,[103] 2009	Longitudinal	Greater brain contraction in R PFC in CHR-t vs CHR over time
	Takahashi et al,[94] 2009	Longitudinal	Smaller baseline insula bilaterally in CHR-t vs CHR-n, and in R insula vs controls Reduced GM of bilateral insula in CHR-t vs CHR-n and controls
	Hannan et al,[96] 2010	Cross-sectional	No differences in caudate volume in CHR at baseline vs controls or in CHR-t vs CHR-n
	Takahashi et al,[79] 2010	Cross-sectional	Smaller STG bilaterally at baseline in CHR vs controls
	Wood et al,[86] 2010	Cross-sectional	Smaller L hippocampal volume in CHR vs controls
	Dazzan et al,[81] 2012	Longitudinal	Smaller frontal cortex volume in CHR-t vs CHR-n at baseline Reduced parietal cortex and temporal cortex (trend) in CHR-t vs CHR-n
	Whitford et al,[95] 2012	Cross-sectional	Smaller cuneus in CHR-HSV-1+ vs CHR-HSV-1− and controls

Site	Study	Design	Findings
Basel	Borgwardt et al,[69] 2007	Cross-sectional	Smaller GM at baseline in posterior cingulate and precuneus bilaterally and L superior parietal lobule in CHR-t vs controls
	Borgwardt et al,[88] 2007	Longitudinal	Smaller L insula, STG, cingulate gyrus, and precuneus in CHR vs controls
	Borgwardt et al,[102] 2008	Longitudinal	Reduced R insula, inferior frontal and STG in CHR-t vs CHR-n Reduced orbitofrontal, superior frontal, inferior temporal, parietal cortex, and cerebellum in CHR-t vs controls over time
	Haller et al,[92] 2009	Cross-sectional	Whole-brain cortical thickness asymmetry in CHR vs controls
	Koutsouleris et al,[73] 2009	Cross-sectional	Smaller GM volume in frontotemporal and limbic structures in CHR-L vs controls Alterations of bilateral temporal and limbic structures in CHR-E vs controls Alterations of PFC in CHR-t vs CHR-n and controls
	Buehlmann et al,[164] 2010	Cross-sectional	Asymmetry between L and R hippocampus in CHR vs controls
	Smieskova et al,[93] 2012	Cross-sectional	Smaller insula GM volume bilaterally in CHR-E at baseline vs CHR-L Insular alterations associated with negative symptoms in CHR
	Walter et al,[165] 2012	Longitudinal	Reduced hippocampal volume in CHR over time vs controls No hippocampal volume differences in CHR-t vs CHR-n
Berlin	Witthaus et al,[85] 2009	Cross-sectional	Smaller GM volume in cingulate gyrus bilaterally, R inferior frontal, R STG, and bilateral cingulate cortex in CHR
	Witthaus et al,[104] 2010	Cross-sectional	Smaller corpus and tail volume of hippocampus bilaterally in CHR vs controls Smaller R hippocampal tail volume in CHR-t vs CHR-n
	Bohner et al,[91] 2012	Cross-sectional	Smaller cingulate gyrus GM in CHR vs controls
Seoul	Choi et al,[98] 2008	Cross-sectional	Higher incidence of cavum septum pellucidum in CHR vs controls
	Jung et al,[72] 2011	Cross-sectional	Reduced cortical thickness in PFC, anterior cingulate cortex, inferior parietal cortex, STG, and parahippocampal cortex vs controls
	Han et al,[97] 2012	Cross-sectional	Smaller ALIC volume in CHR vs controls
	Shin et al,[78] 2012	Cross-sectional	Reduced cortical thickness in L Heschl gyrus in CHR vs controls
Munich	Meisenzahl et al,[75] 2008	Cross-sectional	Smaller GM volume in frontal, lateral temporal, and medial temporal areas in CHR vs controls

(continued on next page)

Table 2
(continued)

Group	Reference	Study Type	Results
London	Fusar-Poli et al,[70] 2011	Longitudinal	Smaller middle and medial frontal gyrus, insula, and anterior cingulate cortex volume in CHR vs controls at baseline No structural differences in CHR and controls at follow-up
Utrecht	Ziermans et al,[101] 2009 Ziermans et al,[80] 2012	Cross-sectional Longitudinal	No structural difference in CHR vs controls Greater loss of total brain volume in CHR-t vs CHR-n and controls Cortical thinning in L anterior cingulate, precuneus, and temporoparietal-occipital areas in CHR-t vs CHR-n and controls
Amsterdam	Meijer et al,[77] 2011	Cross-sectional	Smaller baseline GM density in R STG, MTG, R insula, and L anterior cingulate in CHR-t vs CHR-n GM reductions correlated with semantic fluency in CHR
Bonn	Hurlemann et al,[83] 2008	Cross-sectional	Smaller bilateral hippocampal volume in CHR-L and CHR-E vs controls
Tokyo	Iwashiro et al,[71] 2012	Cross-sectional	Smaller bilateral PT volume in CHR vs controls Reduced PT volume correlated with prodromal symptoms in CHR
Los Angeles	Mittal et al,[106] 2010	Cross-sectional	Smaller baseline striatal GM volume in CHR-t vs CHR-n Trend association between reduced GM volume in CHR-t and increased dyskinetic movements
Multicenter	Mechelli et al,[82] 2011	Cross-sectional	Smaller frontal GM volume in CHR vs controls at baseline Smaller baseline L parahippocampal GM volume in CHR-t vs CHR-n

Abbreviations: ALIC, anterior limb of internal capsule; CHR-E, early course clinical high risk; CHR-HSV-1−, clinical high risk without herpes simplex virus 1; CHR-HSV-1+, clinical high risk with herpes simplex virus 1; CHR-L, clinical high risk of long duration; CHR-n, clinical high risk without transition to psychosis; CHR-t, clinical high risk with transition to psychosis; L, left; MTG, middle temporal gyrus; PT, pars triangularis; R, right.

Structural alterations of limbic brain areas and insula are also among the most consistently reported findings in CHR individuals compared with controls. This finding includes less bilateral[83–85] and ipsilateral[86,87] hippocampal GM volume, aberrant surface morphology[80,87–90] and smaller GM[70,76,82,85,91] in anterior cingulate and paracingulate cortex, as well as asymmetry[92] and smaller GM volume[69,70,93,94] of the insula. In several studies, structural alterations of anterior cingulate[89] and insula[93,94] have been significantly associated with greater negative symptom levels in CHR. Structural abnormalities in CHR involving the cuneus,[95] caudate,[96] anterior limb of the internal capsule,[97] and the presence of cavum septum pellucidum[98,99] are less frequently assessed and less consistently reported. In 1 study,[100] CHR individuals showed less total whole-brain volume compared with controls. Only 1 study[101] has reported no significant differences in any brain structures in CHR persons versus controls.

Cross-sectional comparisons of CHR individuals who transition to psychosis (CHR-t) with nonconverters or controls have provided evidence for smaller GM volume in PFC[102,103] and temporal cortical (STG[69,88]) GM among CHR-t. CHR-t have also shown aberrant anterior cingulate morphology,[89] smaller insula bilaterally[94] and on the right,[69] as well as both greater[84] and smaller[104] hippocampal or parahippocampal[82] GM volume. One study[105] reported greater pituitary volume in CHR-t, which may reflect greater exposure to environmental stress in persons who transition to psychosis. An additional study of dyskinesia in CHR[106] has reported smaller striatal volume in CHR-t with a trend association between less striatal GM and greater dyskinetic symptoms. A study of CHR persons exposed to herpes simplex virus 1 (HSV-1) showed smaller GM volume of the cuneus among HSV-1–positive CHR-t.[106] Overall, cross-sectional studies have shown smaller GM volume in frontal-temporal and medial temporal/limbic structures in CHR individuals compared with controls, with significantly less GM in these brain areas among individuals who transition to psychosis than in nonconverters.

Longitudinal Findings

In longitudinal studies, comparisons of structural brain alterations in CHR compared with controls have shown progressive GM loss in PFC (orbitofrontal cortex[76,102]), lateral temporal cortex (STG[102,107]), parietal cortex,[102] cingulate gyrus,[76] parahippocampus,[76] fusiform cortex,[76] insula,[94] and cerebellum.[76,102] Further, studies comparing structural changes in CHR-t with CHR nonconverters have shown evidence for reductions over time in PFC[81] and temporal cortex,[107] as well as in the cerebellum.[108]

META-ANALYSES OF CHR STRUCTURAL MRI STUDIES

The clinical diversity of CHR youth and the heterogeneity of MRI morphometric techniques used across studies together have posed a challenge to interpreting CHR structural findings regarding the neural alterations most closely linked to the risk for transitioning to psychosis. To shed further light on the neural correlates associated with the transition to psychosis, Smieskova and colleagues[67] conducted a meta-analysis of structural MRI findings in both GHR and CHR, comparing HR individuals who transitioned to psychosis (HR-t) with nonconverters. Overall, HR-t showed significantly decreased GM volume in PFC, temporal cortex, the limbic system, and cerebellum, compared with nonconverters.[67] A subsequent meta-analysis by Fusar-Poli and colleagues[66] of voxel-based morphometric studies in GHR and CHR showed smaller GM volume in the PFC, temporal cortex (STG), anterior cingulate, parahippocampus, and precuneus in HR individuals.[66] In the same meta-analysis, a comparison

Table 3
Structural MRI findings from studies of early-onset and COS individuals

Group	Reference	Study Type	Results
NIMH	Frazier et al,[130] 1996	Cross-sectional	Smaller total brain and thalamic volume and increased basal ganglia volume, as well as increased lateral ventricular volume in COS vs controls
	Jacobsen et al,[126] 1996	Cross-sectional	Smaller total cerebral volume in COS vs controls
	Jacobsen et al,[131] 1997	Cross-sectional	Smaller cerebellar volume in COS vs controls
	Jacobsen et al,[139] 1997	Cross-sectional	Larger corpus callosum volume in COS vs controls
	Rapoport et al,[140] 1997	Longitudinal	Reduced thalamic GM volume and increased lateral ventricular volume over time in COS vs controls
	Jacobsen et al,[120] 1998	Longitudinal	Reduced R temporal lobe, bilateral STG, and L hippocampus volume over time in COS vs controls Reduced R STS volume associated with symptom severity
	Nopoulos et al,[146] 1998	Cross-sectional	Enlarged cavum septum pellucidi in COS vs controls
	Giedd et al,[154] 1999	Longitudinal	Reduced total brain volume and hippocampus and increased lateral ventricular volume over time in COS vs controls
	Rapoport et al,[150] 1999	Cross-sectional	Four times smaller frontotemporal GM volume in COS vs controls
	Kumra et al,[138] 2000	Cross-sectional	Reduced total cerebral volume in COS vs controls
	Thompson et al,[151] 2001	Longitudinal	Smaller parietal cortical GM volume with progressive GM volume loss in temporal cortex, followed by PFC over 5 y in COS vs controls
	Keller et al,[153] 2003	Longitudinal	Reduced cerebellar GM volume over time in COS vs controls
	Keller et al,[156] 2003	Longitudinal	Reduced volume of splenium of corpus callosum in COS over time vs controls
	Greenstein et al,[152] 2006	Longitudinal	Reduced cortical thickness in temporal cortex over time in COS vs controls
	Nugent et al,[129] 2007	Cross-sectional	Smaller bilateral total hippocampal volume in COS vs controls
	Bakalar et al,[166] 2009	Longitudinal	No baseline or follow-up asymmetry of lateral or medial cortical surface in COS vs controls
	Greenstein et al,[137] 2011	Longitudinal	Reduced cerebellar GM at baseline and over time in COS vs controls
	Gogtay et al,[114] 2012	Cross-sectional	Smaller PFC and temporal GM volume in COS vs psychosis NOS
	Johnson et al,[145] 2013	Cross-sectional	No corpus callosum volume differences in COS vs controls
UCLA	Sowell et al,[136] 2000	Cross-sectional	Increased lateral ventricular volume in EOS vs controls
	Levitt et al,[127] 2001	Cross-sectional	Larger L amygdala volume in EOS vs controls
	Marquardt et al,[167] 2005	Cross-sectional	Anterior cingulate asymmetry in EOS vs controls
	Taylor et al,[128] 2005	Cross-sectional	Greater posterior STG in EOS vs controls
Iowa	White et al,[22] 2003	Cross-sectional	Reduced cortical thickness and surface morphology in frontotemporoparietal lobes in EOS vs controls
	Clark et al,[125] 2010	Cross-sectional	Loss of planum temporale asymmetry in EOS vs controls

Minnesota	Kendi et al,[143] 2008	Cross-sectional	Smaller fornix volume in EOS vs controls
	Kumra et al,[123] 2012	Cross-sectional	Smaller L parietal volume in EOS vs controls
Harvard	Frazier et al,[141] 2008	Cross-sectional	Smaller L amygdala volume in males with EOS vs controls
UNC	El-Sayed et al,[113] 2010	Cross-sectional	Smaller whole-brain volume and frontoparietal GM in EOS vs controls
Madrid	Reig et al,[117] 2011	Cross-sectional	Smaller frontal/parietal cortical GM in EOS vs controls
	Arango et al,[149] 2012	Longitudinal	Reduced frontal/parietal GM over time in EOS vs controls
	Janssen et al,[155] 2012	Cross-sectional	Smaller thalamic volume in EOS vs controls
Oxford	Davies et al,[142] 2001	Cross-sectional	Larger fornix in EOS vs controls
	James et al,[147] 2002	Cross-sectional	No GM volume differences in EOS vs controls
	Collinson et al,[133] 2003	Cross-sectional	Smaller total brain volume in EOS vs controls
	James et al,[115] 2004	Cross-sectional	Smaller PFC and thalamic volume in EOS vs controls
London	Matsumoto et al,[121] 2001	Longitudinal	Reduced total and R STG GM in EOS vs controls over time. Severity of symptoms associated with reduced STG volume and correlated with age of onset in EOS
	Matsumoto et al,[132] 2001	Longitudinal	Smaller GM whole-brain volume in EOS vs controls
	Hadjulis et al,[168] 2004	Cross-sectional	No asymmetries of hemispheric lateralization in EOS vs controls
Orsay	Paillère-Martinot et al,[116] 2001	Cross-sectional	Smaller PFC, L insula, parahippocampal, and fusiform GM volume in EOS vs controls
	Penttila et al,[124] 2008	Cross-sectional	Smaller global sulcal indices in both hemispheres in EOS vs controls
Copenhagen	Pagsberg et al,[148] 2007	Cross-sectional	No GM volume differences in EOS vs controls
Oslo	Juuhl-Langseth et al,[135] 2012	Cross-sectional	Bilateral enlargement of lateral and fourth ventricle and bilateral enlargement of caudate in EOS vs controls
Changsha	Tang et al,[122] 2012	Cross-sectional	Smaller L STG/MTG GM volume in EOS vs controls. Smaller L STG/MTG negatively correlated with positive symptoms in EOS
Osaka	Hata et al,[134] 2003	Cross-sectional	Enlargement of lateral ventricles in EOS vs controls. Positive correlation between lateral ventricular enlargement and minor physical abnormalities in EOS
Hamamatsu	Yoshihara et al,[119] 2008	Cross-sectional	Smaller parahippocampal and inferior frontal GM volume in EOS vs controls

Abbreviations: L, left; MTG, middle temporal gyrus; NIMH, National Institute of Mental Health; NOS, not otherwise specified; R, right; UCLA, University of California, Los Angeles; UNC, University of North Carolina.

of HR-t with nonconverters revealed less GM in PFC (inferior frontal gyrus) and temporal cortex (STG) in HR-t. A comparison of CHR to GHR in the same meta-analysis showed smaller GM volume in the anterior cingulate bilaterally in CHR, whereas GHR showed less GM in the left hippocampal gyrus, insula, and right temporal cortex (STG) compared with CHR individuals.[66] Taken together, these meta-analyses show smaller PFC, STG, and medial temporal structures across HR populations, as well as converging evidence for reduced frontotemporal GM volume in HR individuals who develop psychosis.

EOS AND COS

Schizophrenia beginning in adolescence (EOS, age 13–18 years) or childhood (COS, age <13 years) occurs rarely (approximately 4% of cases[109]) but is generally more clinically and neurobiologically severe than the adult-onset illness.[110] In particular, the brain structural abnormalities observed in COS have been shown to be significantly greater than in adults with schizophrenia.[110] Research over the last 2 decades regarding the pattern of neural alterations in COS, premorbid risk factors, and neurocognitive deficits in nonaffected family members has provided strong evidence suggesting the neurobiological continuity between COS/EOS and adult-onset schizophrenia.[111] Further, because of evidence for greater genetic vulnerability[110] in COS (eg, increased familiarity,[110] cytogenetic abnormalities,[112] and copy number variants[112]), it is increasingly believed that studies of brain structural alterations in children and adolescents with schizophrenia may be particularly valuable to understanding the neurobiological basis of the GM abnormalities associated with the illness overall. In the following sections, the findings from structural MRI studies of EOS and COS performed by 15 independent research groups worldwide are summarized (**Table 3**) are summarized. Approximately half of the studies included in this review have been performed by the National Institute of Mental Health (NIMH) research group,[110] which has focused on COS. Further, as with the HR structural MRI literature, there is considerable variability in terms of the MRI morphometric techniques and data analytical methods used across studies.

Cross-Sectional Findings

Similar to findings in adult-onset schizophrenia, structural MRI studies of EOS and COS have consistently shown smaller GM volume in PFC[113–119] and the temporal[114,119–122] and parietal[113,117,123] cortices in EOS and COS compared with controls. Abnormalities of PFC thickness,[22] cortical folding,[124] and asymmetry[125] have also been reported. In addition, less STG volume has been linked with both greater symptom severity as well as earlier age of illness onset.[121] However, several cross-sectional studies have found enlargement of temporal cortical structures,[126–128] raising the possibility that, alternatively, temporal GM volume reduction may occur developmentally later.[128] In contrast to HR and adult-onset schizophrenia, decreased hippocampal GM is less commonly reported in COS,[129] with several studies showing no significant alterations compared with controls in hippocampal volume.[130–132] Other commonly reported structural findings in EOS and COS include smaller whole-brain volume,[113,126,130,132,133] greater lateral ventricular volume,[130,134–136] and smaller GM in the cerebellum[137–139] and thalamus.[115,130,140] Fewer, and less consistent, structural alterations are reported regarding the amygdala,[127,141] parahippocampus,[119] insula,[116] fusiform gyrus,[116] basal ganglia,[130] fornix,[142,143] corpus callosum,[144,145] and cavum septum pellucidum.[146] In 2 studies,[147,148] no structural brain abnormalities in any brain areas in EOS versus controls were found. Thus, cross-sectional EOS and COS studies have provided consistent evidence for smaller whole-brain volume, enlargement of lateral ventricles, in conjunction with smaller PFC and (less consistently) STG GM.

Longitudinal Findings

Longitudinal studies comparing brain structure changes in EOS and COS with controls have shown progressive decreases in GM volume involving PFC[149–151] and the temporal[120,150,151] and parietal[149,151] cortices in conjunction with decreases over time in cortical thickness in PFC[152] and temporal cortex.[152] Particularly noteworthy were results from a 5-year longitudinal study conducted by the NIMH group,[151] which revealed a temporal pattern of significant GM volume loss in COS compared with controls, with the earliest deficits seen in the parietal cortex, followed by progression during adolescence to the temporal lobes and to the PFC. Additional brain regions in which volumetric decrements have been observed over time in EOS and COS compared with controls include the cerebellum,[137,153] hippocampus,[120,154] thalamus,[155] and corpus callosum.[156] Progressive enlargement of the lateral ventricles has also been found in COS compared with controls.[140,154] Across longitudinal studies, EOS and COS individuals have most consistently shown decrements in GM volume in frontotemporal and parietal cortices over time.

SUMMARY

This article reviews the structural neuroimaging literature in youth and young adults at high risk for schizophrenia and in EOS and COS. The most consistent finding was that, compared with normal development, there is accelerated frontotemporal cortical GM volume reduction across the spectrum of schizophrenia risk and in EOS/COS. Specifically, progressive GM decline in these brain regions occurs in HR youth and young adults who transition to psychosis and also occurs during adolescence in persons with EOS/COS. Progressive volumetric decline and morphologic alterations of limbic structures (eg, hippocampus, parahippocampus, anterior cingulate) are also prominent among HR individuals who later develop psychosis. Structural alterations over time in limbic areas are less common in COS, although there is some evidence to suggest that these abnormalities may emerge as COS individuals are followed to the end of adolescence.

Overall, these structural neuroimaging findings are broadly consistent with the hypothesis that schizophrenia involves, at least partly, the disruption of normal neurodevelopment occurring during childhood or adolescence. Structural MRI findings in HR individuals suggest the potential involvement of both early and late brain dysmaturational processes in the trajectory of GM alterations during prepsychosis development. For example, evidence for altered surface morphology of PFC[44] and STG[47] in GHR individuals is believed to potentially reflect abnormalities of neuronal migration and minicolumnar formation during gestation.[2,16] It has been proposed that GM volume loss in frontotemporal brain regions of CHR individuals who transition to psychosis[102,107] could reflect dysregulation of synaptic pruning during adolescence.[68] Further, the progressive reduction in GM from posterior (parietal) to anterior (prefrontal) cortical brain areas over time found in COS follows the pattern of decline in GM observed during typically developing adolescents,[13,14] and, thus, has been interpreted as an indication of aberrant acceleration of normal brain maturational processes.[157] Although speculative, taken together these findings lend support to the 2-hit model proposed by Keshavan and colleagues,[2,7,8] in which neural dysmaturation occurring during early development is believed to produce a vulnerability to later abnormalities of adolescent brain development that result in the emergence of psychosis.

Nevertheless, despite the evolving evidence implicating aberrant neural developmental processes in the pathophysiology of schizophrenia, it is acknowledged that the findings from both GHR and CHR structural MRI studies are variable and difficult to replicate.[35,158] Issues pertaining to the clinical heterogeneity of CHR and GHR subjects, as well as the diversity of neuroimaging methods used for acquisition and analysis of MRI data, have been identified as central to the difficulties of comparing results between research groups.[35,158] As a result, in part, structural MRI findings lack sufficient specificity and sensitivity to be used clinically to identify biomarkers for the prospective identification of individuals at risk for developing schizophrenia.

However, we suggest that future neuroimaging studies of GHR/CHR and EOS/COS populations might take several further steps to address the gaps in current knowledge regarding premorbid and prodromal structural brain alterations preceding schizophrenia onset, and to address the challenges of improving the clinical applicability of structural MRI findings to early intervention and prevention strategies for persons at risk for psychosis. First, the predictive value of structural MRI findings might be enhanced if the volumetric or morphologic alterations observed in CHR and GHR individuals are incorporated within a multivariate approach, in which structural changes are combined with clinical and neurocognitive measures in models to predict later psychopathology.[159] In addition, there is recent evidence suggesting that the use of machine learning techniques to identify patterns of structural abnormalities associated with the transition to psychosis in HR individuals could be used prospectively to improve the predictive specificity of structural MRI findings during the prepsychosis period.[73,160] Second, given the extensive clinical and neurobiological overlap between schizophrenia and bipolar affective disorder,[161] studies of young first-degree relatives of probands across the psychotic spectrum may help determine which structural MRI abnormalities are most specific to schizophrenia risk.[162] Third, although our review is limited to structural MRI findings, how GM alterations develop in conjunction with changes in WM, impairments of brain function, cognitive deficits, as well as other potential markers of schizophrenia risk (eg, inflammatory markers and oxidative stress), all of which seem to evolve during the early phase of schizophrenia,[163] remains to be determined. Future longitudinal studies need to address these questions and control for diagnostic variability, as well as differences of age and gender. Fourth, the potential influence of early (eg, perinatal complications) and later (eg, substance misuse, psychosocial stress) environmental stress on neural development in the context of risk needs to be clarified in an effort to elucidate the neurobiology of schizophrenia and to identify the risk markers that can be most useful to early intervention strategies to preempt illness onset. Given the evidence reviewed here of early developmental pathology underlying schizophrenia risk, future research on younger individuals at GHR (ie, preteen children) will be critical to the further clarification of the origins of brain structural abnormalities associated with the development of schizophrenia.

REFERENCES

1. Shenton ME, Dickey CC, Frumin M, et al. A review of MRI findings in schizophrenia. Schizophr Res 2001;49(1–2):1–52.
2. Keshavan MS, Hogarty GE. Brain maturational processes and delayed onset in schizophrenia. Dev Psychopathol 1999;11(3):525–43.
3. Palaniyappan L, Balain V, Radua J, et al. Structural correlates of auditory hallucinations in schizophrenia: a meta-analysis. Schizophr Res 2012;137(1–3):169–73.

4. Palaniyappan L, Mallikarjun P, Joseph V, et al. Reality distortion is related to the structure of the salience network in schizophrenia. Psychol Med 2011;41(8):1701–8.
5. Seidman LJ, Yurgelun-Todd D, Kremen WS, et al. Relationship of prefrontal and temporal lobe MRI measures to neuropsychological performance in chronic schizophrenia. Biol Psychiatry 1994;35(4):235–46.
6. Mitelman SA, Shihabuddin L, Brickman AM, et al. MRI assessment of gray and white matter distribution in Brodmann's areas of the cortex in patients with schizophrenia with good and poor outcomes. Am J Psychiatry 2003;160(12):2154–68.
7. Cannon TD, van Erp TG, Bearden CE, et al. Early and late neurodevelopmental influences in the prodrome to schizophrenia: contributions of genes, environment, and their interactions. Schizophr Bull 2003;29(4):653–69.
8. Keshavan MS, Anderson S, Pettegrew JW. Is schizophrenia due to excessive synaptic pruning in the prefrontal cortex? The Feinberg hypothesis revisited. J Psychiatr Res 1994;28(3):239–65.
9. Paus T. Mapping brain maturation and cognitive development during adolescence. Trends Cogn Sci 2005;9(2):60–8.
10. Giedd JN, Blumenthal J, Jeffries NO, et al. Brain development during childhood and adolescence: a longitudinal MRI study. Nat Neurosci 1999;2(10):861–3.
11. Sowell ER, Trauner DA, Gamst A, et al. Development of cortical and subcortical brain structures in childhood and adolescence: a structural MRI study. Dev Med Child Neurol 2002;44(1):4–16.
12. Ernst M, Mueller SC. The adolescent brain: insights from functional neuroimaging research. Dev Neurobiol 2008;68(6):729–43.
13. Gogtay N, Giedd JN, Lusk L, et al. Dynamic mapping of human cortical development during childhood through early adulthood. Proc Natl Acad Sci U S A 2004;101(21):8174–9.
14. Sowell ER, Thompson PM, Toga AW. Mapping changes in the human cortex throughout the span of life. Neuroscientist 2004;10(4):372–92.
15. Paus T, Keshavan M, Giedd JN. Why do many psychiatric disorders emerge during adolescence? Nat Rev Neurosci 2008;9(12):947–57.
16. Keshavan MS, Bhojraj T. Gray matter alterations in schizophrenia: are they reversible. New York: Routledge; 2011.
17. Marenco S, Weinberger DR. The neurodevelopmental hypothesis of schizophrenia: following a trail of evidence from cradle to grave. Dev Psychopathol 2000;12(3):501–27.
18. Akbarian S, Bunney WE Jr, Potkin SG, et al. Altered distribution of nicotinamide-adenine dinucleotide phosphate-diaphorase cells in frontal lobe of schizophrenics implies disturbances of cortical development. Arch Gen Psychiatry 1993;50(3):169–77.
19. Bunney WE, Bunney BG. Evidence for a compromised dorsolateral prefrontal cortical parallel circuit in schizophrenia. Brain Res Brain Res Rev 2000; 31(2–3):138–46.
20. Chana G, Landau S, Beasley C, et al. Two-dimensional assessment of cytoarchitecture in the anterior cingulate cortex in major depressive disorder, bipolar disorder, and schizophrenia: evidence for decreased neuronal somal size and increased neuronal density. Biol Psychiatry 2003;53(12):1086–98.
21. Vogeley K, Schneider-Axmann T, Pfeiffer U, et al. Disturbed gyrification of the prefrontal region in male schizophrenic patients: a morphometric postmortem study. Am J Psychiatry 2000;157(1):34–9.
22. White T, Andreasen NC, Nopoulos P, et al. Gyrification abnormalities in childhood- and adolescent-onset schizophrenia. Biol Psychiatry 2003;54(4):418–26.

23. Jou RJ, Hardan AY, Keshavan MS. Reduced cortical folding in individuals at high risk for schizophrenia: a pilot study. Schizophr Res 2005;75(2–3):309–13.

24. Pierri JN, Volk CL, Auh S, et al. Decreased somal size of deep layer 3 pyramidal neurons in the prefrontal cortex of subjects with schizophrenia. Arch Gen Psychiatry 2001;58(5):466–73.

25. Rajkowska G, Selemon LD, Goldman-Rakic PS. Neuronal and glial somal size in the prefrontal cortex: a postmortem morphometric study of schizophrenia and Huntington disease. Arch Gen Psychiatry 1998;55(3):215–24.

26. Bennett MR. Schizophrenia: susceptibility genes, dendritic-spine pathology and gray matter loss. Prog Neurobiol 2011;95(3):275–300.

27. Fatemi SH, Earle JA, McMenomy T. Reduction in Reelin immunoreactivity in hippocampus of subjects with schizophrenia, bipolar disorder and major depression. Mol Psychiatry 2000;5(6):654–63, 571.

28. Gill M, Donohoe G, Corvin A. What have the genomics ever done for the psychoses? Psychol Med 2010;40(4):529–40.

29. Lipska BK, Weinberger DR. Delayed effects of neonatal hippocampal damage on haloperidol-induced catalepsy and apomorphine-induced stereotypic behaviors in the rat. Brain Res Dev Brain Res 1993;75(2):213–22.

30. McGorry P. Transition to adulthood: the critical period for pre-emptive, disease-modifying care for schizophrenia and related disorders. Schizophr Bull 2011; 37(3):524–30.

31. MacDonald AW, Schulz SC. What we know: findings that every theory of schizophrenia should explain. Schizophr Bull 2009;35(3):493–508.

32. Stone WS, Faraone SV, Seidman LJ, et al. Searching for the liability to schizophrenia: concepts and methods underlying genetic high-risk studies of adolescents. J Child Adolesc Psychopharmacol 2005;15(3):403–17.

33. Agnew-Blais J, Seidman LJ. Neurocognition in youth and young adults under age 30 at familial risk for schizophrenia: a quantitative and qualitative review. Cogn Neuropsychiatry 2013;18(1–2):44–82.

34. Keshavan MS, DeLisi LE, Seidman LJ. Early and broadly defined psychosis risk mental states. Schizophr Res 2011;126(1–3):1–10.

35. Thermenos HW, Keshavan MS, Juelich E, et al. Neuroimaging of young relatives of persons with schizophrenia: a developmental perspective from schizotaxia to schizophrenia. Am J Med Genet B Neuropsychiatr Genet 2013. Accepted.

36. Byun MS, Kim JS, Jung WH, et al. Regional cortical thinning in subjects with high genetic loading for schizophrenia. Schizophr Res 2012;141(2–3):197–203.

37. Gogtay N, Greenstein D, Lenane M, et al. Cortical brain development in nonpsychotic siblings of patients with childhood-onset schizophrenia. Arch Gen Psychiatry 2007;64(7):772–80.

38. Mattai AA, Weisinger B, Greenstein D, et al. Normalization of cortical gray matter deficits in nonpsychotic siblings of patients with childhood-onset schizophrenia. J Am Acad Child Adolesc Psychiatry 2011;50(7):697–704.

39. Harms MP, Wang L, Campanella C, et al. Structural abnormalities in gyri of the prefrontal cortex in individuals with schizophrenia and their unaffected siblings. Br J Psychiatry 2010;196(2):150–7.

40. Li X, Alapati V, Jackson C, et al. Structural abnormalities in language circuits in genetic high-risk subjects and schizophrenia patients. Psychiatry Res 2012; 201(3):182–9.

41. Francis AN, Seidman LJ, Jabbar GA, et al. Alterations in brain structures underlying language function in young adults at high familial risk for schizophrenia. Schizophr Res 2012;141(1):65–71.

42. Bhojraj TS, Francis AN, Rajarethinam R, et al. Verbal fluency deficits and altered lateralization of language brain areas in individuals genetically predisposed to schizophrenia. Schizophr Res 2009;115(2–3):202–8.

43. Rosso IM, Makris N, Thermenos HW, et al. Regional prefrontal cortex gray matter volumes in youth at familial risk for schizophrenia from the Harvard Adolescent High Risk Study. Schizophr Res 2010;123(1):15–21.

44. Prasad KM, Sanders R, Sweeney J, et al. Neurological abnormalities among offspring of persons with schizophrenia: relation to premorbid psychopathology. Schizophr Res 2009;108(1–3):163–9.

45. Bhojraj TS, Prasad KM, Eack SM, et al. Do inter-regional gray-matter volumetric correlations reflect altered functional connectivity in high-risk offspring of schizophrenia patients? Schizophr Res 2010;118(1–3):62–8.

46. Rajarethinam R, Sahni S, Rosenberg DR, et al. Reduced superior temporal gyrus volume in young offspring of patients with schizophrenia. Am J Psychiatry 2004;161(6):1121–4.

47. Bhojraj TS, Sweeney JA, Prasad KM, et al. Progressive alterations of the auditory association areas in young non-psychotic offspring of schizophrenia patients. J Psychiatr Res 2011;45(2):205–12.

48. Gogtay N, Sporn A, Clasen LS, et al. Structural brain MRI abnormalities in healthy siblings of patients with childhood-onset schizophrenia. Am J Psychiatry 2003;160(3):569–71.

49. Prasad KM, Goradia D, Eack S, et al. Cortical surface characteristics among offspring of schizophrenia subjects. Schizophr Res 2010;116(2–3): 143–51.

50. Dougherty MK, Gu H, Bizzell J, et al. Differences in subcortical structures in young adolescents at familial risk for schizophrenia: a preliminary study. Psychiatry Res 2012;204(2–3):68–74.

51. Ho BC, Magnotta V. Hippocampal volume deficits and shape deformities in young biological relatives of schizophrenia probands. Neuroimage 2010; 49(4):3385–93.

52. Keshavan MS, Dick E, Mankowski I, et al. Decreased left amygdala and hippocampal volumes in young offspring at risk for schizophrenia. Schizophr Res 2002;58(2–3):173–83.

53. Keshavan MS, Montrose DM, Pierri JN, et al. Magnetic resonance imaging and spectroscopy in offspring at risk for schizophrenia: preliminary studies. Prog Neuropsychopharmacol Biol Psychiatry 1997;21(8):1285–95.

54. Lawrie SM, Whalley H, Kestelman JN, et al. Magnetic resonance imaging of brain in people at high risk of developing schizophrenia. Lancet 1999; 353(9146):30–3.

55. Sismanlar SG, Anik Y, Coskun A, et al. The volumetric differences of the frontotemporal region in young offspring of schizophrenic patients. Eur Child Adolesc Psychiatry 2010;19(2):151–7.

56. Karnik-Henry MS, Wang L, Barch DM, et al. Medial temporal lobe structure and cognition in individuals with schizophrenia and in their non-psychotic siblings. Schizophr Res 2012;138(2–3):128–35.

57. Diwadkar VA, Montrose DM, Dworakowski D, et al. Genetically predisposed offspring with schizotypal features: an ultra high-risk group for schizophrenia? Prog Neuropsychopharmacol Biol Psychiatry 2006;30(2):230–8.

58. Harris JM, Whalley H, Yates S, et al. Abnormal cortical folding in high-risk individuals: a predictor of the development of schizophrenia? Biol Psychiatry 2004; 56(3):182–9.

59. Bhojraj TS, Sweeney JA, Prasad KM, et al. Gray matter loss in young relatives at risk for schizophrenia: relation with prodromal psychopathology. Neuroimage 2011;54(Suppl 1):S272–9.
60. Lymer GK, Job DE, William T, et al. Brain-behaviour relationships in people at high genetic risk of schizophrenia. Neuroimage 2006;33(1):275–85.
61. Job DE, Whalley HC, McIntosh AM, et al. Grey matter changes can improve the prediction of schizophrenia in subjects at high risk. BMC Med 2006;4:29.
62. Job DE, Whalley HC, Johnstone EC, et al. Grey matter changes over time in high risk subjects developing schizophrenia. Neuroimage 2005;25(4):1023–30.
63. McIntosh AM, Owens DC, Moorhead WJ, et al. Longitudinal volume reductions in people at high genetic risk of schizophrenia as they develop psychosis. Biol Psychiatry 2011;69(10):953–8.
64. Wood SJ, Pantelis C, Velakoulis D, et al. Progressive changes in the development toward schizophrenia: studies in subjects at increased symptomatic risk. Schizophr Bull 2008;34(2):322–9.
65. Fusar-Poli P, Bonoldi I, Yung AR, et al. Predicting psychosis: meta-analysis of transition outcomes in individuals at high clinical risk. Arch Gen Psychiatry 2012;69(3):220–9.
66. Fusar-Poli P, Borgwardt S, Crescini A, et al. Neuroanatomy of vulnerability to psychosis: a voxel-based meta-analysis. Neurosci Biobehav Rev 2011;35(5):1175–85.
67. Smieskova R, Fusar-Poli P, Allen P, et al. Neuroimaging predictors of transition to psychosis–a systematic review and meta-analysis. Neurosci Biobehav Rev 2010;34(8):1207–22.
68. Jung WH, Borgwardt S, Fusar-Poli P, et al. Gray matter volumetric abnormalities associated with the onset of psychosis. Front Psychiatry 2012;3:101.
69. Borgwardt SJ, Riecher-Rossler A, Dazzan P, et al. Regional gray matter volume abnormalities in the at risk mental state. Biol Psychiatry 2007;61(10):1148–56.
70. Fusar-Poli P, Broome MR, Woolley JB, et al. Altered brain function directly related to structural abnormalities in people at ultra high risk of psychosis: longitudinal VBM-fMRI study. J Psychiatr Res 2011;45(2):190–8.
71. Iwashiro N, Suga M, Takano Y, et al. Localized gray matter volume reductions in the pars triangularis of the inferior frontal gyrus in individuals at clinical high-risk for psychosis and first episode for schizophrenia. Schizophr Res 2012;137(1–3):124–31.
72. Jung WH, Kim JS, Jang JH, et al. Cortical thickness reduction in individuals at ultra-high-risk for psychosis. Schizophr Bull 2011;37(4):839–49.
73. Koutsouleris N, Schmitt GJ, Gaser C, et al. Neuroanatomical correlates of different vulnerability states for psychosis and their clinical outcomes. Br J Psychiatry 2009;195(3):218–26.
74. Koutsouleris N, Patschurek-Kliche K, Scheuerecker J, et al. Neuroanatomical correlates of executive dysfunction in the at-risk mental state for psychosis. Schizophr Res 2010;123(2–3):160–74.
75. Meisenzahl EM, Koutsouleris N, Gaser C, et al. Structural brain alterations in subjects at high-risk of psychosis: a voxel-based morphometric study. Schizophr Res 2008;102(1–3):150–62.
76. Pantelis C, Velakoulis D, McGorry PD, et al. Neuroanatomical abnormalities before and after onset of psychosis: a cross-sectional and longitudinal MRI comparison. Lancet 2003;361(9354):281–8.

77. Meijer JH, Schmitz N, Nieman DH, et al. Semantic fluency deficits and reduced grey matter before transition to psychosis: a voxelwise correlational analysis. Psychiatry Res 2011;194(1):1–6.

78. Shin KS, Jung WH, Kim JS, et al. Neuromagnetic auditory response and its relation to cortical thickness in ultra-high-risk for psychosis. Schizophr Res 2012; 140(1–3):93–8.

79. Takahashi T, Wood SJ, Yung AR, et al. Superior temporal gyrus volume in antipsychotic-naive people at risk of psychosis. Br J Psychiatry 2010;196(3): 206–11.

80. Ziermans TB, Schothorst PF, Schnack HG, et al. Progressive structural brain changes during development of psychosis. Schizophr Bull 2012;38(3):519–30.

81. Dazzan P, Soulsby B, Mechelli A, et al. Volumetric abnormalities predating the onset of schizophrenia and affective psychoses: an MRI study in subjects at ultrahigh risk of psychosis. Schizophr Bull 2012;38(5):1083–91.

82. Mechelli A, Riecher-Rossler A, Meisenzahl EM, et al. Neuroanatomical abnormalities that predate the onset of psychosis: a multicenter study. Arch Gen Psychiatry 2011;68(5):489–95.

83. Hurlemann R, Jessen F, Wagner M, et al. Interrelated neuropsychological and anatomical evidence of hippocampal pathology in the at-risk mental state. Psychol Med 2008;38(6):843–51.

84. Phillips LJ, Velakoulis D, Pantelis C, et al. Non-reduction in hippocampal volume is associated with higher risk of psychosis. Schizophr Res 2002;58(2–3): 145–58.

85. Witthaus H, Kaufmann C, Bohner G, et al. Gray matter abnormalities in subjects at ultra-high risk for schizophrenia and first-episode schizophrenic patients compared to healthy controls. Psychiatry Res 2009;173(3):163–9.

86. Wood SJ, Kennedy D, Phillips LJ, et al. Hippocampal pathology in individuals at ultra-high risk for psychosis: a multi-modal magnetic resonance study. Neuroimage 2010;52(1):62–8.

87. Wood SJ, Yucel M, Velakoulis D, et al. Hippocampal and anterior cingulate morphology in subjects at ultra-high-risk for psychosis: the role of family history of psychotic illness. Schizophr Res 2005;75(2–3):295–301.

88. Borgwardt SJ, McGuire PK, Aston J, et al. Structural brain abnormalities in individuals with an at-risk mental state who later develop psychosis. Br J Psychiatry Suppl 2007;51:s69–75.

89. Fornito A, Yung AR, Wood SJ, et al. Anatomic abnormalities of the anterior cingulate cortex before psychosis onset: an MRI study of ultra-high-risk individuals. Biol Psychiatry 2008;64(9):758–65.

90. Yucel M, Wood SJ, Phillips LJ, et al. Morphology of the anterior cingulate cortex in young men at ultra-high risk of developing a psychotic illness. Br J Psychiatry 2003;182:518–24.

91. Bohner G, Milakara D, Witthaus H, et al. MTR abnormalities in subjects at ultra-high risk for schizophrenia and first-episode schizophrenic patients compared to healthy controls. Schizophr Res 2012;137(1–3):85–90.

92. Haller S, Borgwardt SJ, Schindler C, et al. Can cortical thickness asymmetry analysis contribute to detection of at-risk mental state and first-episode psychosis? A pilot study. Radiology 2009;250(1):212–21.

93. Smieskova R, Fusar-Poli P, Aston J, et al. Insular volume abnormalities associated with different transition probabilities to psychosis. Psychol Med 2012; 42(8):1613–25.

94. Takahashi T, Wood SJ, Yung AR, et al. Insular cortex gray matter changes in individuals at ultra-high-risk of developing psychosis. Schizophr Res 2009; 111(1–3):94–102.

95. Whitford TJ, Wood SJ, Yung A, et al. Structural abnormalities in the cuneus associated with herpes simplex virus (type 1) infection in people at ultra high risk of developing psychosis. Schizophr Res 2012;135(1–3):175–80.

96. Hannan KL, Wood SJ, Yung AR, et al. Caudate nucleus volume in individuals at ultra-high risk of psychosis: a cross-sectional magnetic resonance imaging study. Psychiatry Res 2010;182(3):223–30.

97. Han HJ, Jung WH, Jang JH, et al. Reduced volume in the anterior internal capsule but its maintained correlation with the frontal gray matter in subjects at ultra-high risk for psychosis. Psychiatry Res 2012;204(2–3):82–90.

98. Choi JS, Kang DH, Park JY, et al. Cavum septum pellucidum in subjects at ultra-high risk for psychosis: compared with first-degree relatives of patients with schizophrenia and healthy volunteers. Prog Neuropsychopharmacol Biol Psychiatry 2008;32(5):1326–30.

99. Takahashi T, Yung AR, Yucel M, et al. Prevalence of large cavum septi pellucidi in ultra high-risk individuals and patients with psychotic disorders. Schizophr Res 2008;105(1–3):236–44.

100. Velakoulis D, Wood SJ, Wong MT, et al. Hippocampal and amygdala volumes according to psychosis stage and diagnosis: a magnetic resonance imaging study of chronic schizophrenia, first-episode psychosis, and ultra-high-risk individuals. Arch Gen Psychiatry 2006;63(2):139–49.

101. Ziermans TB, Durston S, Sprong M, et al. No evidence for structural brain changes in young adolescents at ultra high risk for psychosis. Schizophr Res 2009;112(1–3):1–6.

102. Borgwardt SJ, McGuire PK, Aston J, et al. Reductions in frontal, temporal and parietal volume associated with the onset of psychosis. Schizophr Res 2008; 106(2–3):108–14.

103. Sun D, Phillips L, Velakoulis D, et al. Progressive brain structural changes mapped as psychosis develops in 'at risk' individuals. Schizophr Res 2009;108(1–3):85–92.

104. Witthaus H, Mendes U, Brune M, et al. Hippocampal subdivision and amygdalar volumes in patients in an at-risk mental state for schizophrenia. J Psychiatry Neurosci 2010;35(1):33–40.

105. Garner B, Pariante CM, Wood SJ, et al. Pituitary volume predicts future transition to psychosis in individuals at ultra-high risk of developing psychosis. Biol Psychiatry 2005;58(5):417–23.

106. Mittal VA, Daley M, Shiode MF, et al. Striatal volumes and dyskinetic movements in youth at high-risk for psychosis. Schizophr Res 2010;123(1):68–70.

107. Takahashi T, Wood SJ, Yung AR, et al. Progressive gray matter reduction of the superior temporal gyrus during transition to psychosis. Arch Gen Psychiatry 2009;66(4):366–76.

108. Walterfang M, Yung A, Wood AG, et al. Corpus callosum shape alterations in individuals prior to the onset of psychosis. Schizophr Res 2008;103(1–3):1–10.

109. Cannon M, Jones P, Huttunen MO, et al. School performance in Finnish children and later development of schizophrenia: a population-based longitudinal study. Arch Gen Psychiatry 1999;56(5):457–63.

110. Nicolson R, Rapoport JL. Childhood-onset schizophrenia: rare but worth studying. Biol Psychiatry 1999;46(10):1418–28.

111. Gogtay N. Cortical brain development in schizophrenia: insights from neuroimaging studies in childhood-onset schizophrenia. Schizophr Bull 2008;34(1):30–6.

112. Addington AM, Rapoport JL. The genetics of childhood-onset schizophrenia: when madness strikes the prepubescent. Curr Psychiatry Rep 2009;11(2): 156–61.
113. El-Sayed M, Steen RG, Poe MD, et al. Brain volumes in psychotic youth with schizophrenia and mood disorders. J Psychiatry Neurosci 2010;35(4):229–36.
114. Gogtay N, Weisinger B, Bakalar JL, et al. Psychotic symptoms and gray matter deficits in clinical pediatric populations. Schizophr Res 2012;140(1–3):149–54.
115. James AC, James S, Smith DM, et al. Cerebellar, prefrontal cortex, and thalamic volumes over two time points in adolescent-onset schizophrenia. Am J Psychiatry 2004;161(6):1023–9.
116. Paillère-Martinot M, Caclin A, Artiges E, et al. Cerebral gray and white matter reductions and clinical correlates in patients with early onset schizophrenia. Schizophr Res 2001;50(1–2):19–26.
117. Reig S, Parellada M, Castro-Fornieles J, et al. Multicenter study of brain volume abnormalities in children and adolescent-onset psychosis. Schizophr Bull 2011; 37(6):1270–80.
118. Vidal CN, Rapoport JL, Hayashi KM, et al. Dynamically spreading frontal and cingulate deficits mapped in adolescents with schizophrenia. Arch Gen Psychiatry 2006;63(1):25–34.
119. Yoshihara Y, Sugihara G, Matsumoto H, et al. Voxel-based structural magnetic resonance imaging (MRI) study of patients with early onset schizophrenia. Ann Gen Psychiatry 2008;7:25.
120. Jacobsen LK, Giedd JN, Castellanos FX, et al. Progressive reduction of temporal lobe structures in childhood-onset schizophrenia. Am J Psychiatry 1998; 155(5):678–85.
121. Matsumoto H, Simmons A, Williams S, et al. Superior temporal gyrus abnormalities in early-onset schizophrenia: similarities and differences with adult-onset schizophrenia. Am J Psychiatry 2001;158(8):1299–304.
122. Tang J, Liao Y, Zhou B, et al. Decrease in temporal gyrus gray matter volume in first-episode, early onset schizophrenia: an MRI study. PLoS One 2012;7(7): e40247.
123. Kumra S, Robinson P, Tambyraja R, et al. Parietal lobe volume deficits in adolescents with schizophrenia and adolescents with cannabis use disorders. J Am Acad Child Adolesc Psychiatry 2012;51(2):171–80.
124. Penttila J, Paillere-Martinot ML, Martinot JL, et al. Global and temporal cortical folding in patients with early-onset schizophrenia. J Am Acad Child Adolesc Psychiatry 2008;47(10):1125–32.
125. Clark GM, Crow TJ, Barrick TR, et al. Asymmetry loss is local rather than global in adolescent onset schizophrenia. Schizophr Res 2010;120(1–3):84–6.
126. Jacobsen LK, Giedd JN, Vaituzis AC, et al. Temporal lobe morphology in childhood-onset schizophrenia. Am J Psychiatry 1996;153(3):355–61.
127. Levitt JG, Blanton RE, Caplan R, et al. Medial temporal lobe in childhood-onset schizophrenia. Psychiatry Res 2001;108(1):17–27.
128. Taylor JL, Blanton RE, Levitt JG, et al. Superior temporal gyrus differences in childhood-onset schizophrenia. Schizophr Res 2005;73(2–3):235–41.
129. Nugent TF 3rd, Herman DH, Ordonez A, et al. Dynamic mapping of hippocampal development in childhood onset schizophrenia. Schizophr Res 2007; 90(1–3):62–70.
130. Frazier JA, Giedd JN, Hamburger SD, et al. Brain anatomic magnetic resonance imaging in childhood-onset schizophrenia. Arch Gen Psychiatry 1996;53(7): 617–24.

131. Jacobsen LK, Giedd JN, Tanrikut C, et al. Three-dimensional cortical morphometry of the planum temporale in childhood-onset schizophrenia. Am J Psychiatry 1997;154(5):685–7.
132. Matsumoto H, Simmons A, Williams S, et al. Structural magnetic imaging of the hippocampus in early onset schizophrenia. Biol Psychiatry 2001;49(10):824–31.
133. Collinson SL, Mackay CE, James AC, et al. Brain volume, asymmetry and intellectual impairment in relation to sex in early-onset schizophrenia. Br J Psychiatry 2003;183:114–20.
134. Hata K, Iida J, Iwasaka H, et al. Association between minor physical anomalies and lateral ventricular enlargement in childhood and adolescent onset schizophrenia. Acta Psychiatr Scand 2003;108(2):147–51.
135. Juuhl-Langseth M, Rimol LM, Rasmussen IA Jr, et al. Comprehensive segmentation of subcortical brain volumes in early onset schizophrenia reveals limited structural abnormalities. Psychiatry Res 2012;203(1):14–23.
136. Sowell ER, Levitt J, Thompson PM, et al. Brain abnormalities in early-onset schizophrenia spectrum disorder observed with statistical parametric mapping of structural magnetic resonance images. Am J Psychiatry 2000;157(9): 1475–84.
137. Greenstein D, Lenroot R, Clausen L, et al. Cerebellar development in childhood onset schizophrenia and non-psychotic siblings. Psychiatry Res 2011;193(3): 131–7.
138. Kumra S, Giedd JN, Vaituzis AC, et al. Childhood-onset psychotic disorders: magnetic resonance imaging of volumetric differences in brain structure. Am J Psychiatry 2000;157(9):1467–74.
139. Jacobsen LK, Giedd JN, Berquin PC, et al. Quantitative morphology of the cerebellum and fourth ventricle in childhood-onset schizophrenia. Am J Psychiatry 1997;154(12):1663–9.
140. Rapoport JL, Giedd J, Kumra S, et al. Childhood-onset schizophrenia. Progressive ventricular change during adolescence. Arch Gen Psychiatry 1997;54(10): 897–903.
141. Frazier JA, Hodge SM, Breeze JL, et al. Diagnostic and sex effects on limbic volumes in early-onset bipolar disorder and schizophrenia. Schizophr Bull 2008; 34(1):37–46.
142. Davies DC, Wardell AM, Woolsey R, et al. Enlargement of the fornix in early-onset schizophrenia: a quantitative MRI study. Neurosci Lett 2001;301(3): 163–6.
143. Kendi M, Kendi AT, Lehericy S, et al. Structural and diffusion tensor imaging of the fornix in childhood- and adolescent-onset schizophrenia. J Am Acad Child Adolesc Psychiatry 2008;47(7):826–32.
144. Jacobsen LK, Giedd JN, Rajapakse JC, et al. Quantitative magnetic resonance imaging of the corpus callosum in childhood onset schizophrenia. Psychiatry Res 1997;68(2–3):77–86.
145. Johnson SL, Greenstein D, Clasen L, et al. Absence of anatomic corpus callosal abnormalities in childhood-onset schizophrenia patients and healthy siblings. Psychiatry Res 2013;211(1):11–6.
146. Nopoulos PC, Giedd JN, Andreasen NC, et al. Frequency and severity of enlarged cavum septi pellucidi in childhood-onset schizophrenia. Am J Psychiatry 1998;155(8):1074–9.
147. James AC, Javaloyes A, James S, et al. Evidence for non-progressive changes in adolescent-onset schizophrenia: follow-up magnetic resonance imaging study. Br J Psychiatry 2002;180:339–44.

148. Pagsberg AK, Baare WF, Raabjerg Christensen AM, et al. Structural brain abnormalities in early onset first-episode psychosis. J Neural Transm 2007;114(4): 489–98.
149. Arango C, Rapado-Castro M, Reig S, et al. Progressive brain changes in children and adolescents with first-episode psychosis. Arch Gen Psychiatry 2012;69(1):16–26.
150. Rapoport JL, Giedd JN, Blumenthal J, et al. Progressive cortical change during adolescence in childhood-onset schizophrenia. A longitudinal magnetic resonance imaging study. Arch Gen Psychiatry 1999;56(7):649–54.
151. Thompson PM, Vidal C, Giedd JN, et al. Mapping adolescent brain change reveals dynamic wave of accelerated gray matter loss in very early-onset schizophrenia. Proc Natl Acad Sci U S A 2001;98(20):11650–5.
152. Greenstein D, Lerch J, Shaw P, et al. Childhood onset schizophrenia: cortical brain abnormalities as young adults. J Child Psychol Psychiatry 2006;47(10): 1003–12.
153. Keller A, Castellanos FX, Vaituzis AC, et al. Progressive loss of cerebellar volume in childhood-onset schizophrenia. Am J Psychiatry 2003;160(1):128–33.
154. Giedd JN, Jeffries NO, Blumenthal J, et al. Childhood-onset schizophrenia: progressive brain changes during adolescence. Biol Psychiatry 1999;46(7): 892–8.
155. Janssen J, Aleman-Gomez Y, Reig S, et al. Regional specificity of thalamic volume deficits in male adolescents with early-onset psychosis. Br J Psychiatry 2012;200(1):30–6.
156. Keller A, Jeffries NO, Blumenthal J, et al. Corpus callosum development in childhood-onset schizophrenia. Schizophr Res 2003;62(1–2):105–14.
157. Rapoport JL, Addington AM, Frangou S, et al. The neurodevelopmental model of schizophrenia: update 2005. Mol Psychiatry 2005;10(5):434–49.
158. Fusar-Poli P, Borgwardt S, Bechdolf A, et al. The psychosis high-risk state: a comprehensive state-of-the-art review. JAMA Psychiatry 2013;70(1):107–20.
159. Shah J, Eack SM, Montrose DM, et al. Multivariate prediction of emerging psychosis in adolescents at high risk for schizophrenia. Schizophr Res 2012; 141(2–3):189–96.
160. Koutsouleris N, Gaser C, Bottlender R, et al. Use of neuroanatomical pattern regression to predict the structural brain dynamics of vulnerability and transition to psychosis. Schizophr Res 2010;123(2–3):175–87.
161. Sublette ME, Oquendo MA, Mann JJ. Rational approaches to the neurobiologic study of youth at risk for bipolar disorder and suicide. Bipolar Disord 2006; 8(5 Pt 2):526–42.
162. Ivleva EI, Bidesi AS, Thomas BP, et al. Brain gray matter phenotypes across the psychosis dimension. Psychiatry Res 2012;204(1):13–24.
163. Keshavan MS, Tandon R, Boutros NN, et al. Schizophrenia, "just the facts": what we know in 2008 Part 3: neurobiology. Schizophr Res 2008;106(2–3):89–107.
164. Buehlmann E, Berger GE, Aston J, et al. Hippocampus abnormalities in at risk mental states for psychosis? A cross-sectional high resolution region of interest magnetic resonance imaging study. J Psychiatr Res 2010;44(7):447–53.
165. Walter A, Studerus E, Smieskova R, et al. Hippocampal volume in subjects at high risk of psychosis: a longitudinal MRI study. Schizophr Res 2012;142(1-3): 217–22.
166. Bakalar JL, Greenstein DK, Clasen L, et al. General absence of abnormal cortical asymmetry in childhood-onset schizophrenia: a longitudinal study. Schizophr Res 2009;115(1):12–6.

167. Marquardt RK, Levitt JG, Blanton RE, et al. Abnormal development of the anterior cingulate in childhood-onset schizophrenia: a preliminary quantitative MRI study. Psychiatry Res 2005;138(3):221–33.
168. Hadjulis M, Pipe R, Frangou S. Normal cerebral volume asymmetries in early onset schizophrenia. Biol Psychiatry 2004;55(2):148–53.

Neurocognition in Early-Onset Schizophrenia

Sophia Frangou, MD, PhD

KEYWORDS

- Cognition • Early onset • Schizophrenia • Intelligence • Memory
- Executive function • Attention • Development

KEY POINTS

- Early-onset schizophrenia is characterized by significant impairment in general intellectual ability, which seems to show a deteriorating course before but not after the onset of syndromal psychosis.
- Against this background, there is a degree of differentiation with regards to the magnitude and longitudinal evolution of specific cognitive domains.
- Verbal memory and learning emerge as the most consistently and significantly affected domains in which patients show increased deviance both before and after the onset of syndromal psychosis.
- In contrast, attentional resources seem to be initially preserved but show evidence of deterioration after syndromal onset.
- A common theme in cognitive changes observed after psychosis onset is that they seem to reflect both decline from baseline functioning and failure to show the age-related gains observed in healthy developing youth.

INTRODUCTION

Cognitive dysfunction is a central feature of schizophrenia.[1] The focus of this article is the cognitive profile of individuals who develop schizophrenia during childhood (childhood-onset schizophrenia [COS]) or adolescence (adolescent-onset schizophrenia [AOS]). COS is rare, because less than 1% of cases with schizophrenia present before the age of 13 years.[2] AOS is more common, because approximately 18% of cases present before the age of 18 years.[3] In this article, the term early-onset schizophrenia (EOS) is used when referring collectively to both COS and AOS groups.

EOS lies on the same neurobiological continuum as adult-onset schizophrenia.[4] However, EOS is associated with greater genetic loading,[4] more pronounced

Funding Sources: None.
Conflict of Interest: None.
Department of Psychiatry, Icahn School of Medicine at Mount Sinai, Box 1230, 1425 Madison Avenue, New York, NY 10029, USA
E-mail address: sophia.frangou@mssm.edu

Child Adolesc Psychiatric Clin N Am 22 (2013) 715–726
http://dx.doi.org/10.1016/j.chc.2013.04.007
1056-4993/13/$ – see front matter © 2013 Elsevier Inc. All rights reserved.

childpsych.theclinics.com

developmental and premorbid deviance,[4,5] and worse clinical course and outcome.[6,7] These findings suggest that onset of schizophrenia in youth reflects increased disease severity, which may be related to increased deviance in developmental trajectories compared with the adult-onset form.[8] Neurodevelopmental processes are particularly relevant to cognitive function. During late childhood and adolescence, normally developing youth show performance gains primarily in tasks of executive function, memory, and attention, resulting in subtle improvement in general intellectual ability.[9] In this context, the study of the cognitive abnormalities of patients with EOS offers an opportunity to explore how disease-related mechanisms may affect facets of cognitive development in late childhood and adolescence. This article summarizes and synthesizes available data with regards to the profile of cognitive impairments in patients with EOS and their severity, as well as their timing and evolution over the course of the disorder.

NEUROCOGNITIVE TESTS USED TO ASSESS COGNITION IN EOS

A variety of tests have been used to assess cognitive function in EOS based on investigators' preferences and logistical feasibility. **Table 1** summarizes the most commonly used tasks and assigns them to conventional putative cognitive domains. General intellectual ability in samples derived from clinical settings was typically assessed using different versions of the Wechsler Intelligence Scales, whereas epidemiologic studies used a variety of measures, including parental or teacher reports or academic records or country-specific cognitive screening batteries. Processing speed, which reflects coordinated and speeded performance during scanning and matching,[10] was commonly evaluated using the Wechsler Digit Symbol Test,[10] the Trail Making Test (TMT)[11–13] and Category Fluency.[14,15] Different version of the Continuous Performance Test (CPT)[11,15–19] and a variety of Dual Tasks[11,13] were used to assess cognitive mechanisms respectively relating to sustained and selective attention. Verbal memory and learning were commonly assessed using list learning tasks,[11,12,17–23] whereas the digit and spatial span tests were used to evaluate verbal

Table 1 Cognitive tests commonly used in EOS studies	
Cognitive Domain	**Test**
General intellectual ability	Wechsler Intelligence Scales Academic performance
Processing speed	Trails Making Test Symbol Coding Test Category Fluency
Working memory	Wechsler Digit Span Wechsler Spatial Span
Memory and learning	List Learning Tasks
Attention	Wechsler Attentional Control Index Continuous Performance Tests Dual Tasks
Strategy and problem solving	Tower of London Socks of Cambridge
Rule discovery and perseveration	Wisconsin Card Sorting Test
Response inhibition	Stroop Task Hayling Sentence Completion Task

and spatial working memory, respectively.[13,17,23] Other aspects of executive function examined were strategy and problem solving,[13] rule discovery and perseveration using the Wisconsin Card Sorting Test (WCST),[12,15,17,18] and response inhibition using the Hayling Sentence Completion Test[22] and the Stroop Test.[19,23] Significant variability in test selection has been an inherent feature of the literature on neurocognition, and it is only recently that the National Institute of Mental Health MATRICS (Measurement and Treatment Research to Improve Cognition in Schizophrenia)[24,25] test battery has started being used in adolescent populations.[14,26]

PREMORBID PHASE

Information about cognitive function during the premorbid phase of EOS derives mostly from epidemiologic studies in which the focus has been on general intellectual ability. Despite methodological diversity, available studies have consistently shown that patients with schizophrenia, regardless of age of onset, have lower premorbid IQ scores (effect size –0.43) compared with their healthy counterparts[27,28]; this effect is even more pronounced in patients with EOS.[28,29]

Additional information may be gleaned from studies of youth at clinical high risk of schizophrenia. Several definitions have been used to capture the presentation of high-risk individuals such as at-risk mental states, attenuated psychotic symptoms, brief limited intermittent psychotic symptoms, ultrahigh-risk individuals,[30] early initial prodromal states, late initial prodromal states,[31] and attenuated psychosis syndrome (http://www.dsm5.org). Subthreshold psychotic symptoms combined with functional impairment are the common features of all these definitions. Studies of high-risk youth confirm that lower IQ is a consistent feature of the premorbid phase of schizophrenia[32,33] and suggest that abnormalities in processing speed and visual working memory may be the earliest detectable deficits associated with psychosis[26]; additional impairments in verbal memory and learning may characterize those individuals who convert to syndromal disease.[32,33]

TRANSITION TO SYNDROMAL DISORDER

Longitudinal studies have repeatedly shown that, regardless of age of onset, transition to syndromal psychosis is associated with cognitive decline, as captured by global measures of intellectual ability.[34,35] Decline in cognitive function in preschizophrenic youth, regardless of the age of onset, seems to occur between the ages of 7 and 18 years and is even more pronounced in those individuals with EOS.[34,35]

Further cognitive deterioration has been reported in adult-onset schizophrenia occurring during the prodromal period.[36–38] Similarly, a pattern of marked decline in IQ scores about 2 years before the onset of frank psychosis was reported in the National Institute of Mental Health (NIMH) cohort of patients with COS.[39] This finding was later replicated by Cullen and colleagues[40] in an independent sample of 52 patients with EOS recruited at the University of Minnesota. In this study, cognitive decline was based on parental reports and academic records.

COGNITIVE PROFILE OF SYNDROMAL EOS

The key features of the cognitive profile of patients with EOS are summarized in **Box 1**.

General Intellectual Ability

Mean IQ in patients with EOS after illness onset has been consistently found to be about 1 to 1.5 standard deviations lower than the normative mean[12,13,15,22,41–43]

Box 1
Cognitive profile of EOS

- Deficits of large effect size
  - General intellectual ability
  - Processing speed
  - Working memory
  - Verbal memory and learning
- Deficits of medium effect size
  - Rule discovery and perseveration
  - Planning and problem solving
- Minimal deficit
  - Sustained attention
  - Selective attention

---

and about 0.88 standard deviations lower than the pooled mean of patients with adult-onset schizophrenia.[29]

Processing Speed

The magnitude of impairment in processing speed seems to vary depending on how this measure was derived. Kenny and colleagues[23] reported a medium effect size (0.66) in processing speed measured by the Wechsler Digit Symbol Test and category fluency in 17 patients with AOS recruited at Case Western Reserve University. In a sample of 19 Norwegian patients with EOS, Oie and Rund[11] reported a decrement of about 2 standard deviations lower than the control mean in processing speed assessed by combining the Wechsler Digit Symbol Test with the TMT. A deficit of the same magnitude was also reported by Kumra and colleagues[41] in the NIMH COS cohort based on a similar measure of processing speed.

Working Memory

Brickman and colleagues[19] grouped the Wechsler Digit Span Test and the TMT to form a composite variable of working memory. Their sample of 39 patients with AOS who had never been medicated recruited at Mount Sinai Hospital scored nearly 3 standard deviations lower than normative values. A comparable impairment in the Digit Span Test was reported in a sample of 34 psychotic patients aged 8 to 19 years recruited at the University of Minnesota.[44] In a subsequent study, the same research group used the 1-back task to assess spatial memory in 29 patients with EOS compared with healthy youths. Patients with EOS showed impairments of large effect size (0.78–0.98) on all performance measures and particularly in target sensitivity (1.76).[45]

Memory and Learning

Kenny and colleagues[23] were amongst the first to report significant impairment in verbal memory and leaning (effect size range 0.68–0.96) in patients with AOS compared with healthy adolescents. In their study, verbal learning was assessed using list learning tests, whereas immediate and delayed recall were assessed using the Wechsler Logical Memory I and II subtests. Abnormalities in verbal learning and memory have since been consistently reported in a variety of EOS samples, including patients who have never been medicated [19] and patients with EOS and schizophrenia spectrum disorders.[15,21,46] A study in Norwegian youth with either EOS[11] or schizophrenia spectrum disorders[17] suggested that visual memory, assessed using the Kimura Recurring Figures Test, was also significantly impaired. However, data from the Maudsley Early Onset Schizophrenia Study (Maudsley EOSS), which compared 42 patients with AOS with 43 demographically matched participants showed minimal deficits in the Wechsler Visual Memory Composite Index, whereas significant impairment was again noted for verbal memory.[13]

Attention

In their sample of Norwegian patients with EOS, Oie and Rund[11] did not find significant impairment either in sustained attention, as measured by the Degraded Symbol CPT, or selective attention, as assessed using a dichotic listening task. Similarly, data from the Maudsley EOSS did not reveal attentional deficits in patients with AOS either.[13] Attention in this study was measured using the Wechsler Attentional Control Index and selective attention was evaluated using a dual-task paradigm. However, Groom and colleagues[22] reported significant deficits in the Identical Pairs CPT when they compared 30 patients with EOS recruited from the University of Nottingham with 72 matched healthy participants. Karatekin and colleagues[42] were able to provide a more detailed assessment of sustained attention by using the 0-back spatial task to compare 29 patients with EOS with 56 matched healthy youth recruited at the University of Minnesota. Patients showed significantly greater variability in response time (effect size 1.47), suggestive of greater fluctuation in attentional resource allocation.

Rule Discovery and Perseveration

Impairment of moderate effect size has been reported in both rule discovery and perseveration in 4 independent patient samples from Norway,[11] Denmark,[12] and from the Case Western Reserve University[23] and the NIMH[41] in the United States.

Planning and Problem Solving

In the Maudsley EOSS, this domain was assessed using the Tower of London (TOL) Test,[13] whereas Fagerlund and colleagues[12] (2006) used the Socks of Cambridge task, a nearly identical paradigm from the CANTAB battery (Cambridge Neuropsychological Test Automated Battery), in a Danish sample of 18 patients with EOS and 21 patients with schizophrenia spectrum disorders. In both studies, patients with EOS showed deficits of moderate effect size in planning accuracy and response time.

Response Inhibition

Groom and colleagues[22] reported significant deficits in inhibitory control using the Hayling Sentence Completion Test, although the results of 2 studies using the Stroop Test were conflicting; Kenny and colleagues[23] reported a large deficit (effect size 1.12), whereas Mayoral and colleagues[47] could not detect any difference between patients with EOS and healthy adolescents (effect size 0.02).

EVOLUTION OF COGNITIVE IMPAIRMENT IN EOS AFTER PSYCHOSIS ONSET

The key longitudinal cognitive changes in patients with EOS are summarized in **Box 2**.

General Intellectual Ability

An initial report of IQ decline about 2 years after the onset of psychotic symptoms in the NIMH COS cohort[13] has not been substantiated by subsequent studies. A further

---

Box 2
Evolution of cognitive impairment in EOS after psychosis onset

- Evidence of increasing deviance
  - Verbal memory and learning
  - Attention
  - Perseverative errors
- Evidence of stability
  - General intellectual ability
  - Working memory
  - Rule discovery
- Limited or conflicting evidence
  - Processing speed
  - Planning and problem solving
  - Response inhibition

---

study from a larger sample from the same NIMH COS cohort did not find any evidence of decline after psychosis onset based on repeated biennial IQ assessments over an 8-year period.[48] Patients' IQ scores fluctuated during this period, but there was no substantial overall change over time. This pattern was also observed in 4 other independent samples from the United States,[49] Spain,[47] United Kingdom,[50] and Denmark[51] that followed up patients with EOS over a 1-year, 2-year, 4-year, and 5-year period, respectively.

Processing Speed

Data from a 13-year follow-up of a Norwegian EOS sample suggest that processing speed, measured by the Wechsler Digit Symbol, shows significantly increased deviance in patients over time,[52,53] mostly attributable to patients' failure to show the age-related improvements observed in normally developing participants. However, processing speed assessed with the TMT, in the same study as well as in 2 other studies from Spain and from the Maudsley EOSS cohort, showed either no change[50,52] or marginal improvement.[47] Similar findings were reported for category fluency.[50]

Working Memory

Three independent studies from the United States,[49] Spain,[47] and Norway[52] examined longitudinal changes in working memory as measured by the Wechsler Digit Span over follow-up periods of 1 to 13 years. All 3 reported that patients' deficit in test performance remained stable.

Memory and Learning

Data from the Spanish and the Zucker Hillside Hospital EOS cohorts showed no evidence of decline in verbal learning and memory (as assessed with the California Verbal Learning Test) at 1-year and 2-year intervals, respectively.[47,49] However, in the 4-year follow-up of the Maudsley EOSS sample,[50] patients showed evidence of decline in the Wechsler Verbal Memory Index, whereas healthy adolescents performed at the same level at both assessments. More detailed examination revealed that this decline affected primarily acquisition of new information rather than consolidation and recall.

Moreover, Øie and colleagues[52] found evidence of worsening performance in the California Verbal Learning Test in a Norwegian EOS cohort over a long follow-up period of 13 years, whereas healthy participants showed no change in their performance between assessments.

Attention

Thaden and colleagues[54] administered the Identical Pairs CPT to 59 adolescents with EOS and 55 matched healthy youths recruited at the Zucker Hillside Hospital. Across the age span of the sample (10–20 years of age), healthy adolescents improved in task performance, and this was particularly true for task conditions with high processing load.[54] This finding was not present in patients. Similarly, a 4-year longitudinal examination of the Maudsley EOSS cohort found that patients' deviance in attentional measures based on the Wechsler Attentional Control Index increased over time.[50] This finding reflected both age-related improvements in attentional processing in healthy participants and decline in patients with EOS. Dichotic listening was used in only the Norwegian EOS cohort, in which patients showed deterioration over a 13-year follow-up period, whereas the performance of their healthy counterparts remained unchanged.[52] Studies that used more simple measures of attention, primarily the Wechsler Digit Forward Task, did not report any age-related effects.[47,49]

Rule Discovery and Perseveration

The WCST was used in 3 independent studies from the United States,[49] Spain,[47] and Norway[52] to examine longitudinal changes in rule discovery and perseveration. Deficits in rule discovery remained stable over follow-up periods ranging from 1 to 13 years. In contrast, patients with EOS showed deterioration in terms of perseverative errors, which became statistically significant at 13-year follow-up.[52]

Planning and Problem Solving

Longitudinal data are available only for the TOL Test from the Maudsley EOSS,[50] in which patients' deficit remained stable over the 4-year follow-up period.

Response Inhibition

The available data are limited to a single study by Mayoral and colleagues[47] that found no effect of diagnosis either at baseline or at 2-year follow-up.

THE ROLE OF ANTIPSYCHOTIC TREATMENT

Antipsychotic medication is the mainstay treatment in EOS. The effect of treatment on cognition was examined in the Treatment of Early-Onset Schizophrenia Spectrum Disorders (TEOSS) study, the largest study to directly examine the comparative efficacy and safety of first-generation (molindone) and second-generation antipsychotics (olanzapine and risperidone) in the treatment of 116 young patients with EOS or schizoaffective disorder.[55] Information about cognitive task performance was obtained on 105 patients at baseline.[15] Seventy-seven patients repeated the cognitive assessment at week 8, and 51 of these patients had a further assessment at week 52.[56] There was no significant effect of medication type (molindone, risperidone, olanzapine), which could be a result of insufficient power. However as in previous studies, patients showed modest improvement in terms of global cognitive ability at week 8 and at week 52 compared with baseline.[56] At both postbaseline time points, patients committed fewer errors of omission and commission in a version of the CPT; improvement was also seen in processing speed measured by phonologic, semantic, and figural fluency. Improvement in attention showed a modest correlation with global clinical improvement. Although there is still no mechanistic model for the effect of medication on cognition, the results of the TEOSS study suggest that antipsychotic treatment does not impede and may facilitate neurocognitive improvement over time.

CONCLUDING REMARKS

This article examines the cognitive profile of patients with EOS and its longitudinal evolution. Despite significant differences in sample characteristics and cognitive tests used, there are several areas of convergence. EOS is characterized by significant impairment in general intellectual ability, which seems to show a deteriorating course before but not after the onset of syndromal psychosis. Against this background, there is a degree of differentiation with regards to the magnitude and longitudinal evolution of specific cognitive domains. Verbal memory and learning emerge as the most consistently and significantly affected domains in which patients show increased deviance both before and after the onset of syndromal psychosis. In contrast, attentional resources seem to be initially preserved but show evidence of deterioration after syndromal onset. A common theme in cognitive changes observed after psychosis onset is that they seem to reflect both decline from baseline functioning and failure to show the age-related gains observed in healthy developing youth.

Neuroimaging studies of normally developing youth and of patients provide a general framework for understanding the neural underpinnings of the cognitive profile of EOS. During normal development, improvement in higher cognitive function has been associated with increased recruitment of frontoparietal regions[57,58] and enhanced white matter connectivity between the superior frontal and parietal cortices.[59] These findings suggest that during adolescence, there is significant remodeling and strengthening of neural circuits subserving higher cognitive functions. In patients with EOS, there is evidence of an interaction between these developmental changes and disease-related mechanisms. Functional imaging studies have identified progressive deviance in prefrontal recruitment as patients with EOS progress from adolescence to young adulthood.[60] These functional changes resonate with anatomic findings from studies in EOS documenting progressive loss in prefrontal gray volume and white matter integrity throughout adolescence and into young adulthood.[61–64] Further research is required to explore the relationship between cognitive and brain functional and structural changes, particularly in connection with newly identified genetic variants conferring risk for EOS.

REFERENCES

1. Reichenberg A, Harvey PD. Neuropsychological impairments in schizophrenia: integration of performance-based and brain imaging findings. Psychol Bull 2007;133:833–58.
2. Beitchman JH. Childhood schizophrenia. A review and comparison with adult-onset schizophrenia. Psychiatr Clin North Am 1985;8:793–814.
3. Hafner H, Nowotny B. Epidemiology of early-onset schizophrenia. Eur Arch Psychiatry Clin Neurosci 1995;245:80–92.
4. Rapoport JL, Addington AM, Frangou S. The neurodevelopmental model of schizophrenia: update 2005. Mol Psychiatry 2005;10:434–49.
5. Vourdas A, Pipe R, Corrigall R, et al. Increased developmental deviance and premorbid dysfunction in early onset schizophrenia. Schizophr Res 2003;62:13–22.

6. Schimmelmann BG, Conus P, Cotton S, et al. Pre-treatment, baseline, and outcome differences between early-onset and adult-onset psychosis in an epidemiological cohort of 636 first-episode patients. Schizophr Res 2007;95:1–8.
7. Remschmidt H, Martin M, Fleischhaker C, et al. Forty-two-years later: the outcome of childhood-onset schizophrenia. J Neural Transm 2007;114:505–12.
8. Shaw P, Gogtay N, Rapoport J. Childhood psychiatric disorders as anomalies in neurodevelopmental trajectories. Hum Brain Mapp 2010;31:917–25.
9. Waber DP, Forbes PW, Almli CR, et al. Four-year longitudinal performance of a population-based sample of healthy children on a neuropsychological battery: the NIH MRI study of normal brain development. J Int Neuropsychol Soc 2012;18:179–90.
10. Dickinson D, Ramsey ME, Gold JM. Overlooking the obvious: a meta-analytic comparison of digit symbol coding tasks and other cognitive measures in schizophrenia. Arch Gen Psychiatry 2007;64:532–42.
11. Oie M, Rund BR. Neuropsychological deficits in adolescent-onset schizophrenia compared with attention deficit hyperactivity disorder. Am J Psychiatry 1999;156:1216–22.
12. Fagerlund B, Pagsberg AK, Hemmingsen RP. Cognitive deficits and levels of IQ in adolescent onset schizophrenia and other psychotic disorders. Schizophr Res 2006;8:30–9.
13. Kravariti E, Morris RG, Rabe-Hesketh S, et al. The Maudsley Early-Onset Schizophrenia Study: cognitive function in adolescent-onset schizophrenia. Schizophr Res 2003;61:137–48.
14. Holmén A, Juuhl-Langseth M, Thormodsen R, et al. Neuropsychological profile in early-onset schizophrenia-spectrum disorders: measured with the MATRICS battery. Schizophr Bull 2010;36:852–9.
15. Hooper SR, Giuliano AJ, Youngstrom EA, et al. Neurocognition in early-onset schizophrenia and schizoaffective disorders. J Am Acad Child Adolesc Psychiatry 2010;49:52–60.
16. Rund BR, Zeiner P, Sundet K, et al. No vigilance deficit found in either young schizophrenic or ADHD subjects. Scand J Psychol 1998;39:101–7.
17. Ueland T, Øie M, Landrø IN, et al. Cognitive functioning in adolescents with schizophrenia spectrum disorders. Psychiatry Res 2004;126:229–39.
18. Rhinewine JP, Lencz T, Thaden EP, et al. Neurocognitive profile in adolescents with early-onset schizophrenia: clinical correlates. Biol Psychiatry 2005;58:705–12.
19. Brickman AM, Buchsbaum MS, Bloom R, et al. Neuropsychological functioning in first-break, never-medicated adolescents with psychosis. J Nerv Ment Dis 2004;192:615–22.
20. McClellan J, Prezbindowski A, Breiger D, et al. Neuropsychological functioning in early onset psychotic disorders. Schizophr Res 2004;68:21–6.
21. Roofeh D, Cottone J, Burdick KE, et al. Deficits in memory strategy use are related to verbal memory impairments in adolescents with schizophrenia-spectrum disorders. Schizophr Res 2006;85:201–12.
22. Groom MJ, Jackson GM, Calton TG, et al. Cognitive deficits in early-onset schizophrenia spectrum patients and their non-psychotic siblings: a comparison with ADHD. Schizophr Res 2008;99:85–95.
23. Kenny JT, Friedman L, Findling RL, et al. Cognitive impairment in adolescents with schizophrenia. Am J Psychiatry 1997;154:1613–5.
24. Nuechterlein KH, Green MF, Kern RS, et al. The MATRICS consensus cognitive battery, part 1: test selection, reliability, and validity. Am J Psychiatry 2008;165:203–13.

25. Kern RS, Nuechterlein KH, Green MF, et al. The MATRICS consensus cognitive battery, part 2: co-norming and standardization. Am J Psychiatry 2008;165: 214–20.

26. Kelleher I, Clarke MC, Rawdon C, et al. Neurocognition in the extended psychosis phenotype: performance of a community sample of adolescents with psychotic symptoms on the MATRICS neurocognitive battery. Schizophr Bull 2012. http://dx.doi.org/10.1093/schbul/sbs086.

27. Woodberry KA, Giuliano AJ, Seidman LJ. Premorbid IQ in schizophrenia: a meta-analytic review. Am J Psychiatry 2008;165:579–87.

28. Khandaker GM, Barnett JH, White IR, et al. A quantitative meta-analysis of population-based studies of premorbid intelligence and schizophrenia. Schizophr Res 2011;132:220–7.

29. Rajji TK, Ismail Z, Mulsant BH. Age at onset and cognition in schizophrenia: meta-analysis. Br J Psychiatry 2009;195:286–93.

30. Fusar-Poli P, Borgwardt S, Bechdolf A, et al. The psychosis high-risk state: a comprehensive state-of-the-art review. Arch Gen Psychiatry 2012. http://dx.doi.org/10.1001/jamapsychiatry.2013.269.

31. Ruhrmann S, Schultze-Lutter F, Klosterkötter J. Early detection and intervention in the initial prodromal phase of schizophrenia. Pharmacopsychiatry 2003;36: S162–7.

32. Brewer WJ, Wood SJ, Phillips LJ, et al. Generalized and specific cognitive performance in clinical high-risk cohorts: a review highlighting potential vulnerability markers for psychosis. Schizophr Bull 2006;32:538–55.

33. Seidman LJ, Giuliano AJ, Meyer EC, et al. Neuropsychology of the prodrome to psychosis in the NAPLS consortium: relationship to family history and conversion to psychosis. Arch Gen Psychiatry 2010;67:578–88.

34. Fuller R, Nopoulos P, Arndt S, et al. Longitudinal assessment of premorbid cognitive functioning in patients with schizophrenia through examination of standardized scholastic test performance. Am J Psychiatry 2002;159:1183–9.

35. Maccabe JH, Wicks S, Löfving S, et al. Decline in cognitive performance between ages 13 and 18 years and the risk for psychosis in adulthood: a Swedish longitudinal cohort study in males. JAMA Psychiatry 2013;70:261–70.

36. Cosway R, Byrne M, Clafferty R, et al. Neuropsychological change in young people at high risk for schizophrenia: results from the first two neuropsychological assessments of the Edinburgh High Risk Study. Psychol Med 2000;30:1111–21.

37. Zanelli J, Reichenberg A, Morgan K, et al. Specific and generalized neuropsychological deficits: a comparison of patients with various first-episode psychosis presentations. Am J Psychiatry 2010;167:78–85.

38. Caspi A, Reichenberg A, Weiser M, et al. Cognitive performance in schizophrenia patients assessed before and following the first psychotic episode. Schizophr Res 2003;65:87–94.

39. Bedwell JS, Keller B, Smith AK, et al. Why does postpsychotic IQ decline in childhood-onset schizophrenia? Am J Psychiatry 1999;156:1996–7.

40. Cullen K, Guimaraes A, Wozniak J, et al. Trajectories of social withdrawal and cognitive decline in the schizophrenia prodrome. Clin Schizophr Relat Psychoses 2011;4:229–38.

41. Kumra S, Wiggs E, Bedwell J, et al. Neuropsychological deficits in pediatric patients with childhood-onset schizophrenia and psychotic disorder not otherwise specified. Schizophr Res 2000;42:135–44.

42. Karatekin C, White T, Bingham C. Divided attention in youth-onset psychosis and attention deficit/hyperactivity disorder. J Abnormal Psychol 2008;117:881–95.

43. White T, Ho BC, Ward J, et al. Neuropsychological performance in first-episode adolescents with schizophrenia: a comparison with first-episode adults and adolescent control subjects. Biol Psychiatry 2006;60:463–71.
44. Karatekin C, White T, Bingham C. Divided attention in youth-onset psychosis and attention deficit/hyperactivity disorder. J Abnorm Psychol 2008;117:881–95.
45. Karatekin C, Bingham C, White T. Regulation of cognitive resources during an n-back task in youth-onset psychosis and attention-deficit/hyperactivity disorder (ADHD). Int J Psychophysiol 2009;73:294–307.
46. Landrø NI, Ueland T. Verbal memory and verbal fluency in adolescents with schizophrenia spectrum disorders. Psychiatry Clin Neurosci 2008;62:653–61.
47. Mayoral M, Zabala A, Robles O, et al. Neuropsychological functioning in adolescents with first episode psychosis: a two-year follow-up study. Eur Psychiatry 2008;23:375–83.
48. Gochman PA, Greenstein D, Sporn A, et al. IQ stabilization in childhood-onset schizophrenia. Schizophr Res 2005;77:271–7.
49. Cervellione KL, Burdick KE, Cottone JG, et al. Neurocognitive deficits in adolescents with schizophrenia: longitudinal stability and predictive utility for short-term functional outcome. J Am Acad Child Adolesc Psychiatry 2007;46: 867–78.
50. Frangou S, Hadjulis M, Vourdas A. The Maudsley early onset schizophrenia study: cognitive function over a 4-year follow-up period. Schizophr Bull 2008;34:52–9.
51. Jepsen JR, Fagerlund B, Pagsberg AK, et al. Course of intelligence deficits in early onset, first episode schizophrenia: a controlled, 5-year longitudinal study. Eur Child Adolesc Psychiatry 2010;19:341–51.
52. Øie M, Sundet K, Rund BR. Neurocognitive decline in early-onset schizophrenia compared with ADHD and normal controls: evidence from a 13-year follow-up study. Schizophr Bull 2010;36:557–65.
53. Øie M, Hugdahl K. A 10-13 year follow-up of changes in perception and executive attention in patients with early-onset schizophrenia: a dichotic listening study. Schizophr Res 2008;106:29–32.
54. Thaden E, Rhinewine JP, Lencz T, et al. Early-onset schizophrenia is associated with impaired adolescent development of attentional capacity using the identical pairs continuous performance test. Schizophr Res 2006;81:157–66.
55. Sikich L, Frazier JA, McClellan J, et al. Double-blind comparison of first and second-generation antipsychotics in early-onset schizophrenia and schizoaffective disorder: findings from the treatment of early-onset schizophrenia spectrum disorders (TEOSS) study. Am J Psychiatry 2008;165:1420–31.
56. Frazier JA, Giuliano AJ, Johnson JL, et al. Neurocognitive outcomes in the treatment of early-onset schizophrenia spectrum disorders study. J Am Acad Child Adolesc Psychiatry 2012;51:496–505.
57. Klingberg T, Forssberg H, Westerberg H. Increased brain activity in frontal and parietal cortex underlies the development of visuospatial working memory capacity during childhood. J Cogn Neurosci 2002;14:1–10.
58. Kwon H, Reiss AL, Menon V. Neural basis of protracted developmental changes in visuo-spatial working memory. Proc Natl Acad Sci U S A 2002;99:13336–41.
59. Nagy Z, Westerberg H, Klingberg T. Maturation of white matter is associated with the development of cognitive functions during childhood. J Cogn Neurosci 2004;16:1227–33.
60. Kyriakopoulos M, Dima D, Roiser JP, et al. Abnormal functional activation and connectivity in the working memory network in early-onset schizophrenia. J Am Acad Child Adolesc Psychiatry 2012;51:911–20.

61. Thompson PM, Vidal C, Giedd JN, et al. Mapping adolescent brain change reveals dynamic wave of accelerated gray matter loss in very early-onset schizophrenia. Proc Natl Acad Sci U S A 2001;98:11650–5.
62. Giedd JN, Jeffries NO, Blumenthal J, et al. Childhood-onset schizophrenia: progressive brain changes during adolescence. Biol Psychiatry 1999;46:892–8.
63. Arango C, Moreno C, Martínez S, et al. Longitudinal brain changes in early-onset psychosis. Schizophr Bull 2008;34:341–53.
64. Kyriakopoulos M, Perez-Iglesias R, Woolley JB, et al. Effect of age at onset of schizophrenia on white matter abnormalities. Br J Psychiatry 2009;195:346–53.

Psychopharmacologic Treatment of Psychosis in Children and Adolescents: Efficacy and Management

Harvey N. Kranzler, MD*, Sarah D. Cohen, MD

KEYWORDS

- Psychopharmacology • Psychosis • Schizophrenia • Children • Adolescents
- Antipsychotic medication • Clozapine • Antipsychotic side effects

KEY POINTS

- Antipsychotic medications are effective in controlling psychosis in children and adolescents.
- Children and adolescents have a higher risk than adults for developing side effects from antipsychotic medications.
- Treatment strategies include minimizing the use of polypharmacy and basing choice of antipsychotic on risk for specific side effects.
- Monitoring and managing side effects of antipsychotic medication allows a more successful treatment plan.
- Clozapine should be part of the menu of options for treatment-resistant psychosis including schizophrenia, schizoaffective disorder, and bipolar disorder with psychosis and mania.
- The management of side effects of clozapine is not as daunting as many clinicians think.

INTRODUCTION

The psychopharmacologic treatment of psychosis in children and adolescents has been scrutinized for both efficacy and safety because of concerns about their increasing use,[1–3] especially with the advent of second-generation antipsychotics (SGAs) as well as aripiprazole, a third-generation antipsychotic (TGA) that is a dopamine agonist in low doses in addition to being a dopamine antagonist at higher doses. There is little controversy that medication treatment is an essential modality in the treatment of psychotic symptoms and prevention of recurrence within the context of psychotherapy, family, social, and cognitive interventions.

Disclosures: Dr Harvey N. Kranzler and Dr Sarah D. Cohen both report no funding sources or conflicts of interest.

Division of Child and Adolescent Psychiatry, Department of Psychiatry, Albert Einstein College of Medicine, 1300 Morris Park Avenue, Bronx, NY 10461, USA
* Corresponding author. 451 West End Avenue #2H, New York, NY 10024.
E-mail address: Harvey.Kranzler@gmail.com

Child Adolesc Psychiatric Clin N Am 22 (2013) 727–744
http://dx.doi.org/10.1016/j.chc.2013.06.002
childpsych.theclinics.com

There have been an increasing number of randomized controlled trials (RCTs) that have been the impetus for the US Food and Drug Administration (FDA) to approve the use of aripiprazole, olanzapine, quetiapine, and risperidone for ages 10 to 17 years (olanzapine 13–17 years) for schizophrenia, schizoaffective disorder, and bipolar mania.[4–6] The use of antipsychotic medication for bipolar mania, aggression in autistic spectrum disorders, disruptive behavior disorders, and tic disorders is not reviewed here but the same concerns about efficacy and safety are relevant in these populations.

Efficacy

In 7 RCT studies in a pediatric population with schizophrenia aged 13 to 17 years all the SGAs were superior to placebo in changes in the Positive and Negative Syndrome Scale (PANSS) scores except for ziprasidone and paliperidone.[7] These studies had small sample sizes and short duration and there was no difference in efficacy among nonclozapine antipsychotics.[8] Clozapine was superior in efficacy in 3 RCT trials compared with haloperidol,[9] olanzapine,[10] and high-dose olanzapine.[11] Although clozapine is not considered a first-line antipsychotic, it is still an important medication and clinicians should be comfortable with its use. The efficacy of this oldest SGA has particular benefit for treatment-resistant youth when at least 2 antipsychotics have been tried.[12]

In early onset schizophrenia (EOS), it is important to initiate antipsychotic medication as quickly as possible to ameliorate positive and negative symptoms, as well as impairments in motor, language, social, and cognitive development. The pathophysiology of schizophrenia is still unclear and the dopamine hypothesis has been proposed to explain the efficacy of antipsychotic medication by blocking the dopamine D2 receptors in the mesolimbic system. However, there is increasing evidence that antipsychotic medication, especially SGAs, affect multiple neuroreceptors including serotonin, alpha-adrenergic, histaminic, muscarinic, and glutaminergic receptors, which also have potential therapeutic as well as adverse effects.[6,7]

Given that EOS is a chronic condition that requires long-term medication management, it is important that there is ongoing monitoring of any changes in positive and negative symptoms, cognitive functioning, social interactions and side effects.

Side Effects

Children and adolescents are at a higher risk than adults for developing side effects including sedation, extrapyramidal side effects (EPS), withdrawal dyskinesias, increased prolactin levels, weight gain, and other metabolic abnormalities.[13–17] Tardive dyskinesia and diabetes mellitus were more likely to occur in adults than in youth.[16] Given that these children may require chronic long-term medication treatment, the concern for efficacy and safety of antipsychotic medication increases the importance of continuous close monitoring of side effects.[16,17] The hope was that the advantage of the SGAs compared with the first-generation antipsychotics (FGAs) with their potential for decreased EPS and withdrawal or tardive dyskinesias would make them more tolerable and safer for youth. However, the cardiometabolic side effects of SGAs have been an increasing concern. In a comprehensive review of prospective head-to-head and placebo-controlled studies,[8] there were relevant differences between SGAs in weight gain (olanzapine>clozapine>risperidone>quetiapine>aripiprazole), increased prolactin levels (risperidone>olanzapine, with clozapine being prolactin neutral and aripiprazole causing decrease in prolactin) and there were no significant differences between SGAs in neuromotor side effects. Except for clozapine, the heterogeneity within SGAs is mainly caused by differences in the rates and severity of adverse effects, especially in weight gain, which is a marker for potential cardiometabolic disturbance. In the Treatment of Early Onset Schizophrenia Spectrum Disorders Study (TEOSS)[5] comparing risperidone, olanzapine, and the FGA molindone, there were no significant differences in response rates or degree of symptom reduction after 8 weeks of treatment. There was significantly greater risk for weight gain, fasting glucose, fasting cholesterol, low-density lipoproteins, and insulin and liver transaminase levels (olanzapine>risperidone and molindone significantly less). A review of only short-term SGA studies in youth (41 studies between 1996 and 2010) found significant frequent treatment-related increases in weight gain (olanzapine>clozapine>risperidone>quetiapine>aripiprazole), glucose levels (risperidone>olanzapine), cholesterol levels (quetiapine>olanzapine), triglyceride levels (olanzapine>quetiapine), prolactin levels (risperidone>olanzapine>ziprasidone), and EPS (ziprasidone>olanzapine>aripiprazole>risperidone).[18] De Hert and colleagues[19] conducted a systematic review of randomized, placebo-controlled trials of SGAs in pediatric populations and, similar to adults, clozapine and olanzapine were associated with the most weight gain, whereas risperidone, quetiapine, aripiprazole, and ziprasidone followed in that order. A child's individual risk for weight gain may be influenced by environmental as well as genetic factors,[20] not just the choice of antipsychotic, as shown by the high interindividual variability in weight gain among patients treated with any given agent. Analyses of prospective and retrospective clinical reports reveal the possibility that a child's risk of weight gain might be related to a synergistic interaction between age and polypharmacy.[21,22]

Reviews of adult data examining the incidence of glycemic abnormalities from antipsychotic use have found inconsistent results, suggesting that associations with adverse effects depend on the patient population and the mental illnesses being studied.[23] However, there is some evidence of an increased risk of diabetes mellitus from antipsychotic use, particularly in patients less than 24 years old.[24] Panagiotopoulos and colleagues[25] also found that 21.5% of pediatric patients taking SGA medications (n = 65) had glycemic abnormalities (increased fasting plasma glucose or type 2 diabetes), compared with 7.5% of antipsychotic-naive individuals (P = .01). A prospective large-scale pharmacoepidemiologic study followed previously antipsychotic-naive patients after their first episode of schizophrenia and treatment with antipsychotic medications (n = 7139).[26] During the first year of treatment, time to onset of diabetes mellitus was significantly shorter during use with olanzapine and midpotency FGAs, including perphenazine, compared with patients not on antipsychotics. Olanzapine, clozapine, and low-potency FGAs including chlorpromazine were associated with diabetes arising early in treatment.[26] More recently, a study examining antipsychotic medication use in children enrolled in Health Maintenance Organization (HMO) plans (n = 9636) found a potential 4-fold increase in the rate of diabetes compared with nonpsychotropic medication users.[27] However, this increase was not significant compared with a group taking antidepressant medications, suggesting that, as in adult studies, associations with adverse effects depend on other factors.

In an attempt to translate the data in the literature into an evidence-based clinically useful tool, we merged all the review data and latest original data into simplified tables using the categories of "strong", "some", "less likely", "less likely?", and question mark.[8,15,17–19,28–30] "Strong" was used for a data point that has repeatedly shown up as significant in the publications cited earlier, as well as in clinical practice. "Some" was used when a data point had either had weak significance or only showed up in a portion of the studies. "Less likely" was used when the data point was never (or almost never) significant both in the studies and in clinical practice. We chose not to use a category of never because it seems that, particularly in this category of medication, any side effect is possible and we did not want to mislead the patient or the

Table 1
Risk for neuromotor adverse events of antipsychotics in youth

Antipsychotic	EPS	Akathisia	Withdrawal Dyskinesia	Tardive Dyskinesia	Seizures
First Generation					
Chlorpromazine	Some	Some	Less likely	Less likely	Less likely
Haldol	Strong	Strong	Some	Some	Less likely
Molindone	Some	Some	Some	Some	Less likely
Perphenazine	Some	Some	Some	Some	Less likely
Second Generation					
Clozapine	Less likely	Some	Less likely	Least likely	Some
Iloperidone	Less likely	Less likely	Some	?	Less likely
Olanzapine	Some	Some	Less likely	Less likely	Less likely
Paliperidone	Some	Some	Some	?	Less likely
Quetiapine	Some	Some	Less likely	Less likely	Less likely
Risperidone	Some	Some	Less likely	Less likely	Less likely
Ziprasidone	Strong	Some	Some	Less likely	Less likely
Third Generation					
Aripiprazole	Some	Some	Some	Less likely	Less likely

Table 2
Risk of metabolic adverse effects of antipsychotics in youth

Antipsychotic	Weight Gain	Increased Glucose	Increased Cholesterol	Increased Triglycerides	Prolactin Change
First Generation					
Chlorpromazine	Strong	Strong	Some	Less likely	Some
Haldol	Some	Less likely?	Less likely?	Less likely	Some
Molindone	Less likely	Less likely?	Less likely?	Less likely?	Some
Perphenazine	Some	Some	Some	Less likely	Some
Second Generation					
Clozapine	Strong	Strong	Some	Strong	Least likely
Iloperidone	Some	Less likely?	Less likely?	Less likely?	Less likely
Olanzapine	Strong	Some	Strong	Strong	Strong
Paliperidone	Some	Less likely?	Less likely?	Less likely?	Strong
Quetiapine	Some	Some	Strong	Strong	Less likely
Risperidone	Some	Strong	Some	Strong	Strong
Ziprasidone	Less likely	Less likely	Some	Less likely	Some
Third Generation					
Aripiprazole	Some	Some	Some	Less likely	Least likely[a]

[a] Clinical experience suggests that aripiprazole may lower increased prolactin levels.

Table 3
Risk for miscellaneous adverse effects of antipsychotics in youth

Antipsychotic	Liver Toxicity	Neutropenia	Agranulocytosis	Orthostasis	QTc Prolongation	Myocarditis	Sedation	Constipation	Dry Mouth
First Generation									
Chlorpromazine	Less likely	Less likely	Some	Some	Less likely	Less likely	Some	Some	Some
Haldol	Less likely	Less likely	Less likely	Less likely	Less likely	Less likely	Less likely	Less likely	Less likely
Molindone	Less likely	Less likely	Less likely	Some	Some	Less likely	Some	Less likely	Less likely
Perphenazine	Less likely	Less likely	Less likely	Some	Some	Less likely	Some	Less likely	Less likely
Second Generation									
Clozapine	Less likely	Some	Some	Strong	Some	Some	Strong	Strong	Some
Iloperidone	?	Less likely	Less likely	Strong	Some	Less likely	?	?	?
Olanzapine	Some	Less likely	Less likely	Some	Less likely	Less likely	Some	Strong	Less likely
Paliperidone	?	Less likely	Less likely	Some	Some	Less likely	?	?	?
Quetiapine	Less likely	Some	Less likely	Some	Some	Less likely	Some	Less likely	Less likely
Risperidone	Less likely	Some	Less likely	Some	Some	Less likely	Some	Less likely	Less likely
Ziprasidone	Less likely	Less likely	Less likely	Less likely	Some	Less likely	Some	Less likely	Less likely
Third Generation									
Aripiprazole	Less likely	Less likely	Less likely	Less likely	Less likely	Less likely	Some	Less likely	Less likely

practitioner into thinking otherwise. "Less likely?" was used when the study data were slightly mixed or lacking, but clinical practice suggests that it is a very low chance. A question mark implies that there are not enough published data or that there is insufficient clinical experience to make an appropriate estimate of risk. The authors present[19,31]:

- Generalized risks for FGA, SGA, and TGA for neuromotor adverse events (**Table 1**)
- Risk for metabolic adverse effects (**Table 2**)
- Risk for miscellaneous adverse effects (**Table 3**)
- Definitions of metabolic syndrome (**Table 4**)

Management of Side Effects

As discussed earlier, when children and adolescents take antipsychotic medications, they usually experience some unwanted side effects. Most of these, such as sedation and nausea, remit with time and should not be considered a reason to stop the treatment. There are some serious adverse events that demand immediate cessation of treatment, such as neuroleptic malignant syndrome (NMS), agranulocytosis, myocarditis and cardiomyopathy, and severe allergic reactions (**Table 5**). There are some conflicting data on whether SGAs are less likely to cause NMS than FGAs, as originally thought.[32,33] However the most recent review suggests that SGAs have a less permanent and lethal course of NMS than do the FGAs.[33] There are other serious adverse effects that most often require a change in choice of antipsychotic, including persistent hypertension or tachycardia, excessive weight gain, hyperglycemia, dyslipidemia, and electrolyte changes (**Table 6**). There are also adverse effects that demand some clinical management to continue with treatment (**Table 7**). We have created a 1-page pediatric antipsychotic tracking sheet to help clinicians monitor and track side effects (**Table 8**).

Healthy habits should be encouraged in all youth being given antipsychotic medications, including diet changes (lower fat/cholesterol, smaller portions, increased fiber, increased water) and increased aerobic exercise (30–60 minutes per day), which helps prevent weight gain, constipation, blood pressure changes, and glucose abnormalities. Youth should be encouraged to be free of substance abuse and develop healthy sleep habits. Parents and guardians should follow the same advice to enhance patient success.[34] There has been success in introducing weight gain prevention agents into this population, including metformin[35,36] and topiramate,[37] although the best data are found in the adult literature.[38,39]

Table 4
Metabolic syndrome in children and adolescents defined

Component	Definition
Obesity	Waist circumference ≥90th percentile, BMI ≥95th percentile
Increased triglyceride levels	Less than 10 y: fasting serum triglycerides ≥110 mg/dL More than 10 y (same as adults): fasting serum triglycerides ≥150 mg/dL
Low HDL levels	Fasting HDL cholesterol <40 mg/dL
High blood pressure	Blood pressure ≥90th percentile (based on age and gender)
Increased glucose	Prediabetes: fasting glucose ≥l00 mg/dL. Impaired glucose tolerance: 2 h post glucose load >149–199 mg/dL Diabetes: repeated fasting glucose ≥126 mg/dL 2-h post glucose load ≥200 mg/dL

Abbreviations: BMI, body mass index; HDL, high-density lipoprotein.

Table 5
Rare adverse events requiring immediate cessation of antipsychotic in children and adolescents

Serious Adverse Event	Definition	Action
Agranulocytosis	Laboratory tests: ANC <500/mm^3	Stop medication Consider granulocyte colony-stimulating factor Monitor until restoration to baseline Reassess need for antipsychotic and choose lower risk drug
NMS	Symptoms: marked motor rigidity, fever, tachycardia, hypotension, or hypertension Laboratory tests: increased CPK (>1000) and increased WBC count	Stop medication and hydrate Medical supportive treatment (often in ICU) Consider amantadine, bromocriptine, dantrolene, ECT Consider clozapine for psychotic symptoms (does not cause NMS)
Myocarditis/ cardiomyopathy	Symptoms: palpitations, chest pain, shortness of breath, and syncope Characteristic ECG changes: atrial or ventricular fibrillation, ectopic beats, atrioventricular block, atrial flutter, ventricular tachycardia, low QRS voltages, and intraventricular conduction disturbance Echocardiogram changes: thickening of intraventricular muscle	Stop medication Reassess need for antipsychotic and choose lower risk drug
Severe allergic reaction	Anaphylaxis Stevens-Johnson syndrome	Stop medication Supportive medical treatment Switch to a different antipsychotic

Abbreviations: ANC, absolute neutrophil count; CPK, creatine phosphokinase; ECG, electrocardiogram; ECT, electroconvulsive therapy; ICU, intensive care unit; WBC, white blood cell.

Treatment Strategies

It is an open question whether the first or second choice of antipsychotic should include an FGA such as molindone, as was used in the TEOSS study.[5] Since molindone is no longer available as an option because of manufacturing difficulties, a potential other FGA to consider is perphenazine. Molindone, as well as perphenazine, manifest greater EPS and akathisia than the SGAs. Based on the increased efficacy of clozapine compared with all other antipsychotic medications in children and adults, the recommendation is that if 2 SGAs, or 1 SGA and 1 FGA, have not provided sufficient symptom relief after at least 6 to 8 weeks at therapeutic dosages, a trial of clozapine should be initiated.[12,40]

When there is treatment resistance, there is some evidence in the adult literature that using 2 antipsychotics at the same time may be beneficial.[41] This may also be necessary with children and adolescents who do not respond to therapeutic dosages of 1

Table 6
Serious adverse effects suggesting a need for switch to a lower risk drug

Serious Adverse Effect	Recommended Response
Hypertension, tachycardia	Lower the dose and titrate more slowly Consider switch to lower risk drug Healthy habits Add weight loss agents Add antihypertensive agents
ECG changes	Lower the dose and titrate more slowly Consider switch to lower risk drug (aripiprazole or olanzapine) Lower dose and reassess
Excessive weight gain	Consider switch to lower risk drug Healthy habits Add weight loss agents
Electrolyte abnormalities	Lower the dose and reassess Consider switch to lower risk drug Address specific abnormality as needed
Increased liver enzymes	Consider switch to lower risk drug Lower dose and reassess
Glucose abnormalities	Consider switch to lower risk drug Healthy habits Add weight loss agents Add antihyperglycemic agents
Symptomatic hyperprolactinemia (galactorrhea, breast tenderness, menses changes, gynecomastia)	Consider switch to lower risk drug (aripiprazole, quetiapine, or clozapine) Rule out common causes (hormonal contraception, pregnancy, hypothyroidism, renal failure) Endocrine consultation only if symptoms persist or increase is >200 ng/mL Consider MRI of sella turcica (looking for pituitary adenoma or parasellar tumor) Add full (bromocriptine, amantidine) or partial dopamine agonists (aripiprazole)
Withdrawal dyskinesia	Taper and discontinue Switch to lower risk drug (clozapine)
Tardive dyskinesia	Taper and discontinue Switch to lower risk drug (clozapine) Add vitamin E

Abbreviation: MRI, magnetic resonance imaging.

antipsychotic, but it is preferable whenever possible to limit the use of 2 antipsychotics at the same time. There is also evidence that polypharmacy in youth increases the risk for obesity, cardiovascular and hypertensive adverse events.[42,43] During a cross titration between 2 antipsychotic medications there is the potential for a worsening of symptoms if the first antipsychotic has been tapered too quickly and the new antipsychotic has been titrated up too slowly or because differences in absorption, receptor binding affinity, and half-life contribute to insufficient dopamine blockade and dopamine rebound. This increase in symptoms may result in the child or adolescent continuing to be treated with both antipsychotics without complete crossover to the second antipsychotic, at times increasing the potential for greater side effects. The recommendation is for overlapping plateau switch strategies that take the

Table 7
Management of the more common side effects of antipsychotics in children and adolescents

Side Effect	Recommended Management
Akathisia	Slow titration Reduce dose Switch to lower risk drug Add benzodiazepine, β-blocker, antihistamine, or anticholinergic agent
Asymptomatic hyperprolactinemia	Reassess value because it often normalizes over time Rule out common causes (hormonal contraception, pregnancy hypothyroidism, renal failure) Reduce dose Consider adding low-dose aripiprazole Monitor for symptoms
Constipation	Behavioral changes (increase exercise and monitor bowel movements) Increase fluid and fiber in diet Add stool softeners, laxatives, motility agent; (Senokot, Miralax) Switch to lower risk drug
Dizziness Orthostatic hypotension Syncope	Reduce dose (except with quetiapine, which has less orthostasis ≥300 mg/d) Slow titration Increase fluid intake Encourage getting up slowly Switch to lower risk drug
Enuresis (secondary nocturnal)	Reduce dose of antipsychotic or other agent (lithium) Behavioral changes (no fluid after dinner, midnight wake-up, Bell and Pad) Add DDAVP, Ditropan, or oxybutynin
Neutropenia	Assess history for baseline benign ethnic neutropenia Redo laboratory tests later in the day (to avoid morning pseudoneutropenia) Redo laboratory tests after exercise (tends to increase the WBC count) Switch to lower risk drug Add lithium low dose (boosts WBC count)
Parkinsonism	Slow titration Reduce dose Switch to lower risk drug Add anticholinergic, antihistamine, benzodiazepine
Sedation	Wait; tolerance often develops after a few days Reduce dose (except with quetiapine, which has less orthostasis ≥300 mg/d) Switch to lower risk drug
Sialorrhea	Wait; tolerance often develops after a few weeks Behavioral changes (towel on pillow, chew gum) Add guanfacine, fluticasone, clonidine, scopolamine patch, or sublingual atropine (1% eye drops)

Abbreviation: DDAVP, desamino-ᴅ-arginine vasopressin.

pharmacokinetic and pharmacodynamic profiles of each antipsychotic into consideration.[44] Especially with a cross titration to aripiprazole, which requires higher receptor occupancy to achieve therapeutic dopamine blockade, there is a greater potential for rebound symptoms if the first FGA or SGA is removed too quickly. Once the second

Table 8
Pediatric antipsychotic tracking sheet
Directions: fill in date and document relevant results or abnormalities. Continue with original chart even if antipsychotic medication is changed. For BMI and percentile calculations, use www.cdc.gov, and for blood pressure percentile calculations use pediatric.aappublications.org. If any values are abnormal, monitor more frequently in consultation with primary care doctor. This table may be copied, enlarged and placed in medical record.

Parameter	Baseline	1 mo	2 mo	3 mo	6 mo	9 mo	1 y	2 y
Date of office assessment								
Personal and family history		X	X	X	X	X		
Healthy lifestyle reviewed								
Assess for symptoms of side effects								
Sedation								
Constipation								
Enuresis								
Sialorrhea or dry mouth								
Height								
Weight								
BMI and percentile (indicate trend)								
Blood pressure and percentile								
AIMS		X	X					
Name of medication								
Date of laboratory assessment								
Fasting serum glucose		X	X			X		
Fasting total cholesterol		X	X			X		
Fasting LDL		X	X			X		
Fasting HDL		X	X			X		
Fasting triglycerides		X	X			X		
Aspartate aminotransferase		X	X	X		X		
Alanine aminotransferase		X	X	X		X		
Prolactin (only when symptomatic)								
CBC (for clozapine follow FDA guidelines)		X	X			X		
Electrolytes (document abnormalities)		X	X			X		
HbA1c		X	X			X		
Date of ECG		X	X	X		X		
QTC		X	X	X		X		
PR interval		X	X	X		X		
Echocardiogram for clozapine	X	X			X	X		
CK-MB and troponin levels for clozapine		X	X					
Consultations (only as needed)								

Abbreviations: AIMS, abnormal involuntary movement scale; CBC, complete blood count; CK-MB, creatine kinase myocardial band; HbA1c, hemoglobin A1c; LDL, low-density lipoprotein.

Table 9 Selected CYPP450 drug interactions for atypical antipsychotics		
Drug	**CYP Isoenzyme**	**Effect on Plasma Concentration**
Carbamazepine	CYP1A2, CYP3A4	↓↓CLZ ↓ OLZ ↓QTP
Cigarette Smoking	CYP1A2	↓↓CLZ ↓↓OLZ
Cimetadine	CYP inhibitor	↑↑CLZ ↑↑OLZ ↑↑RISP ↑QTP
Ciprofloxacin	CYP1A2	↑↑CLZ ↑OLZ
Erythromycin	CYP3A4	↑↑CLZ ↑OLZ
Fluoxetine	CYP2D6, CYP2DC, CYP3A4	↑↑CLZ ↑RISP ↑QTP
Fluvoxamine	CYP1A2, CYP2C, CYP3A4	↑↑↑CLZ ↑↑OLZ ↑QTP
Ketoconazole	CYP3A4	↑↑CLZ ↑OLZ ↑QTP
Paroxetine	CYP2D6	↑CLZ ↑RISP
Quinidine	CYP2D6	↑CLZ ↑RISP
Risperidone	CYP2D6	↑CLZ

Abbreviations: CLZ, clozapine; CYP, cytochrome P 450; OLZ, olanzapine; RISP, risperidone; QTP, quetiapine.
Data from Brown CS, Markowitz JS, Moore TR, et al. Atypical antipsychotics: part II: adverse effects, drug interactions, and costs. Ann Pharmacother 1999;33:210–7.

antipsychotic has achieved therapeutic dose, an effort should be made to fully taper the first antipsychotic.

When initiating antipsychotic treatment or switching to a different antipsychotic, the goal is to start low and titrate up as slowly as the acute symptoms tolerate. The maintenance dosage should be determined by either the therapeutic response or adverse effects. Some children and adolescents require higher or lower dosages than usual to achieve therapeutic response because of variable absorption, poor or ultrarapid metabolism,[45] cytochrome P (CYP) 450 interactions with other medications (**Table 9**), and medical comorbidities.[46] The best strategy is to choose the antipsychotic that has the least metabolic risk and the side effect profile that provides therapeutic response with ongoing monitoring of physical health and recommendations for healthy lifestyle.

Augmentation Strategies

There are no published data at present on augmentation strategies for children and adolescents on antipsychotic medication who have only partial response. In the adult literature no augmentation strategies have provided a significant level of evidence of efficacy, although there is a high prevalence of the use of more than one antipsychotic simultaneously.[61] A meta-analysis of 19 RCTs showed only weak evidence for the benefit of using 2 antipsychotics simultaneously in adults.[41] A second meta-analysis of 21 studies of augmentation of clozapine with another antipsychotic suggested some benefit when there is only a partial response to clozapine.[62] There is no evidence from the adult literature that augmenting antipsychotic medication with the mood stabilizers valproate[63,64] or carbamazepine[65] is beneficial. Likewise, the addition of lithium to an antipsychotic medication did not show any augmentation superior to placebo on meta-analysis[66] except for individuals with a diagnosis of schizoaffective disorder or the use of lithium to increase the WBC and ANC in cases of neutropenia.[58,59] There is mixed evidence in adults about augmenting antipsychotic medication with lamotrigine[67] but in a meta-analysis of augmenting clozapine with lamotrigine there is some suggestion that there may be benefit, but this needs further study.[68] There are a few studies on the benefit of augmenting antipsychotic medication with topiramate with equivocal results,[69] but the added benefit of decreased weight is countered with its potential for increased cognitive blunting. Other strategies such as augmenting with benzodiazepines and β-blockers did not show any benefit and the addition of polyunsaturated fatty acids to antipsychotic medication needs further study. A trial of clozapine is still the best strategy for partial or no response to antipsychotic medication and there is a need for new RCTs in the augmentation of partial response to clozapine in children and adolescents.

CLINICAL VIGNETTE: ANTIPSYCHOTIC MEDICATION ADJUSTMENT IN A 13-YEAR-OLD GIRL

S is a 13-year-old African American girl referred for medication reevaluation by her psychiatrist because of a poor response to risperidone, olanzapine, and aripiprazole at therapeutic doses for more than 1 year. She manifested symptoms of auditory and visual hallucinations, thought racing, grandiosity, decreased need for sleep, and intense preoccupation with her inner fantasy life that interfered with her ability to function in school and with peers despite being bright and sociable. She is the only child of older professional parents who were devastated by their exemplary daughter's deterioration. They denied any family psychiatric history or traumatic events in S's childhood until the gradual onset of symptoms around puberty, which they initially attributed to adolescent preoccupation. She was in therapy with a psychologist who was using cognitive behavioral approaches to help her manage her internal stimuli. She had a significant deterioration in her grades and was having difficulty remaining in school. Peers noted that something was seriously wrong with her despite her being well liked and she became increasingly isolated, spending most of her time in her room alone. At the time of referral she was being treated with aripiprazole 15 mg/d and lithium 1200 mg/d with little change in her symptoms. She had significant EPS including tremors, akathisia, and some muscle rigidity. Parents and S agreed to a trial of clozapine after the potential benefits and side effects were explained. Baseline fasting CBC and differential, comprehensive metabolic panel, lipid panel, thyroid profile, ECG, and EEG were all normal. A slow titration of clozapine 25 mg/wk was initiated while maintaining her previous medication. The goal was to attain a therapeutic response and then try to slowly taper the aripiprazole as well as her lithium. Initial sedation resolved and there was some fluctuation in her WBC/ANC, which was prevented by having the blood drawn in the afternoon after exercise (see **Table 7**).[59] When clozapine dosage reached 100 mg/d, a slow taper of aripiprazole was initiated at 2.5 mg every 2 to 3 weeks with a decrease and elimination of her EPS symptoms as the aripiprazole was discontinued. She became more alert and less preoccupied with her auditory hallucinations, noting that the voices were now thoughts that were there but could be controlled. She was able to differentiate between fantasy and reality, increasingly focusing on her school work and extracurricular activities. An echocardiogram was taken at 8 weeks after the initiation of clozapine and was normal. Lithium was tapered to 600 mg/d, which reduced the tremors but was maintained at this dosage to help support the WBC/ANC as well as to treat underlying affective symptoms. She did gain weight, especially in the abdominal area, which was disturbing to her and her parents but they were committed to continuing the clozapine because of its significant benefits. S and her parents together embarked on a healthy diet and vigorous exercise schedule, which allowed her to lose weight, decrease her abdominal circumference, as well as enhance her mood. She has been maintained on clozapine 200 mg/d and lithium 600 mg/d with a clozapine blood level of 367 ng/mL. She was able to finish junior high school and enroll in an excellent local high school where she is functioning well, making new friends, and is involved in both team sports and the high school newspaper.

Clozapine

Clozapine, which was the first SGA, has the advantage of being more effective for refractory symptoms than both FGAs and SGAs both in the adult[47,48] and pediatric literature.[9–11,49,50] Despite its efficacy, clozapine is underused both in adults and children because of concerns about managing the side effect profile, in particular the hematological side effects, which require frequent blood testing, and the rare potential cardiac side effects, which can be life threatening. With careful monitoring, the risks associated with clozapine can be minimized, thereby enabling the benefits of its use in severely ill children and adolescents who have treatment-resistant psychotic symptoms.

In adult studies the incidence of clozapine-induced agranulocytosis is between 0.7% and 1%, mostly occurring between 6 weeks and 6 months, and after the first year decreases to 0.38%.[51–54] The FDA mandated weekly blood tests for the first 6 months, biweekly for the next 6 months, and monthly blood tests thereafter has further reduced the potential for agranulocytosis. An incidence of clozapine-induced neutropenia of up to 22% has been found in adults.[55] However, 4% to 8% of African Americans and people of Middle Eastern origin have benign ethnic neutropenia in which their white blood cell (WBC) count is chronically between 2500/mm^3 and 3500/mm^3 and their absolute neutrophil count (ANC) is between 1300/mm^3 and 1700/mm^3. The data are clear that adults with benign ethnic neutropenia are not at greater risk for agranulocytosis than the general population, and a baseline low WBC and ANC should not be a contraindication for using clozapine.[56,57] Neutropenia in children and adolescents is also more frequent[58,59] and can be managed as described in **Table 7** and rechallenged as per FDA guidelines (ie, ANC <2000/mm^3, repeat complete blood count [CBC] within the week; ANC <1500/mm^3, stop clozapine and repeat CBC within the week). In children and adolescents, if clozapine is reinitiated after a few days, the ANC usually rebounds and clozapine treatment can be continued.[59] Fear of hematological adverse effects should not be a reason to avoid the use of clozapine.

Cardiomyopathy, myocarditis, and other cardiac and QTc changes need to be monitored with preclozapine family history, personal history for cardiovascular risk factors, full blood work including baseline troponin and creatine kinase myocardial band (CK-MB) levels, baseline electrocardiogram (ECG), baseline vital signs, and ongoing monitoring.[29] Ongoing pulse and blood pressure monitoring until the therapeutic dose of clozapine is achieved is recommended. An echocardiogram between 4 and 8 weeks after the initiation of clozapine may show signs of cardiac muscle thickening, which can be an early silent indicator of cardiomyopathy (unpublished clinical experience with more than 300 children and adolescents treated with clozapine in an inpatient setting at the New York City Children's Center, Bronx Campus). Regular monitoring of eosinophilia, troponin, and CK-MB levels is also recommended.

Because there is an increased risk of clozapine lowering the seizure threshold,[60] it is recommended that a preclozapine electroencephalogram (EEG) be obtained and repeated if the dosage of clozapine reaches 600 mg/day or the clozapine blood level (clozapine + norclozapine) is more than 600 ng/mL (based on the authors' clinical experience). If a seizure does occur and clozapine has been beneficial in ameliorating and treating the symptoms of psychosis, an antiseizure medication such as lamotrigine or topiramate may be used with the added advantage of potentially augmenting the efficacy of clozapine and decreasing weight gain as well as preventing a recurrence of seizures. In general, clozapine blood levels can be helpful to determine compliance, poor or ultrarapid metabolism, and interactions with other medications and foods, which can potentiate side effects. Other side effects of clozapine such as weight gain, metabolic changes, tachycardia, hypotension, sialorrhea, sedation, constipation, and enuresis can be managed as described in **Tables 5–7**.

In our clinical experience, the therapeutic dosage of clozapine in children and adolescents can range between 150 and 600 mg/day. It is important to titrate up slowly to minimize side effects, and the response to clozapine tends to increase over time, often requiring a wait of 3 to 6 months to achieve full benefit.

Future Directions

There is a need for more RCTs and cohort studies that examine the long-term efficacy and safety of antipsychotics in children, which include long-term quality-of-life issues, school performance, and developmental outcomes.[70] These studies need larger samples that can be generalized and that track therapeutic and adverse effects at different stages of development.[7] Further studies of head-to-head drug comparisons will help clinicians to determine the relative benefits of each antipsychotic and further elucidate their side effect profiles. Given the current evidence, clozapine still remains the gold standard for refractory psychosis in both adults and children.[71]

REFERENCES

1. Olfson M, Blanco C, Liu L, et al. National trends in the outpatient treatment of children and adolescents with antipsychotic drugs. Arch Gen Psychiatry 2006;63(6):679–85.
2. Olfson M, Crystal S, Huang C, et al. Trends in antipsychotic drug use by very young, privately insured children. J Am Acad Child Adolesc Psychiatry 2010; 1:13–23.
3. Olfson M, Blanco C, Liu S, et al. National trends in the office-based treatment of children, adolescents, and adults with antipsychotics. Arch Gen Psychiatry 2012;69(12):1247–56.
4. Sikich L. Efficacy of atypical antipsychotics in early-onset schizophrenia and other psychotic disorders. J Clin Psychiatry 2008;69(4):21–5.
5. Sikich L, Frazier JA, McClellan J, et al. Double-blind comparison of antipsychotics in early-onset schizophrenia and schizoaffective disorder: findings from the Treatment of Early-Onset Schizophrenia Spectrum Disorders (TEOSS). Am J Psychiatry 2008;165:1420–31.
6. Kumra S, Oberstar JV, Sikich L, et al. Efficacy and tolerability of second-generation antipsychotics in children and adolescents with schizophrenia. Schizophr Bull 2008;34(1):60–71.
7. Correll CU, Kratochvil CJ, March JS. Developments in pediatric psychopharmacology: focus on stimulants, antidepressants, and antipsychotics. J Clin Psychiatry 2011;72(5):655–70.
8. Fraguas D, Correll C, Merchan-Naranjo J, et al. Efficacy and safety of second generation antipsychotics in children and adolescents with psychotic and bipolar spectrum disorders: comprehensive review of prospective head-to-head and placebo-controlled comparisons. Eur Neuropsychopharmacol 2011;21(8): 621–45.
9. Kumra S, Frazier JA, Jacobsen LK, et al. Childhood-onset schizophrenia: a double-blind clozapine-haloperidol comparison. Arch Gen Psychiatry 1996;53: 1090–7.
10. Shaw P, Sporn A, Gogtay N, et al. Childhood-onset schizophrenia: a double-blind randomized clozapine-olanzapine comparison. Arch Gen Psychiatry 2006;63(7):721–30.
11. Kumra S, Kranzler HN, Gerbino-Rosen G, et al. Clozapine and "high-dose" olanzapine in refractory early-onset schizophrenia: a 12-week randomized and double-blind comparison. Biol Psychiatry 2008;63(5):524–9.
12. Kranzler H, Kester HM, Gerbino-Rosen G, et al. Treatment-refractory schizophrenia in children and adolescents: an update on clozapine and other pharmacological interventions. Child Adolesc Psychiatr Clin N Am 2006;15:135–59.

13. Correll CU, Penzner JB, Parikh UH, et al. Recognizing and monitoring adverse events of second generation antipsychotics in children and adolescents. Child Adolesc Psychiatr Clin N Am 2006;15(1):177–206.

14. Correll CU, Carlson HE. Endocrine and metabolic adverse effects of psychotropic medications in children and adolescents. J Am Acad Child Adolesc Psychiatry 2006;45(7):771–91.

15. Correll CU. Weight gain and metabolic effects of mood stabilizers and antipsychotics in pediatric bipolar disorders: a systematic review and pooled analysis of short-term trials. J Am Acad Child Adolesc Psychiatry 2007;46(6):687–700.

16. Correll CU. Antipsychotic use in children and adolescents: minimizing adverse effects to maximize outcomes. J Am Acad Child Adolesc Psychiatry 2008;47(1): 9–20.

17. Correll CU, Manu P, Olshanskiy V, et al. Cardiometabolic risk of second generation antipsychotic medications during first-time use in children and adolescents. JAMA 2009;302(16):1765–73.

18. Cohen D, Bonnot O, Bodeau N, et al. Adverse effects of second-generation antipsychotics in children and adolescents: a Bayesian meta-analysis. J Clin Psychopharmacol 2012;32(3):309–16.

19. De Hert M, Dobbelaere M, Sheridan EM, et al. Metabolic and endocrine adverse effects of second generation antipsychotics in children and adolescents: a systematic review of randomized, placebo controlled trials and guidelines for clinical practice. Eur Psychiatry 2011;26(3):144–58.

20. Malhotra AK, Correll CU, Chowdhury NI, et al. Association between common variants near the melanocortin 4 receptor gene and severe antipsychotic drug-induced weight gain. Arch Gen Psychiatry 2012;69(9):904–12.

21. Coccurello R, Moles A. Potential mechanisms of atypical antipsychotic-induced metabolic derangement: clues for understanding obesity and novel drug design. Pharmacol Ther 2010;127(3):210–51.

22. Correll CU, Lencz T, Malhotra AK. Antipsychotic drugs and obesity. Trends Mol Med 2011;17(2):97–107.

23. Bushe CJ, Leonard BE. Blood glucose and schizophrenia: a systematic review of prospective randomized clinical trials. J Clin Psychiatry 2007;68:1682–90.

24. Hammerman A, Dreiher J, Klang SH, et al. Antipsychotics and diabetes: an age-related association. Ann Pharmacother 2008;42(9):1316–22.

25. Panagiotopoulos C, Ronsley R, Davidson J. Increased prevalence of obesity and glucose intolerance in youth treated with second generation antipsychotic medications. Can J Psychiatry 2009;54(11):743–9.

26. Nielsen J, Skadhede S, Correll CU. Antipsychotics associated with the development of type 2 diabetes in antipsychotic-naïve schizophrenia patients. Neuropsychopharmacology 2010;35(9):1997–2004.

27. Andrade SE, Lo JC, Roblin D, et al. Antipsychotic medication use among children and risk of diabetes mellitus. Pediatrics 2011;128(6):1135–41.

28. Pringsheim T, Panagiotopoulos C, Davidson J, et al. Evidence-based recommendations for monitoring safety of second generation antipsychotics in children and youth. J Can Acad Child Adolesc Psychiatry 2011;20(3):218–33.

29. De Hert M, Detraux J, van Winkel R, et al. Metabolic and cardiovascular adverse effects associated with antipsychotic drugs. Nat Rev Endocrinol 2012;8:114–26.

30. Correll CU. Antipsychotic agents: traditional and atypical. In: Martin A, Scahill L, editors. Pediatric psychopharmacology. New York, NY: Oxford University Press; 2011. p. 312–37.

31. Zimmet P, Alberti G, Kaufman F, et al. The metabolic syndrome in children and adolescents. Lancet 2007;369:2059–61.
32. Ananth J, Parameswaran S, Gunatilake S. Side effects of atypical antipsychotic drugs. Curr Pharm Des 2004;10:2219–29.
33. Neuhut R, Lindenmayer JP, Silva R. Neuroleptic malignant syndrome in children and adolescents on atypical antipsychotic medication: a review. J Child Adolesc Psychopharmacol 2009;19(4):415–22.
34. Bartlow S, et al. Expert committee recommendations regarding the prevention, assessment, and treatment of child and adolescent overweight and obesity: Summary report. Pediatrics 2007;120:S164.
35. Klein DJ, Cottingham EM, Sorter M, et al. A randomized, double-blind, placebo-controlled trial of metformin treatment of weight gain associated with initiation of atypical antipsychotic therapy in children and adolescents. Am J Psychiatry 2006;163(12):2072–9.
36. Shin L, Bregman H, Breeze JL, et al. Metformin for weight control in pediatric patients on atypical antipsychotic medication. J Child Adolesc Psychopharmacol 2009;19:275–9.
37. Tramontina S, Zeni CP, Pheula G, et al. Topiramate in adolescents with juvenile bipolar disorder presenting weight gain due to atypical antipsychotics or mood stabilizers: an open clinical trial. J Child Adolesc Psychopharmacol 2007;17(1):129–34.
38. Das C, Mendez G, Jagasia S, et al. Second-generation antipsychotic use in schizophrenia and associated weight gain: a critical review and meta-analysis of behavioral and pharmacologic treatments. Ann Clin Psychiatry 2012;24(3):225–39.
39. Fiedorowicz JG, Miller DD, Bishop JR, et al. Systematic review and meta-analysis of pharmacological interventions for weight gain from antipsychotics and mood stabilizers. Curr Psychiatry Rev 2012;8(1):25–36.
40. Findling RL, Frazier JA, Gerbino-Rosen G, et al. Is there a role for clozapine in the treatment of children and adolescents? Psychopharmacology perspectives column. J Am Acad Child Adolesc Psychiatry 2007;46:423–8.
41. Correll CU, Rummel-Kluge C, Corves C, et al. Antipsychotic combinations vs monotherapy in schizophrenia: a meta-analysis of randomized controlled trials. Schizophr Bull 2009;35(2):443–57.
42. Jerrell JM, McIntyre RS. Adverse events in children and adolescents treated with antipsychotic medications. Hum Psychopharmacol 2008;23:283–90.
43. McIntyre RS, Jerrell JM. Metabolic and cardiovascular adverse events associated with antipsychotic treatment in children and adolescents. Arch Pediatr Adolesc Med 2008;162:929–35.
44. Correll CU. From receptor pharmacology to improved outcomes: individualizing the selection, dosing, and switching of antipsychotics. Eur Psychiatry 2010;25(2):S12–21.
45. Zhang JP, Malhotra AK. Pharmacogenetics and antipsychotics: therapeutic efficacy and side effects prediction. Expert Opin Drug Metab Toxicol 2011;7(1):9–37.
46. Correll CU. Real-life dosing with second-generation antipsychotics. J Clin Psychiatry 2005;66:1610–1.
47. Kane J, Honigfeld G, Singer J, et al. Clozapine for the treatment-resistant schizophrenic. A double-blind comparison with chlorpromazine. Arch Gen Psychiatry 1988;45(9):789–96.
48. Meltzer HY, Okayli G. Reduction of suicidality during clozapine treatment of neuroleptic-resistant schizophrenia: impact on risk benefit assessment. Am J Psychiatry 1995;152(2):183–90.

49. Kranzler H, Roofeh D, Gerbino-Rosen G, et al. Clozapine: its impact on aggressive behavior among children and adolescents with schizophrenia. J Am Acad Child Adolesc Psychiatry 2005;44(1):55–63.

50. Sporn AL, Vermani A, Greenstein DK, et al. Clozapine treatment of childhood-onset schizophrenia: evaluation of effectiveness, adverse effects, and long-term outcome. J Am Acad Child Adolesc Psychiatry 2007;46(10):1349–56.

51. Honigfeld G, Arellano F, Sethi J, et al. Reducing clozapine-related morbidity and mortality: 5 years of experience with the Clozaril National Registry. J Clin Psychiatry 1998;59(Suppl 3):3–7.

52. Schulte PF. Risk of clozapine-associated agranulocytosis and mandatory white blood cell monitoring. Ann Pharmacother 2006;40(4):683–8.

53. Alvir JM, Lieberman JA, Safferman AZ, et al. Clozapine-induced agranulocytosis: incidence and risk factors in the United States. N Engl J Med 1993;329: 204–5.

54. Cohen D, Bogers JP, van Dijk D, et al. Beyond white blood cell monitoring: screening in the initial phase of clozapine therapy. J Clin Psychiatry 2012; 73(10):1307–12.

55. Hummer M, Kurz M, Barnas C, et al. Clozapine-induced white blood count disorders. J Clin Psychiatry 1994;55:429–32.

56. Kelly DL, Kreyenbuhl J, Dixon L, et al. Clozapine underutilization and discontinuation in African Americans due to leucopenia. Schizophr Bull 2007;33(5): 1221–4.

57. Blackman G. Benign ethnic neutropenia and clozapine monitoring. J Am Acad Child Adolesc Psychiatry 2008;47(8):967–8.

58. Sporn A, Gogtay N, Ortiz-Aguayo R, et al. Clozapine-induced neutropenia in children: management with lithium carbonate. J Child Adolesc Psychopharmacol 2003;13:401–4.

59. Gerbino-Rosen G, Roofeh D, Tompkins A, et al. Hematological adverse events in clozapine-treated children and adolescents. J Am Acad Child Adolesc Psychiatry 2005;44(10):1024–31.

60. Centorrino F, Price BH, Tuttle M, et al. EEG abnormalities during treatment with typical and atypical antipsychotics. Am J Psychiatry 2002;159(1):109–15.

61. Zink M, Englisch S, Meyer-Lindenberg A. Polypharmacy in schizophrenia. Curr Opin Psychiatry 2010;23:103–11.

62. Barbui C, Signoretti A, Mule S, et al. Does the addition of a second antipsychotic drug improve clozapine treatment? Schizophr Bull 2009;35(2):458–68.

63. Schwarz C, Volz A, Li C, et al. Valproate for schizophrenia. Cochrane Database Syst Rev 2008;(3):CD004028.

64. Casey DE, Daniel DG, Tamminga C, et al. Divalproex ER combined with olanzapine or risperidone for treatment of acute exacerbations of schizophrenia. Neuropsychopharmacology 2009;34:1330–8.

65. Leucht S, McGrath J, White P, et al. Carbamazepine augmentation for schizophrenia: how good is the evidence? J Clin Psychiatry 2002;63(3):218–24.

66. Leucht S, Kissling W, McGrath J. Lithium for schizophrenia. Cochrane Database Syst Rev 2007;(3):CD003834.

67. Goff DC, Keefe R, Citrome L, et al. Lamotrigine as add-on therapy in schizophrenia: results of 2 placebo-controlled trials. J Clin Psychopharmacol 2007; 27:582–9.

68. Tiihonen J, Wahlbeck K, Kiviniemi V. The efficacy of lamotrigine in clozapine-resistant schizophrenia: a systematic review and meta-analysis. Schizophr Res 2009;109:10–4.

69. Muscatello M, Bruno A, Pandolfo G, et al. Topiramate augmentation of clozapine in schizophrenia: a double-blind placebo-controlled study. J Psychopharmacol 2011;25(5):667–74.
70. Seida JC, Schouten JR, Boylan K, et al. Antipsychotics for children and young adults: a comparative effectiveness review. Pediatrics 2012;128(3):771–84.
71. Kane JM, Correll CU. Past and present progress in the pharmacologic treatment of schizophrenia. J Clin Psychiatry 2010;79:1115–24.

Community Rehabilitation and Psychosocial Interventions for Psychotic Disorders in Youth

Eóin Killackey, D. Psych.[a,b,]*, Mario Alvarez-Jimenez, PhD[a,b],
Kelly Allott, PhD[a,b], Sarah Bendall, PhD[a,b],
Patrick McGorry, MD, PhD[a,b]

KEYWORDS

- Psychosis • Psychosocial rehabilitation • Recovery • Vocational • Physical health

KEY POINTS

- The functional outcomes for people with psychosis have been very poor in a range of domains.
- In the vocational domain, individual placement and support help young people with psychosis to return to school or work successfully.
- Addressing the physical health of people with early psychosis is important.
- Addressing functional domains such as vocation and physical health needs to be as important as medication in the treatment of early psychosis.

INTRODUCTION

Community rehabilitation of people with psychotic disorders can mean one of two things. In the first instance it can refer simply to the provision in the community rather than in an inpatient setting of some of the interventions such as pharmacologic and psychological therapies discussed elsewhere in this issue. More broadly, it can refer to the interventions that assist in the recovery of a young person with psychosis so

Disclosures: Ronald Phillip Griffith Fellowship from the Faculty of Medicine at The University of Melbourne, Australian Research Council Linkage Grant LP0883237, Australian Rotary Health Research Grant (E. Killackey); Postdoctoral Clinical Research Fellowship from the National Health and Medical Research Council (NHMRC) of Australia (#628884) (K. Allott); Early Career Research Fellowship from the NHMRC of Australia (#1036425), Australian Rotary Health Research Grant (S. Bendall); Colonial Foundation (M. Alvarez-Jimenez); Colonial Foundation (P. McGorry).
[a] Orygen Youth Health Research Centre, 35 Poplar Road, Parkville, Victoria 3052, Australia;
[b] Centre for Youth Mental Health, The University of Melbourne, 35 Poplar Road, Parkville, Victoria 3052, Australia
* Corresponding author. Orygen Youth Health Research Centre, 35 Poplar Road, Parkville, Victoria 3052, Australia.
E-mail address: eoin@unimelb.edu.au

that, in addition to achieving a symptomatic recovery, he or she achieves a functional recovery, which included specifics such as a return to school or work, having a place to live, and addressing physical health needs. In considering this latter definition of community rehabilitation in psychotic disorders in young people, it is worth starting by revisiting the World Health Organization (WHO) definition of mental health.[1]

> *Mental health is not just the absence of mental disorder. It is defined as a state of well-being in which every individual realizes his or her own potential, can cope with the normal stresses of life, can work productively and fruitfully, and is able to make a contribution to her or his community.*

The broader definition, as well as being congruent with the WHO's, is closely aligned to the stated aims of people with psychotic illness who rate positive functional outcomes as being more important than symptomatic remission.[2] While this was found to be the case in persons with schizophrenia, it has recently been found to be equally so in young people being treated for their first psychotic episode in both the United States[3] and India.[4] Ramsay and colleagues[3] found that the top 5 life goals of young people with first-episode psychosis (FEP) were (in descending order) employment, education, relationships, housing, and general health. Recovery from the current episode was rated ninth. In India, Iyer and colleagues[4] found an almost identical list (work, interpersonal, school, symptom relief, living situation).

Despite research in populations separated both geographically and in stage of illness showing highly similar wishes to address functioning, and despite improvements in psychiatric medication and psychological interventions for people with psychotic illnesses leading to better symptomatic prognoses,[5] persons with psychosis are still overrepresented among those with a poor functional outcome.[6] Compared with the general community, people with a psychotic illness experience more unemployment,[7] experience more physical ill health and die earlier,[8] and experience greater homelessness.[9] Consequently, people with psychosis are among the most socially excluded in the community. Furthermore, the economic impact of poor functional outcomes is enormous and is responsible for more than half of the total costs associated with psychotic illnesses.[10] Largely because of neglect, stigma, and a view of inevitable deterioration, intervention in psychotic illness tended to happen only after illness was well established.[11] The early intervention paradigm aimed to change this. Pioneered in Melbourne, Australia in the 1990s,[12] this paradigm aimed to reduce the duration of untreated psychosis, maximize symptomatic and functional recovery, prevent the development of disability, and prevent or minimize the impact of relapse.[11]

The promise of early intervention in psychosis is that it offers a unique opportunity to intervene to improve functional outcome before disability has developed or has become entrenched. However, symptom-focused early intervention alone is not enough. It has recently been found that functional recovery at 7.5 years posttreatment was not predicted by symptomatic recovery at 14 months posttreatment, but by functional recovery at 14 months,[13] emphasizing the need for evidence-based functional recovery to be a central part of early intervention. In this study, although short-term symptomatic remission (at 7 months) predicted functional recovery at 14 months, symptom remission at 7 or 14 months had limited predictive value for long-term recovery, meaning that if early symptom remission does not lead to early functional gains it is unlikely that long-term functional recovery will occur.

This article reviews 2 key areas of functioning in relation to early psychosis: employment and education, and physical health. What is known in these areas in terms of the scale of the problem is discussed. The article then highlights some of the research evidence that is available for interventions in each of these areas. Finally, the implications for research and clinical practice with respect to these domains of functioning in young people with early psychosis are discussed.

EMPLOYMENT AND EDUCATION: THE PROBLEM

Psychotic illnesses have their peak onset in the ages 15 to 25 years,[14] which is also the stage of life at which people normally finish school/tertiary education and enter the workforce. The onset of psychosis at this time can be extremely disruptive, often derailing the vocational development process completely. This disruption means that basic employment skills such as job searching and interviewing are not learned, nor are required qualifications gained. At the same time, people in this situation develop no employment history. These factors may explain why, even after eventual symptomatic remission, people with psychotic illnesses tend not to achieve good vocational outcomes. It should also be mentioned that there is a potential protective value in having a job because of the meaning, purpose in life, and valued social role that are intrinsic to being employed. This corollary of employment can buffer against the development of chronic disability. There is a window of opportunity to minimize or prevent vocational disability in this group by applying evidence-based vocational interventions earlier rather than later.

Whereas general unemployment in most developed economies is between 5% and 10%, youth unemployment (15–24 years) is usually between 2 and 3 times higher. Even allowing for high youth unemployment, the level of unemployment among young people with psychosis is even higher. At the onset of illness an average of 50% of people with psychosis are unemployed,[7] which rises quickly[15] to up to 95%.[16] Unemployment is the main functional disability of people with psychotic illness, despite employment being a primary goal of people with early[3,4] and chronic[6] psychotic illnesses. In the general community, being unemployed predisposes people to a greater risk of a range of poor outcomes such as substance abuse, homelessness, poor physical and mental health, and social and economic exclusion.[17,18] It is also known that for the majority, these poor outcomes follow unemployment.[18] For those with psychotic illness unemployment reinforces marginalization, has the potential to exacerbate symptoms, increases the risk of homelessness, and often persists after symptoms have resolved. Over and above the individual consequences of unemployment in psychosis, there are significant economic costs, which equate to half of the total costs of illness.[10]

Education is the foundation of employment, with increased education leading to less unemployment and higher wages in the general population.[19] This observation is also true in relation to employment for people with schizophrenia, with those who have completed high school more likely to be employed than those who have not.[20] Unfortunately, there are low levels of people with FEP completing high school. In a study of vocational recovery conducted by the authors, only about one-quarter of participants with psychosis had completed high school,[21] compared with 84% of their same-age peers in the community.[22] In the same study, more than 50% of young people with psychosis had less than a year-10 education. Although there is limited research to guide answering questions of cause and effect in relation to education, it is reasonable to suppose that the early development of illness and the onset of prodrome is related to this reduction in academic functioning. However, even in the absence of a mental illness, this low level of education would mitigate against successful vocational outcomes in life. Therefore it is imperative that in addressing the vocational functioning of young people with psychosis, education is considered on equal terms with employment.

Interventions for Employment and Education in Youth with Psychosis

Addressing the vocational domain of functioning in recovery is not new.[23] However, a consequence of the increasing medicalization of mental illness was the neglect of the vocational elements of recovery.[24] The period following the World War II saw the advent of Clubhouses and Social Firms as a means to address unemployment among those with mental illness. The literature for both of these approaches suggests that they do not usually lead to gaining a job in the competitive labor market.[7] Conversely, supported employment, an intervention whereby a person is assisted to gain a job in the open labor market and is supported to stay in that position, has been very successful.[25] Individual Placement and Support (IPS) is the most defined form of supported employment, which has been found to be superior to a range of control interventions in populations with schizophrenia in 14 randomized controlled trials (RCTs).[26] These studies have occurred in a range of countries with a range of economic and labor market conditions. IPS has 8 principles (**Box 1**). Given its success in populations with chronic illness, it is appropriate to ask to what degree this approach can be applied to early intervention in psychosis.

IPS in Early Psychosis

In addition to an earlier uncontrolled study in the United Kingdom,[27] there have now been 2 published RCTs of IPS in early psychosis.[21,28] In their RCT (n = 41) with participants aged between 15 and 25 (mean 21.3) years in Australia, Killackey and colleagues[21] found that over 6 months, more people in the IPS group obtained employment (13 vs 2), gained significantly more jobs in total (23 vs 4), earned significantly more money ($2432 vs $0), and worked longer (45 vs 19 days) than those who did not receive IPS. Four people in each group engaged in educational courses. This finding means that 17 (85%) of those in the IPS group had a positive vocational outcome compared with only 6 (29%) in the control group. The percentage of those dependent on government benefits decreased significantly in the IPS group, whereas there was no change in the control group. As a point of comparison, 10 participants in the control group accessed federally funded employment agencies, if whom 1 had a single interview. None obtained employment.

Box 1
Eight principles of IPS

1. Every person with severe mental illness who wants to work is eligible for IPS supported employment

2. Employment services are integrated with mental health treatment services

3. Competitive employment is the goal

4. Personalized benefits counseling is provided

5. The job search starts soon after a person expresses interest in working

6. Employment specialists systematically develop relationships with employers based on their client's work preferences

7. Job supports are continuous

8. Client preferences are honored

From Dartmouth IPS Supported Employment Center. Core Principles of IPS Supported Employment. 2012 [updated January 17, 2012; cited 2012 November 26]. Available at: http://www.dartmouth.edu/~ips/page29/page31/page31.html. Accessed November 26, 2012.

Another RCT (n = 69) conducted in FEP (age range 18–45, mean 25.1 years) by Nuechterlein and colleagues[28] at the University of California Los Angeles found very similar results, with 83% of people receiving IPS having a good vocational outcome (returning to either work or study). Across all of the IPS studies (RCTs and others) in early psychosis, 69% have a successful vocational outcome, compared with 35% in those not receiving IPS.[15]

A key difference between the studies conducted in early psychosis and those conducted in populations with more established illness is the equal focus on achieving educational outcomes for those for whom education is the most appropriate vocational outcome. This approach fits with the developmental and recovery orientations of early intervention, and in this way introduces the concept of career rather than job as an outcome. In a study conducted in the United Kingdom, Rinaldi and colleagues[27] showed that with IPS the enrollment of all those involved in education was maintained until their courses were complete. Most of these people then transitioned to employment.

Clinical Lessons

There is some evidence that one of the barriers to vocational success for young people with psychosis is the attitude of clinicians and carers about both the ability of the person with psychosis to work and the impact that work is likely to have on them.[15] It is often thought that people with psychosis are not able to work, or that work will be a stressful experience leading to an exacerbation of symptoms and relapse. In fact recently published evidence shows that, in line with the general population, work is less stressful than unemployment for people with psychosis.[29] Therefore, clinicians need to work with clients and their families toward vocational recovery. An important element of this is in helping to overcome the powerful effects of self-directed stigma, which may encourage people with psychosis to not bother looking for work in the belief that it will be too stressful or that they will be discriminated against.[30] Having a job is likely to lead to more positive experiences, increased social networks, and increased social support, all of which may protect against relapse and promote full functional recovery.

A further lesson is the need for specialist employment input. IPS works through a specialist employment worker being part of the clinical mental health program. In addition to providing direct services to clients, this person often "up-skills" other clinicians about employment and helps raise the profile of employment as a possible outcome for clients.

A final lesson is that there must be a focus on career rather than jobs. This approach may mean that the most appropriate first step is the completion of secondary education or the attainment of some other qualification.

Research Lessons

The results from IPS trials in early psychosis are consistently good, although more work is needed in understanding the predictors of success in both obtaining and keeping a job or completing a course of education. Vocational success requires cognitive and social cognitive skills that are known to be affected with the onset of psychosis. There has been a lack of research examining social and neurocognitive interventions and vocational functioning in the early phases of psychotic illness.[31] Although the specific degree of overlap between general neurocognitive (eg, attention, memory, executive functioning) and social cognitive processes remains unclear, research supports these 2 domains as independent constructs that contribute unique variance to the prediction of social functioning and interpersonal skills in both chronic schizophrenia and early psychosis.[32-37] Furthermore, social cognition has been shown to have a greater impact than neurocognition on work-related social skills and work outcomes,[34,38,39] with a recent meta-analysis confirming that social cognition, particularly theory of mind, was a stronger predictor of overall community functioning, incorporating social and work functioning, than general neurocognition.[40] The studies that have examined the relationship between social cognition and functional outcome in FEP support the findings of chronic schizophrenia research indicating that this relationship exists at the earliest stages of the illness. A recent 12-month follow-up study in individuals with FEP highlighted the significant negative impact of baseline social cognitive deficits on prospective work, independent living, and social functioning.[41] Schizophrenia studies comparing IPS with IPS plus neurocognitive training have shown the latter to be superior with respect to employment outcomes such as competitive jobs attained, hours worked, and wages earned.[42-44] However, no study to date has examined this in early psychosis. Future research needs to determine whether remediation in these domains improves vocational outcome.

PHYSICAL HEALTH: THE PROBLEM

The physical health outcomes of people with psychosis are very poor,[2,45] resulting in a 20-year decrease in life expectancy.[46] The majority of the excess morbidity and mortality is accounted for by obesity (particularly that induced as a medication side effect) and tobacco smoking, and their various related illnesses.[46] Although this may not seem to be the most important issue in early psychosis, the evidence indicates that declining physical health is a process that starts very early in mental illness.[47] The physical health of people with FEP has fallen into the gap between physical and mental health care systems. For example, studies have shown that people with psychotic illnesses use primary care providers to a greater extent than the general community. However, they have higher rates of preventable illness, with lower rates of investigations, early detection, and early intervention. This finding is demonstrated by data showing that people with schizophrenia have the same incidence of cancer as the general population, but significantly higher mortality.[48] With respect to smoking, studies have shown that although people with mental illness make up about 25% of the population, they smoke nearly 50% of all cigarettes.[49] In Australia 71% of males and 58% of females with psychosis smoke, compared with 20% in the general population,[2] and, remarkably, Australians with mental illness pay more in excise on tobacco than the government pays them in disability support pensions.[49] Data from the long-running British General Practitioners study show that if smoking is ceased before age 30 years, the long-term risk levels recede to those of nonsmokers.[50]

Addressing Weight Gain in Early Psychosis

To date, only one RCT has shown the effectiveness of preventive strategies in attenuating antipsychotic-induced weight gain in a young cohort with early psychosis.[47] This study showed the feasibility and effectiveness of preventive strategies, which comprised dietary counseling, exercise increase, and behavioral techniques, for early psychosis patients who commenced antipsychotic treatment.[47]

However, although the behavioral intervention was effective in reducing weight gain in early psychosis patients during the 3-month intervention period, treatment effects were no longer significant by 12 months' follow-up.[51] These results are in agreement with previous findings that behavioral interventions lead to significant short-term weight-loss benefits in nonpsychiatric populations, whereas intervention effects erode over longer periods of time.[52] The extant literature on the general population further shows that significant predictors of long-term success include continuous adherence to diet and exercise strategies, internal motivation to control weight, social support, more adaptive coping strategies, and maintenance of weight loss for at least 2 years.[53,54] In addition, some studies have suggested that energy restriction might lead to short-term weight control, and that a regular exercise regime might be required to maintain the long-term achievements.[55] As a result, most experts argue that extended treatment and booster sessions are necessary to stabilize behavioral modification changes, and studies are now under way to determine their long-term effectiveness.[52]

Although there are few studies, it seems apparent that there is great potential for interventions aimed at the early stages before weight gain takes place. Weight gain is arguably a greater problem for young people experiencing early psychosis. This group is considered to be especially susceptible to substantial weight gain[56] that could interfere with the early recovery process. First, younger populations are already less disposed to adhering to medication regimens,[57] and potential weight gain might exacerbate nonadherence. Second, the physical changes produced by weight gain might result in social discrimination and stigma, as young patients are more sensitive to issues of body image and self-esteem than their older counterparts.[58] Early interventions could prevent or attenuate weight gain as well as the adverse consequences derived from it.

Smoking

As there are no studies in early psychosis that address tobacco smoking, it is worth considering what is known about smoking cessation and mental illness in general.

Interventions for smoking for people with mental illness

There are several important considerations in relation to examining what might work for people with mental illness who wish to stop smoking. First, do people with mental illness want to stop smoking? Second, what is already known about interventions to stop smoking for people with mental illness? Third, if people with a mental illness want to stop smoking and there are effective interventions, what are the barriers to them doing so?

Do people with a mental illness want to stop smoking? One of the common observations of people in the general community who smoke is that the majority would like to quit.[59] Studies that have examined the rate of desire to quit smoking among those with mental illness find that there is no difference in motivation to quit between those with and without mental illness.[60] The implication of this finding is that if there are effective interventions to quit, people with mental illness are likely to avail themselves of them. However, most are not made aware of or referred to such services,[61] make fewer attempts to quit, and have a higher level of tobacco use from which to quit.[62] Not surprisingly, the rate of quitting is lower in the population with mental illness than in the general population.[63]

Interventions There are 3 kinds of intervention to assist people to stop smoking: pharmacologic (a nicotine replacement treatment, a nicotine antagonist such as bupropion, or a nicotine partial agonist such as varenicline), psychological/psychosocial (eg, cognitive behavioral therapy [CBT], supportive counseling or education), or a combination of the two. The most recent review of smoking cessation strategies in mental illness included only 8 RCTs.[64] A Cochrane review on smoking cessation and reduction in people with schizophrenia found 11 trials focused on cessation and 4 focused on reduction.[65] Both reviews pointed to the generally small nature of the trials and the heterogeneous measures used as well as the variable follow-up periods. However, they report that interventions that used bupropion alone, or in combination with a psychological intervention such as CBT, achieved better end-of-treatment outcomes in terms of quitting and reducing than interventions that used other pharmacologic agents such as replacement therapies or other psychosocial interventions,[64,65] such as self-help or purely educational programs.[62] The gains made through the interventions did diminish over time.[64] However, this is something also found in the general population.[62] The general understanding is that giving up smoking generally takes several attempts.

Given the suggestion that having smoked longer or more heavily makes quitting more difficult,[62] it is at first surprising that none of the studies to date have attempted to study a tobacco cessation intervention in younger people earlier in the course of mental illness. However, it is less surprising when it is discovered that there is an acknowledged paucity of research on smoking cessation in young people in general, despite this being the phase of life when smoking is initiated.[66] Such studies are an area that cessation research needs to engage in, both in the general youth population and in the population of young people with mental illness.

Barriers Smoking has been, and arguably still is, part of the culture of mental health treatment settings.[67] One effect of this has been that clinicians have seen the provision of information and support for quitting as being of low priority.[61,68] Clinicians believe that there is no evidence that interventions can work for people with mental illness,[69] or that people with mental illness do not want to quit.[70] Because there has been a long history of detecting lower rates of cancer in populations of people with mental illness,[71] there is a belief that smoking is not harmful to people with mental illness. There is also a misguided belief that smoking is one of the few comforts enjoyed by people with mental illness. Consumers of mental health services report that one of the most powerful arguments against quitting is witnessing clinical staff themselves smoking.[69]

Clinical Lessons

The important clinical lesson with respect to physical health of young people with early psychosis is that it cannot be ignored. The development of poor physical health starts with the onset of mental illness, and it is in this early stage that it needs to be vigorously addressed. The basics that must be conducted include baseline and regular metabolic monitoring to identify any of these issues at their earliest point. Services need to see weight gain and metabolic side effects of medication as the iatrogenic problems that they are, and their prevention and remediation as being as much a part of treatment as the prescription of antipsychotic medication in the first place. Unfortunately, metabolic monitoring is not done well, but can be improved[72] by following guideline recommendations (**Box 2**).

It is noteworthy that even the guidelines for early psychosis[73] make no mention of smoking reduction or cessation. This attitude toward smoking must change. Although there is currently little evidence as to what works, there is evidence that people with psychosis want to stop smoking. Therefore, given the tremendous health damage that smoking can cause, it is incumbent on clinicians to provide access to and support for interventions that may help with quitting.

Research Lessons

While a great deal of research, over a very long period, has illustrated the prevalence of poor physical health in people with psychotic illness, there has been very little

---

Box 2
Interventions to monitor and prevent metabolic side effects

- Baseline
  - Weight measures including weight, body mass index, and waist/hip circumference
  - Blood pressure
  - Fasting blood glucose
  - Fasting blood lipid (full profile)
  - Smoking status
  - Exercise status
- Monitoring at 1, 3, 6, 12, and 18 months and then yearly
- Interventions
  - Dietary advice/exercise and lifestyle education, and behavioral interventions (possible with specialist dietician involvement)
  - Consider change to less "metabologenic" antipsychotic medications
  - Consider other pharmacotherapy (eg, statins) with primary care provider/specialist input

From ORYGEN Youth Health. The Australian Clinical Guidelines for Early Psychosis. Melbourne: ORYGEN Youth Health; 2010; with permission.

---

research in developing and trialing preventive physical health interventions for this group. Consequently there is a lack of clear guidelines detailing appropriate interventions for the management of the physical health of people with a mental illness.[74] There is an urgent need for research in this domain to establish effective interventions that would reduce the burden of physical ill health and contribute to the overall functional recovery of young people with early psychosis. This approach may involve thinking more broadly about solutions to the problem. For example, although the evidence suggests that a mixture of caloric restriction and exercise may help to control weight gain, it is well known in the general community that achieving this is difficult. Instead of pursuing this alone, thinking broadly may see the addition of theory-driven interventions aimed at enhancing intrinsic motivation and social support in interventions for both weight management and smoking cessation.

SUMMARY

Outpatient care of people with psychiatric illness is now more than 100 years old.[75] Since the advent of pharmacologic treatment the focus of attention has been on symptom reduction, with a view that this would lead to reengagement with community function. Unfortunately, the evidence suggests that this has not happened. Early intervention in psychosis is a paradigm that has developed over the last 20 years. A fundamental element of its rationale is that people with psychosis will avoid the development of disability and will achieve a full recovery in terms of their functioning in the community. This article considers 2 key areas of functioning: vocation and physical health. In both of these areas there is a long-standing acknowledgment of poor outcome for people with mental illness in general and people with psychotic illness specifically.

With respect to vocational recovery, IPS has the capacity to help a significant proportion of young people with psychosis return to full vocational functioning. The potential personal and economic benefit of this is considerable. The impact on illness of having a valued social role, social contact, and income is also potentially significant. To realize these potentials some changes in clinical practice are necessary, and an increasing number of early psychosis services worldwide are engaging with this issue. There is an international consensus statement that may also be useful for clinicians who wish to involve their clinics in this practice.[76] Despite progress in this area there is still a need for further development, particularly in relation to understanding the neurocognitive and social cognitive predictors of vocational success.

The urgency of addressing physical health among those with early psychosis cannot be overstated. The evidence suggests significant life-expectancy gaps for people with psychotic illness in comparison with the general population, owing to largely preventable illnesses that arise as side effects of medication as well as lifestyle choices such as smoking. The evidence also suggests that for both metabolic syndrome and smoking, the earlier the intervention, the better. Addressing these problems has not traditionally been seen as the domain of mental health services. Given the evidence, it is imperative that this is seen as part of the mandate of early psychosis services. The pressing need here is for evidence of treatments that work. Research in this area has concentrated on documenting the extent of the problem rather than evaluating potential solutions, but it is now time for this focus to shift.

The onset of psychotic illness was once synonymous with a bleak future, unemployment, poor physical health, potential homelessness, and social marginalization. Community-focused treatment of psychosis ensures that this need not be the case. Along with evidence-based pharmacologic and psychological treatment, the treatments discussed herein have the capacity to restore hope and optimism. The challenge now is for their implementation and for the pursuit of further research in these domains.

REFERENCES

1. World Health Organization. Mental health: a state of well-being. World Health Organization; 2011 [cited 2012 November 19]. Available at: http://www.who.int/features/factfiles/mental_health/en/index.html. Accessed November 19, 2012.
2. Morgan VA, Waterreus A, Jablensky A, et al. People living with psychotic illness 2010. In: Department of Health and Ageing. Canberra (Australia): Commonwealth of Australia; 2011.
3. Ramsay CE, Broussard B, Goulding SM, et al. Life and treatment goals of individuals hospitalized for first-episode nonaffective psychosis. Psychiatry Res 2011;189(3):344–8.
4. Iyer SN, Mangala R, Anitha J, et al. An examination of patient-identified goals for treatment in a first-episode programme in Chennai, India. Early Interv Psychiatry 2011;5(4):360–5.
5. Killackey E. Something for everyone: employment interventions in psychotic illness. Acta Neuropsychiatr 2008;20:277–9.
6. Galletly C. People living with psychosis: the good news and the bad news. Aust N Z J Psychiatry 2012;46(9):803–7.
7. Killackey EJ, Jackson HJ, Gleeson J, et al. Exciting career opportunity beckons! Early intervention and vocational rehabilitation in first episode psychosis: employing cautious optimism. Aust N Z J Psychiatry 2006;40(11–12): 951–62.
8. Mai Q, Holman CD, Sanfilippo FM, et al. Do users of mental health services lack access to general practitioner services? Med J Aust 2010;192(9):501–6.

9. Herrman H, Evert H, Harvey C, et al. Disability and service use among homeless people living with psychotic disorders. Aust N Z J Psychiatry 2004;38(11–12): 965–74.

10. Wu EQ, Birnbaum HG, Shi L, et al. The economic burden of schizophrenia in the United States in 2002. J Clin Psychiatry 2005;66(9):1122–9.

11. McGorry PD, Killackey E, Yung A. Early intervention in psychosis: concepts, evidence and future directions. World Psychiatry 2008;7(3):148–56.

12. Killackey E, Nelson B, Yung A. Early detection and intervention in psychosis in Australia: history, progress and potential. Clinical Neuropsychiatry 2008;5(6): 279–85.

13. Alvarez-Jimenez M, Gleeson JF, Henry LP, et al. Road to full recovery: longitudinal relationship between symptomatic remission and psychosocial recovery in first-episode psychosis over 7.5 years. Psychol Med 2012;42(3):595–606.

14. Vos T, Begg S. Victorian burden of disease study: morbidity. Melbourne (Australia): Public Health Division, Department of Human Services; 2003.

15. Rinaldi M, Killackey E, Smith J, et al. First episode psychosis and employment: a review. Int Rev Psychiatry 2010;22(2):148–62.

16. Marwaha S, Johnson S. Schizophrenia and employment: a review. Soc Psychiatry Psychiatr Epidemiol 2004;39(5):337–49.

17. Creed P. Improving the mental and physical health of unemployed people: why and how? Med J Aust 1998;168(4):177–8.

18. Mathers C, Schofield D. The health consequences of unemployment: the evidence. Med J Aust 1998;168(4):178–82.

19. Australian Bureau of Statistics. Education and training experience. Canberra (Australia): Australian Bureau of Statistics; 2010.

20. Waghorn G, Chant D, Whiteford H. The strength of self-reported course of illness in predicting vocational recovery for persons with schizophrenia. J Vocat Rehabil 2003;18(1):33–41.

21. Killackey E, Jackson HJ, McGorry PD. Vocational intervention in first-episode psychosis: a randomised controlled trial of individual placement and support versus treatment as usual. Br J Psychiatry 2008;193:114–20.

22. Department of Education and Training. Department of education and training: annual report. Melbourne (Australia): Department of Education and Training; Victorian Government; 2006.

23. Amariah Brigham. The moral treatment of insanity. Am J Psychiatry 1844;4(1): 1–15.

24. Briggs LV. Occupational and industrial therapy: how can this important branch of treatment of our mentally ill be extended and improved? Am J Psychiatry 1918;74(3):459–79.

25. Crowther RE, Marshall M, Bond GR, et al. Vocational rehabilitation for people with severe mental illness [review]. Cochrane Database Syst Rev 2001;(2):1–55.

26. Bond G. Evidence for the effectiveness of the individual placement and support model of supported employment. 2012 [updated October 23, 2012; cited 2012 November 20]. Available at: http://www.dartmouth.edu/~ips2/resources/12-ips-evidence-10-23.pdf. Accessed November 20, 2012.

27. Rinaldi M, McNeil K, Firn M, et al. What are the benefits of evidence-based supported employment for patients with first-episode psychosis? Psychiatr Bull 2004;28(8):281–4.

28. Nuechterlein KH, Subotnik KL, Turner LR, et al. Individual placement and support for individuals with recent-onset schizophrenia: integrating supported education and supported employment. Psychiatr Rehabil J 2008;31(4):340–9.

29. Allott KA, Yuen HP, Garner B, et al. Relationship between vocational status and perceived stress and daily hassles in first episode psychosis: an exploratory study. Soc Psychiatry Psychiatr Epidemiol 2012. [Epub ahead of print].

30. Thornicroft G, Brohan E, Rose D, et al. Global pattern of experienced and anticipated discrimination against people with schizophrenia: a cross-sectional survey. Lancet 2009;373(9661):408–15.

31. Bartholomeusz CF, Allott K. Neurocognitive and social cognitive approaches for improving functional outcome in early psychosis: theoretical considerations and current state of evidence. Schizophr Res Treatment 2012;2012:815315.

32. Addington J, Saeedi H, Addington D. Facial affect recognition: a mediator between cognitive and social functioning in psychosis? Schizophr Res 2006; 85(1–3):142–50.

33. Allen DN, Strauss GP, Donohue B, et al. Factor analytic support for social cognition as a separable cognitive domain in schizophrenia. Schizophr Res 2007; 93(1–3):325–33.

34. Bell M, Tsang HW, Greig TC, et al. Neurocognition, social cognition, perceived social discomfort, and vocational outcomes in schizophrenia. Schizophr Bull 2009;35(4):738–47.

35. Brune M. Emotion recognition, 'theory of mind,' and social behavior in schizophrenia. Psychiatry Res 2005;133(2–3):135–47.

36. Pinkham AE, Penn DL. Neurocognitive and social cognitive predictors of interpersonal skill in schizophrenia. Psychiatry Res 2006;143(2–3):167–78.

37. Williams LM, Whitford TJ, Flynn G, et al. General and social cognition in first episode schizophrenia: identification of separable factors and prediction of functional outcome using the IntegNeuro, test battery. Schizophr Res 2008; 99(1–3):182–91.

38. Brekke J, Kay DD, Lee KS, et al. Biosocial pathways to functional outcome in schizophrenia. Schizophr Res 2005;80(2–3):213–25.

39. Vauth R, Rusch N, Wirtz M, et al. Does social cognition influence the relation between neurocognitive deficits and vocational functioning in schizophrenia? Psychiatry Res 2004;128(2):155–65.

40. Fett AK, Viechtbauer W, Dominguez MD, et al. The relationship between neurocognition and social cognition with functional outcomes in schizophrenia: a meta-analysis. Neurosci Biobehav Rev 2011;35(3):573–88.

41. Horan WP, Green MF, Degroot M, et al. Social cognition in schizophrenia, Part 2: 12-month stability and prediction of functional outcome in first-episode patients. Schizophr Bull 2012;38(4):865–72.

42. Bell MD, Zito W, Greig T, et al. Neurocognitive enhancement therapy with vocational services: work outcomes at two-year follow-up. Schizophr Res 2008; 105(1–3):18–29.

43. McGurk SR, Mueser KT, Feldman K, et al. Cognitive training for supported employment: 2-3 year outcomes of a randomized controlled trial. Am J Psychiatry 2007;164(3):437–41.

44. Vauth R, Corrigan PW, Clauss M, et al. Cognitive strategies versus self-management skills as adjunct to vocational rehabilitation. Schizophr Bull 2005;31(1):55–66.

45. Lawrence D, Holman C, Jablensky A. Preventable physical illness in people with mental illness. Perth (Australia): The University of Western Australia; 2001.

46. De Hert M, Correll C, Bobes J, et al. Physical illness in patients with severe mental disorders. I. Prevalence, impact of medications and disparities in health care. World Psychiatry 2011;10(1):52–77.

47. Alvarez-Jiménez M, González-Blanch C, Vázquez-Barquero JL, et al. Attenuation of antipsychotic-induced weight gain with early behavioral intervention in drug-naive first-episode psychosis patients: a randomized controlled trial. J Clin Psychiatry 2006;67(8):1253–60.
48. Lawrence D, D'Arcy C, Holman J, et al. Excess cancer mortality in Western Australian psychiatric patients due to higher case fatality rates. Acta Psychiatr Scand 2000;101(5):382–8.
49. SANE Australia. Smoking and mental illness: costs. Melbourne (Australia): SANE; 2007.
50. Doll R, Peto R, Boreham J, et al. Mortality in relation to smoking: 50 years' observations on male British doctors. BMJ 2004;328(7455):1519.
51. Alvarez-Jimenez M, Martinez-Garcia O, Perez-Iglesias R, et al. Prevention of antipsychotic-induced weight gain with early behavioural intervention in first-episode psychosis: 2-year results of a randomized controlled trial. Schizophr Res 2010;116(1):16–9.
52. Aronne LJ, Wadden T, Isoldi KK, et al. When prevention fails: obesity treatment strategies. Am J Med 2009;122(4 Suppl 1):S24–32.
53. Rossner S, Hammarstrand M, Hemmingsson E, et al. Long-term weight loss and weight-loss maintenance strategies. Obes Rev 2008;9(6):624–30.
54. Wing RR, Hill JO. Successful weight loss maintenance. Annu Rev Nutr 2001;21: 323–41.
55. McGuire MT, Wing RR, Klem ML, et al. Behavioral strategies of individuals who have maintained long-term weight losses. Obes Res 1999;7(4):334–41.
56. Alvarez-Jimenez M, Gonzalez-Blanch C, Crespo-Facorro B, et al. Antipsychotic-induced weight gain in chronic and first-episode psychotic disorders: a systematic critical reappraisal. CNS Drugs 2008;22(7):547–62.
57. Coldham EL, Addington J, Addington D. Medication adherence of individuals with a first episode of psychosis. Acta Psychiatr Scand 2002;106(4): 286–90.
58. Gortmaker SL, Must A, Perrin JM, et al. Social and economic consequences of overweight in adolescence and young adulthood. N Engl J Med 1993;329(14): 1008–12.
59. Malarcher A, Dube S, Shaw L, et al. Quitting smoking among adults—United States, 2001-2010. Centers for Disease Control and Prevention. MMWR Morb Mortal Wkly Rep 2011;60(44):1513–6.
60. Siru R, Hulse GK, Tait RJ. Assessing motivation to quit smoking in people with mental illness: a review. Addiction 2009;104(5):719–33.
61. Prochaska JJ. Integrating tobacco treatment into mental health settings. JAMA 2010;304(22):2534–5.
62. Campion J, Checinski K, Nurse J. Review of smoking cessation treatments for people with mental illness. Adv Psychiatr Treat 2008;14:208–16.
63. Lasser K, Boyd JW, Woolhandler S, et al. Smoking and mental illness: a population-based prevalence study. JAMA 2000;284(20):2606–10.
64. Banham L, Gilbody S. Smoking cessation in severe mental illness: what works? Addiction 2010;105(7):1176–89.
65. Tsoi DT, Porwal M, Webster AC. Interventions for smoking cessation and reduction in individuals with schizophrenia. Cochrane Database Syst Rev 2010;(6):CD007253.
66. Fiore M, Jaén C, Baker T, et al. Treating tobacco use and dependence: 2008 update. Clinical practice guideline. Rockville (MD): U.S. Department of Health and Human Services. Public Health Service; 2008.

67. Ratschen E, Britton J, McNeill A. The smoking culture in psychiatry: time for change. Br J Psychiatry 2011;198(1):6–7.
68. Williams JM, Ziedonis D. Addressing tobacco among individuals with a mental illness or an addiction. Addict Behav 2004;29(6):1067–83.
69. Morris CD, Waxmonsky JA, May MG, et al. What do persons with mental illnesses need to quit smoking? Mental health consumer and provider perspectives. Psychiatr Rehabil J 2009;32(4):276–84.
70. Association American of Medical Colleges. Physician behavior and practice patterns related to smoking cessation summary report. Washington, DC: Association of American Medical Colleges; 2007.
71. Coghlan R, Lawrence D, Holman CD, et al. Duty to care. Physical illness in people with mental illness. Perth: The University of Western Australia; 2001.
72. Hetrick S, Alvarez-Jimenez M, Parker A, et al. Promoting physical health in youth mental health services: ensuring routine monitoring of weight and metabolic indices in a first episode psychosis clinic. Australas Psychiatry 2010;18(5): 451–5.
73. ORYGEN Youth Health. The Australian clinical guidelines for early psychosis. Melbourne (Australia): ORYGEN Youth Health; 2010.
74. Citrome L, Yeomans D. Do guidelines for severe mental illness promote physical health and well-being? J Psychopharmacol 2005;19(Suppl 6):102–9.
75. Stearns A. The value of out-patient work among the insane. Am J Psychiatry 1918;74(4):595–602.
76. International First Episode Vocational Recovery (iFEVR) Group. Meaningful lives: supporting young people with psychosis in education, training and employment: an international consensus statement. Early Interv Psychiatry 2010;4(4):323–6.

Index

Note: Page numbers of article titles are in **boldface** type.

Child Adolesc Psychiatric Clin N Am 22 (2013) 759–768
http://dx.doi.org/10.1016/S1056-4993(13)00069-2
1056-4993/13/$ – see front matter © 2013 Elsevier Inc. All rights reserved.

childpsych.theclinics.com

United States Postal Service

Statement of Ownership, Management, and Circulation
(All Periodicals Publications Except Requester Publications)

1. Publication Title	2. Publication Number	3. Filing Date
Child and Adolescent Psychiatric Clinics of North America	0 1 1 1 - 3 6 8	9/14/13

4. Issue Frequency	5. Number of Issues Published Annually	6. Annual Subscription Price
Jan, Apr, Jul, Oct	4	$297.00

7. Complete Mailing Address of Known Office of Publication (Not printer) (Street, city, county, state, and ZIP+4®)

Elsevier Inc.
360 Park Avenue South
New York, NY 10010-1710

Contact Person
Stephen R. Bushing
Telephone (Include area code)
215-239-3688

8. Complete Mailing Address of Headquarters or General Business Office of Publisher (Not printer)

Elsevier Inc., 360 Park Avenue South, New York, NY 10010-1710

9. Full Names and Complete Mailing Addresses of Publisher, Editor, and Managing Editor (Do not leave blank)

Publisher (Name and complete mailing address)

Linda Belfus, Elsevier, Inc., 1600 John F. Kennedy Blvd. Suite 1800, Philadelphia, PA 19103-2899

Editor (Name and complete mailing address)

Joanne Husovski, Elsevier, Inc., 1600 John F. Kennedy Blvd. Suite 1800, Philadelphia, PA 19103-2899

Managing Editor (Name and complete mailing address)

Barbara Cohen-Kligerman, Elsevier, Inc., 1600 John F. Kennedy Blvd. Suite 1800, Philadelphia, PA 19103-2899

10. Owner (Do not leave blank. If the publication is owned by a corporation, give the name and address of the corporation immediately followed by the names and addresses of all stockholders owning or holding 1 percent or more of the total amount of stock. If not owned by a corporation, give the names and addresses of the individual owners. If owned by a partnership or other unincorporated firm, give its name and address as well as those of each individual owner. If the publication is published by a nonprofit organization, give its name and address.)

Full Name	Complete Mailing Address
Wholly owned subsidiary of	1600 John F. Kennedy Blvd, Ste. 1800
Reed/Elsevier, US holdings	Philadelphia, PA 19103-2899

11. Known Bondholders, Mortgagees, and Other Security Holders Owning or Holding 1 Percent or More of Total Amount of Bonds, Mortgages, or Other Securities. If none, check box → ☐ None

Full Name	Complete Mailing Address
N/A	

12. Tax Status (For completion by nonprofit organizations authorized to mail at nonprofit rates) (Check one)
The purpose, function, and nonprofit status of this organization and the exempt status for federal income tax purposes:
☐ Has Not Changed During Preceding 12 Months
☐ Has Changed During Preceding 12 Months (Publisher must submit explanation of change with this statement)

PS Form 3526, September 2007 (Page 1 of 3 Instructions Page 3) PSN 7530-01-000-9931 PRIVACY NOTICE: See our Privacy policy in www.usps.com

---

13. Publication Title		14. Issue Date for Circulation Data Below
Child and Adolescent Psychiatric Clinics of North America		July 2012

15. Extent and Nature of Circulation			Average No. Copies Each Issue During Preceding 12 Months	No. Copies of Single Issue Published Nearest to Filing Date
a. Total Number of Copies (Net press run)			561	526
b. Paid Circulation (By Mail and Outside the Mail)	(1)	Mailed Outside-County Paid Subscriptions Stated on PS Form 3541 (Include paid distribution above nominal rate, advertiser's proof copies, and exchange copies)	337	315
	(2)	Mailed In-County Paid Subscriptions Stated on PS Form 3541 (Include paid distribution above nominal rate, advertiser's proof copies, and exchange copies)		
	(3)	Paid Distribution Outside the Mails Including Sales Through Dealers and Carriers, Street Vendors, Counter Sales, and Other Paid Distribution Outside USPS®	65	64
	(4)	Paid Distribution by Other Classes Mailed Through the USPS (e.g. First-Class Mail®)		
c. Total Paid Distribution (Sum of 15b (1), (2), (3), and (4))			402	379
d. Free or Nominal Rate Distribution (By Mail and Outside the Mail)	(1)	Free or Nominal Rate Outside-County Copies Included on PS Form 3541	70	72
	(2)	Free or Nominal Rate In-County Copies Included on PS Form 3541		
	(3)	Free or Nominal Rate Copies Mailed at Other Classes Through the USPS (e.g. First-Class Mail)		
	(4)	Free or Nominal Rate Distribution Outside the Mail (Carriers or other means)		
e. Total Free or Nominal Rate Distribution (Sum of 15d (1), (2), (3) and (4))			70	72
f. Total Distribution (Sum of 15c and 15e)			472	451
g. Copies not Distributed (See instructions to publishers #4 (page #3))			89	75
h. Total (Sum of 15f and g)			561	526
i. Percent Paid (15c divided by 15f times 100)			85.17%	84.04%

16. Publication of Statement of Ownership

If the publication is a general publication, publication of this statement is required. Will be printed in the October 2013 issue of this publication. ☐ Publication not required.

17. Signature and Title of Editor, Publisher, Business Manager, or Owner

Stephen R. Bushing

Stephen R. Bushing – Inventory Distribution Coordinator

Date
September 14, 2013

I certify that all information furnished on this form is true and complete. I understand that anyone who furnishes false or misleading information on this form or who omits material or information requested on the form may be subject to criminal sanctions (including fines and imprisonment) and/or civil sanctions (including civil penalties)

PS Form 3526, September 2007 (Page 2 of 3)

Moving?

Make sure your subscription moves with you!

To notify us of your new address, find your **Clinics Account Number** (located on your mailing label above your name), and contact customer service at:

Email: journalscustomerservice-usa@elsevier.com

800-654-2452 (subscribers in the U.S. & Canada)
314-447-8871 (subscribers outside of the U.S. & Canada)

Fax number: 314-447-8029

**Elsevier Health Sciences Division
Subscription Customer Service
3251 Riverport Lane
Maryland Heights, MO 63043**

Printed and bound by CPI Group (UK) Ltd, Croydon, CR0 4YY

03/10/2024

01040489-0006